Poultry Production

Poultry Production

R. M. Acharya
B.V.Sc. & A.H. (Pb), M.S. (Ohio), Ph.D. (Iowa)
Former Deputy Director General (Animal Science) ICAR
784, Sector-9, Faridabad (Haryana)

and

Puneet Kumar, Ph.D.
Principal Scientist (Animal Physiology)
Indian Veterinary Research Institute, Izatnagar (UP)

SATISH SERIAL PUBLISHING HOUSE
403, Express Tower, Commercial Complex
Azadpur, Delhi-110033 (India)
Phone : 011-27672852, Fax : 91-11-27672046
e-mail : info@satishserial.com, hkjain1975@yahoo.com
Website : www.satishserial.com

Published by :

SATISH SERIAL PUBLISHING HOUSE

403, Express Tower, Commercial Complex, Azadpur, Delhi-110033 (INDIA)
Phone : 011-27672852 Fax : 91-11-27672046
E-mail : info@satishserial.com, hkjain1975@yahoo.com

ISBN 978-93-86200-15-0

Composed, Designed & Printed in India

Preface

Avian species especially chicken has played an important role in food and nutrition, and employment and incomes, particularly in urban and peri-urban areas since 1970s. Chicken was first domesticated in India, where the progenitors of the modern day chicken still exist in wild. The chicken from India spread both eastward and westward. The major research for improving egg and poultry production through evolving new breeds and strains within breeds started in European countries and later spread to North America comprising USA and Canada when the Europeans migrated to the region. Canada and USA have established large commercial Research and Development facilities supported by their Agricultural Research and Educational Institutions specially the Land Grant University in USA. The North America has done large Research Development and have evolved both technologies and germ plasm for producing high yielding broiler and layer stocks. The layers have reached in excess of 320 eggs in 365 days and broilers more than 3.0 kg live weight at six weeks with a very high efficiency of feed conversion and survival. In addition to chicken; ducks, quails, turkeys have been reared for eggs and meat and have not achieved commercial importance as in chicken except in a few countries.

India has been a pioneer among Asian countries to initiate research almost in the beginning of 20th century and had undertaken a large number of research and development projects both with the indigenous and exotic breeds. Inspite in 1950s and 60s, ICAR had supported a large number of projects for improving layer and broiler production using indigenous and exotic stocks, however; it was in 1970-71, that a large initiative was taken to make country free from continuous imports of grandparent lines/ commercial stocks from large poultry breeding farms in Europe and America for establishing franchise hatcheries for production of commercial layer and broiler chicks. This had to be allowed considering the demand of the industry.

The All India Coordinated Research Projects (AICRPs) on Poultry for Egg and Poultry for Meat were initiated in 1971 and were allowed to import best pure lines of layers and broilers which were maintained at the Division of Poultry Science of the Indian Veterinary Research Institute (IVRI) and supplied to various centers of the AICRPs located in different agro-ecological regions and the research was thus initiated in various State Agricultural Universities and IVRI. The coordinating units of the two projects were located at IVRI, to maintain pure lines and also had research units of both the projects. Considering the importance of poultry research and development, the ICAR had established the Central Avian Research Institute in upgrading the facility and man power of the Division of Poultry Science of IVRI. The Institute subsequently started research on other avian species and considering large expansion of mandate and research programmes, it was decided in 2005 to establish a Project Directorate on Poultry (PDP) at Rajendranagar, Hyderabad utilizing initially some of the facilities of office and laboratories and poultry sheds from AICRP on broiler unit located in the University. It had to coordinate AICRP on layers and broilers, maintaining of pure lines and also random bred control population of layers and broilers. In addition, research related to Genetics, Nutrition, Management, Health and Poultry Products Technology were allocated to CARI which also provided data regularly to cooperating units so that the comparison could be made among centers maintain the same lines. The institute has also mandated to conduct post graduate education in Poultry Science and take Transfer of Technology Programmes. The PDP has to maintain pure lines without causing any genetic change as well as to maintain the random bred control population of layers and broilers and supply these stocks to each of the cooperating center.

Extensive research and development, both under the aegis of ICAR at CARI and PDP and various State Agricultural / Veterinary Universities and the research done by private large poultry breeding farms specially Venkateshwra Hatcheirs and Kegg Farms and few other commercial poultry breeding farms has led to the generation of large knowledge on various aspects of poultry production, health and product processing technology. The research on socio-economic aspects has been relatively week, although with the establishment of National Center of Agricultural Economic Research, some work has been initiated.

Considering extensive R&D on poultry production, health and products technology, which has primarily served urban poultry production and consumption of eggs and meat products, the Union Ministry of Agriculture has directed both the Department of Animal Husbandry, Dairying and Fisheries (DAHD &F) and Department of Agricultural Research and Education (DARE) through the Indian Council of Agricultural Research (ICAR) to strengthen research and development on poultry production in rural areas so that it can create self employment, provide food and nutrition for rural masses which still comprise of 68.5% of the total human population and have relatively lower consumption of animal protein so important for pregnant and lactating mothers, young children and ailing and old people. Poultry eggs and meat are the cheapest source of animal protein and can be very easily produced in rural areas both under extensive and intensive production systems. The present programmes are however directed towards extensive systems essentially using indigenous or improved indigenous birds with relatively low production. Considering the experience of Cooperative Dairy Farming and now Dairy Producer Companies which are collectively providing inputs and services for production, collection, processing and marketing of milk and dairy products, a similar approach if taken on rural commercial poultry production for eggs and meat can help in generating large employment and incomes and provide the rural people with better nutrition.

The senior author has a long experience of national and international research, education and development in the areas of domestic animal production, animal health, animal products technologies, fisheries, social sciences and forage production as he had held teaching, research and research management positions, and had been associated with a large number of international organizations such as UNDP, FAO, World Bank, IDRC, Ford Foundation, Rock Feller Foundation and has served on a number of national and international organizations as a member. He was UNDP/ FAO advisor in buffalo breeding and later served as Advisor, Animal Husbandry in Iran. He has already published a number of books by the ICAR, FAO and on his own, the latter through Indian leading publishers. The senior author was principal investigator for the project on improving poultry production under a number of projects funded by PL-480 and the ICAR involving both indigenous non-descript and exotic descript breeds used for egg and meat production.

The co-author has a long experience in research and education particularly in Animal Physiology and Climatology. The authors have tried to collect the latest information on the world and Indian poultry production scenario and the state of knowledge generated and how it is being or can further be profitably used in enhancing poultry production in the country through proper direction of research and development both in the public and the private sector. The publication has paid a greater attention to the rural poultry production which should not be confined to backyard production system but more intensive system with relatively smaller units, supported by their own organization for provision of inputs and services and undertaking collective processing and marketing of produce so that not only the rural areas benefit from the availability of cheaper eggs and broiler meat but also have increased opportunities for employment and incomes.

The authors are grateful to the ICAR and its institutes related to poultry (CARI and PDP) in providing both published and unpublished information on all aspects of poultry production involving chicken, quail, ducks, turkey and emu. These institutes also provided library facilities. This information alongwith the published information in the international journals related to animal science and particularly to poultry science has been critically reviewed and recommendations have been made for further research, technology transfer and other related aspects of production of avian species both under urban and peri-urban, intensive poultry production, and under rural poultry production both having small and extensively reared units as well as relatively larger units raising layers and broilers collectively as is in co-operative dairy farming and now also under producer companies. There are serious differences in poultry production, processing and marketing of products compared to dairy and suitable modifications in the approach to the rural poultry producer have been suggested to become economically vaiable and competitive production system. The authors are grateful to the Directors of CARI and PDP for providing not only the requisite information both published and unpublished but also interaction with the scientists, which is greatefully acknowledged.

Dr. R.M.Acharya
Dr. Puneet Kumar

Contents

CHAPTER-1

Historical Background of Avian Production, Health and Product Technology in India and its Critical Analysis and Projections for Future Research, Education, Training and Development

1.1 Early History of Poultry Development in India

Poultry rearing in India dates back to 2000-2500 BC with the evidence for domestication of chicken in the form of seals found at Mohenjo-Daro depicting fighting cocks. Collection of chicken made of clay including one of a hen with a feed dish, chicken bones (Femur ~ 130 mm in size) which was much larger than that of jungle fowl (~ 69 mm) and other chicken that existed in India at that time. Till 1900s, the poultry rearing remained restricted to indigenous birds under free range backyard rearing system. Presently, poultry farming has taken a shape of an organized industry. The history of poultry development may be divided into two periods *i.e.* pre and post 1950.

1.1.1 Pre 1950s period

i) It is only in the early 1900s, the initiative was taken for organized poultry farming with improved birds. In 1907, the then most reputed British Poultry Firm "Sperrin" established its business in India, but did not have much success. During the early 1900s, some European Christian Missionaries started importing purebred European stocks in the then provinces of Agra and Oudh and the Madras Presidency. The birds came from UK, USA and Australia and were given to poor people for improving their economic and nutritional conditions, however this made little impact.

ii) A mission's poultry breeding farm was established at Etah in UP in 1912 and maintained Rhode Island Red (RIR), White Leghorn (WLH) and Black Minorca breeds. In 1919, another important development took place when Sir Harcourt Butler, the Governor of UP, advised the provincial government on improving poultry production and engaged a British expert Mrs Fawkes. She organized UP Poultry Association and set up a state poultry farm at Lucknow. Training in Poultry farming was also initiated by her. She also wrote a book "Poultry Farming in the East" in 1933.

iii) In 1932, a grant of Rs 32,000 was sanctioned by Royal Commission on Agriculture (RCA) to Mission Farm in Etah for breeding experiments on chicken. One major step towards the scientific poultry management was taken in 1939 with the establishment of the Poultry Research Section at the Imperial and now Indian Veterinary Research Institute (IVRI), Izatnagar in UP, where organized poultry research and training started. Later this section was upgraded to the Poultry Research Division. It recruited experts from UK and also deputed Indian scientists for training in UK and this led to initiation of systematic research on poultry production and health. Ministry of Defense started a number of poultry farms at its cantonment for supply of eggs and chicken to MilPersonal. However, after the second world war these were dismantled. These farms, however, served as a model for starting small commercial poultry farms in the country.

1.1.2 Post 1950s period

iv) Till 1950s no organized poultry breeding efforts were made by the poultry industry in India and most egg production was only in free range maintained indigenous birds. Even in First Five Year Plan (1951-56), poultry development did not get priority except a launching of pilot project in Orissa to establish 33 extension centers.

v) During the Second Five Year Plan (1956-61), poultry as a commercial venture took roots and an All India Poultry Development scheme was launched. Five regional poultry farms at Bangalore, Bombay, Bhubaneswar, Delhi and Shimla were established to acclimatize imported genetically superior stock and to popularize them along with to provide training to state Government Officers. Purebred exotic stocks including 30,000 White Leghorn (WLH) and Rhode Island Red (RIR) chicks were imported from USA under Technical Cooperation Mission (TCM) and were supplied to the Central and State poultry farms along with poultry equipments. A network of 269 Poultry Extension-cum-Demonstration Centers was established for multiplication and distribution of exotic layer and broiler chicken.

vi) A new approach was tried in Third Five Year Plan with remarkable success. The Intensive Poultry Development Programme (1961-66) was organized along the lines of Intensive Agriculture District Programme. About 80 Poultry Development Projects were established for bringing to the door of the small farmers with all the essential inputs such as chicks, feed, medicines, equipments, credit and marketing assistance in the form of a package. In support of this programme, 5 regional farms, 79 State farms and 43 Extension centers were expended. About 83 feed manufacturing units were started in public and private sectors. Two large-scale poultry processing plants for dressing chicken were started at Pune and Chandigarh. A scientific breeding programme was taken-up at three Regional Farms to make country self-sufficient in hybrid chicken.

vii) During Fourth Five Year Plan (1969-1974), emphasis was on better breeding stocks, dissemination of latest scientific farming practices and extension of intensive production in new areas. In private sectors, the four hatcheries imported the original breeding stocks from foreign sources. These hatcheries were Rani Shaver, Uni Chix Hi-bred and Arbor Acre. These hatcheries started to reproduce the exotic breeds and multiply the hybrid chicks. A High Level In-service Training (Poultry) Institute was established in Hesaraghatta in Bangalore with the assistance of FAO. At IVRI, Izatnagar a Centre of Excellence was established under the aegis of UNDP. Five hatcheries each of 50,000 eggs capacity were established at Bangalore, Bombay, Calcutta, Chandigarh and Delhi with the assistance of Australian "Freedom from Hunger" campaign channeled through FAO, SFDA (Small Farmers' Development Agencies) and MFAL (Marginal Farmers and Agricultural Labours Development Agencies). The government of India established two large broiler dressing plants at Chandigarh and Pune to assist the private broiler farmers in selling their live birds at remunerative price as well as provide healthy, dressed broiler chicken to the consumers.

viii) In Fourth Five Year Plan, Departments of Poultry Science were established in a number of State Agricultural Universities and in 1970-71, All India Coordinated Research Projects (AICRPs) on Poultry for Egg and Poultry for Meat were started by the ICAR with coordinating unit at the Division of Avian Research of IVRI and a number of research centers at IVRI and a number of SAUs by importing pure lines from America and European countries. The Poultry Section in Animal Husbandry in the Ministry of Food and Agriculture was upgraded and a Joint Commissioner (Poultry) was appointed to look after poultry development in the country. A number of pure lines were brought into the country for research and development to avoid its dependence on foreign poultry breeding farms. Four large poultry breeding farms with hatcheries were also established by the Union Department of Agriculture at Mumbai, Bengaluru, Chandigarh and Bhubaneswar. A high level Central Poultry Production and Management Institute was established at Bangalore with the assistance of FAO of UN. It also had a large feed analytical laboratory and facilities for random sample testing commercial stocks produced by the Government of India and private organizations. The results of such tests were published annually by the Ministry of Agriculture. This period also saw a large development of indigenous poultry equipment manufacturing. As mentioned earlier, the random sample testing scheme started at IVRI in 1955 which did not make any impact was shifted to Bangalore as a random sample testing scheme with additional centers at Bhubaneswar and Mumbai. The education in poultry science not only got a fillip at the SAUs but also at IVRI with the starting of an UNDP Advanced Centre for Poultry Science. The efforts of the CARI and subsequently establishment of two AICRPs and Project Direct on Poultry (PDP) centers on poultry for egg and meat and of the Central Poultry Breeding Farms had a large impact on research and development through the supply of superior layer and broiler germplasm, production technologies and training personnel at different levels in poultry production. This led to availability of a large trained manpower not only in India but a large part of South and South-East Asia.

ix) In addition to R & D in poultry breeding, a large research effort on poultry feed and nutrition was made at a number of newly established State Agricultural Universities and at IVRI. A number of new cheaper and readily available agro-industrial processing by-products and non-conventional feed recourses were identified for incorporation in poultry compounded feeds. An AICRP on identifying newer feed resources and evaluating their nutritive value and incriminating factors, if any, and their ameliorative measures were instituted. In addition to research on breeding and nutrition, large efforts on developing poultry shelters both for commercial and semi-commercial poultry units were made. This led not only in developing suitable designs but also identifying materials which will reduce heat stress as well as make farm operation more labour efficient. Health continued to receive important attention and a number of new diagnostics and vaccines for control and eradication of avian diseases were developed.

x) Punjab had given particular importance to poultry developments during the period when the late Sardar Partap Singh Kairon was the Chief Minister. A separate unit for promoting poultry production was created in the Department of Animal Husbandry. The Punjab Agricultural University started a two years specialized course in poultry production. The ICAR supported research on layer and broiler production through a number of *ad hoc* research schemes. Two PL-480 projects on studies in indigenous poultry germplasm especially with respect to heat and disease resistance and its incorporation in breeding high producing layer and broiler strains using exotic high producing layer and broiler stocks were also started.

Studies were carried out on comparative performance with respect to body weight at different ages, carcass yield and quality. The indigenous breed involved were Deshi, generally known as non-descript, Black Bengal, Nacked Neck and Aseel with exotic layer (WLH) and broiler breeds (White Rock and Cornish). Both purebreds and their reciprocal crosses were studied for egg production, egg quality in terms of egg weight, shell thickness, haugh units and yolk index. There were some improvements in percent egg production and in laying house mortality. There were also significant differences in other economic traits viz. egg size and efficiency of feed conversion and daily feed consumption among desi and its reciprocal crosses with exotic layer and broiler breeds.

Some studies were also carried out on resistance of Desi and its reciprocal crosses with exotic layer breeds (White Leg Horn). The chicks of purebreds and reciprocal crosses were hatched and raised under disease free conditions and 50% chicks were exposed to Ranikhet and Spirochaetosis diseases. The crosses involving the native males and exotic females had higher resistance when exposed to 50% lethal dose of live infectious agents. In addition, extensive work was done on the genetic aspects of egg production in White Leg Horn. This involved estimation of heritabilities of production and egg quality traits and developing selection indices for maximizing genetic gain and studying the relative efficiency of individual, family and combined selection.

In general, it was observed that an index incorporating age at first egg and 70 day egg production, the former given a negative weightage of 1.5 will be twice as effective in reducing age at first egg and 2 to 3 times more effective in increasing 70 day egg production compared to selection based on individual trait. Effect of diurnal variation and other environmental factors on egg production in Desi and its reciprocal crosses with RIR were also studied. The Desi and Desi x RIR had higher tolerance to the temperature. Sex chromatin studies for sex differentiation were also carried out. The incidence of drum sticks and sessile bodies were higher in males than in females.

Efficiency of selection for egg production showed that an index incorporating individual own egg production that of full sibs and progeny would provide maximum genetic gain per year.

A significant heterosis was observed in 10 week body weight of crosses involving four exotic breeds viz White Plymouth Rock, White Cornish and New Hampshire. The difference among pure bred were not significant but all crossbred were superior to purebreds. New Hampshire crosses with White Cornish had significantly better performances than other crosses.

xi) For Fifth Five Year Plan (1974-1978), annual egg production in the country crossed 13,000 million mark, while the annual broiler production reached to 30 millions. The facilities were created for establishment of new Central Breeding Farms under GOI, expansion of 17 breeding farms and 55 IPDP units. A new commercial hybrid was released from Hesaraghatta with a brand name HH-260. The new marketing arrangements were tried out by NAFED, State Poultry Cooperation of Andhra Pradesh, Tamil Nadu and Eggs Authorities of Gujarat and Maharashtra. Modern vaccine units in private sectors were putting in production. The basic breeding projects were started in private sectors under collaboration with foreign breeding farms. This five year plan was succeeded by two annual plans. The Sixth Five Year Plan (1980-1985) witnessed the broiler boom, which was reflected from increased production from 30 million in 1980 to 75 million in 1985. The emphasis was made to open the way for importing pure line poultry stocks and poultry vaccines. A network of more than 330 hatcheries (approx. 173 in public and 158 in private sector), feed plants, veterinary pharmacological and biological and equipment industries have made the country self sufficient in almost all aspects of inputs, needed by the poultry industry. Some 66 members of Compound Livestock Feed Manufacturers Associations of India (CLFMA) with 98 production units produced about 0.4 million tones of poultry feed which constituted about 15% of the total output of poultry feed in the country.

xii) The Government of India has entrusted the responsibilities for marketing of eggs and meat at the regional and national level to the National Agricultural Cooperative Marketing Federation India Ltd

(NAFED). The National Egg Coordination Committee (NECC) was established in 1982 to control the egg prices. Another major steps to bring farmers together was formation of a public limited company "Agro-CorpeX Ltd." in Bombay for procurement, storage and marketing of eggs. The other cooperation federations such as Gujarat State Poultry Farms Cooperative Federation Ltd, Bangalore Egg Promotion Associations were also active in Egg marketing.

xiii) The Central Avian Research Institute (C.A.R.1.) was established at Izatnagar in IVR1 Campus on 2nd November 1979 to undertake the basic and applied research in all aspects of poultry production. Four strains crosses namely ILI-80 (Layer) and B-77 (Broiler) from CARI, IBL-80 (Broiler) from Punjab Agricultural University (PAU) and IBB-83 from Karnatake Agricultural University, Bangalore were released. One major setback during 1980 was the imposition of income tax that hit the big farmers rather badly and resulted in a setback to their extension Plan.

xiv) In the Seventh Five Year Plan (1985-1990), the regional laboratories devoted to poultry feed were set-up by the Union Ministry of Agricultural in Bhubneshwar, Bombay and Chandigarh with the facilities for analyzing amino acids. Government of India initiated a new scheme of registration of hatcheries during this plan. A noteworthy development was introduction of the Specific Pathogen Free (SPF) eggs from the production of vaccines in private sectors-Bhartiya Agro-Industries Foundation (BAIF) and Venkateshwara Hatcheries Pvt. Ltd. at Pune. To develop the self-sufficiency in high yielding germ-plasm of egg and meat type, the All India Coordination Research Project programme of Indian Council of Agricultural Research (ICAR) and Central Poultry Farm of Ministry of Agriculture were strengthened. The Project Directorate on Poultry (PDP) came in operation in 1988 at Hyderabad with the objectives of monitoring and coordinating the research programmes of All India Coordinated Research Project (AICRP) on Poultry Breeding, Poultry Nutrition, Poultry Housing and Management being carried out both at State Agricultural Universities and at the CARI and Directorate of Poultry Research (DPR). ICAR initiated projects on developing systems of surveillance, monitoring and forecasting of important diseases.

xv) The fast food waves gained momentum in various parts of the country. As a result of which the number of branded chicken products such a Venky's, Al-Kabeer, Lazis, All Man's, Tasty Bites etc. came in the market. India's first automatic plant handling about three lakhs broilers per month came in operation in 1986 at Pune. Another automatic plant was set-up at Agra in UP. In Southern India, the process of integration began in the mid-1990s and accelerated rapidly as independent growers found the guaranteed returns of contract farming preferable to the vagaries of market returns. Integration has brought two important changes to the poultry industry in south India: lower average costs of production through improved technology and management practices and, particularly, a collapsing of the margins previously commanded for the various production inputs; and smaller producer-retail margins and lower retail prices for poultry meat, which has been a key demand stimulus in the southern and western regions.

xvi) During Eighth Five Year Plan (1992-1997), the poultry farming has been identified as one of the thrust areas. The plan envisaged an annual growth target of 7 percent in egg and 18 to 20 percent in broilers. The number of Poultry States were established to ensure easy access to all the necessary facilities including inputs, credit and marketing. They collaborated with agencies like National Cooperative Development Corporation (NCDC), National Bank for Agricultural and Rural Development (NABARD), State Government and Non-Government Organization (NGO). The poultry production suffered badly due to of Gumboro disease. In Namakkal, more than 15 to 20 lakhs starter and grower chicks died due to Gumboro disease. In 1995, the policies such as liberalization of grandparent imports was implemented, which subsequently resulted in presence of almost all the reputed brands of layer and broilers in India.

xvii) During Ninth Five Year Plan (1997-2002), integrated poultry farming was extended to the Western India also especially in Pune and Nashik areas and also to the other cities of Southern India such as Bangalore and Hyderabad and also to Eastern region such as Calcutta. In 2000s, the only major region where large integrators have not yet made significant inroads was North India. This period also felt the threats to domestic poultry due to liberalization of import of poultry meat products. It was felt that full liberalization of imports of poultry meat could be disastrous to the domestic poultry industry as the production would fall by 29 percent.

xviii) During the Tenth Five Year Plan (2002-2007), integrated farming system of poultry strengthened. In late 2000s, proportion of poultry farming under integrated system were 80% in South, 70% in West, 50% in East and 10% in North. Till 2006, India remained free of the disease, but between 27th January and 18th April, outbreaks of HPAI virus subtype H5N1 were reported in two districts (Navapur and Jalgaon) of Maharashtra and adjoining areas in Gujarat and Madhya Pradesh. On August 11, 2006, the government declared that India had regained its notifiable AI-free country status as per the regulations of the World Organization for Animal Health (OIE).

xix) Poultry production is further shifting from Western to Eastern countries and South and South East Asia are becoming large centers for production of eggs and broilers. Nearly one-third of the world wide broiler stock, placement is in Asian countries such as India and China which are emerging as important locations for production and consumption in poultry products considering the size of the human population, increasing urbanization, education, employment and incomes. The chicken meat has higher nutritional value in terms of protein and low fat content, lower cost and wider acceptability. The major problem with modern day broiler stocks is their adaptation to higher ambient temperature requiring expensive shelters with cooling arrangements. With high ambient temperature and humidity, alternative genetic resources which may be as efficient as the current day broilers which are better adapted to tropical climate with high ambient temperature and humidity and thus increasing growth and efficiency of feed conversion and meat yield, are required. India is an important center for genetic resources of heterogeneous avian species and genetic variants within such populations and has unique major genes such as naked neck which can allow adaptation to unforeseen and unexpected environmental circumstances. There is a further likelihood of a change in environment due to global warming resulting from GHG emissions arising from use of fossil fuels especially coal and petroleum products, which will require breeding livestock with higher resistance to environmental stresses. Lack of resistance to infectious diseases and genotype x environment interaction and in general sub-optimal production condition in rural and peri-urban areas, it is desirable to have a bird which has more resistance to stressful environment and diseases and yet has a competitive edge.

1.2 Critical Analysis and Projections for Future Research, Education, Training and Development in Avian production

i) The importance of the world biodiversity- the variety of its plants, animals, aquatic organisms, other micro-organisms and ecosystems of which they form an integral part is increasingly recognized for the very sustainability of human life on earth. Agricultural biodiversity includes domestic animal (DA) species which are extremely important for sustainability of production, product quality and environmental integrity. Over ages nature and man have been involved in evolving different types of living organisms, best suited to the changing physical, economic and social environments created by man and nature. Genetically diverse DA populations provide a great range of options for meeting the present and future challenges, whether associated with environmental changes, emerging diseases threats, new knowledge of human nutritional requirement, fluctuating market conditions, or changes in socio-economic and cultural conditions and desire for foods with better nutrition and taste. The role of Domestic Animal Diversity (DAD) in meeting these goals is enormous in DAs and extremely difficult to be understood and efforts must be made to fully appreciate the existing Farm Animal Genetic Resources (FAnGR), their diversity by species, production types, breeds/strains within a production and genetic variances in and co-variances among various economic characters related to production / productivity, health and products quality.

ii) The human population in the world is growing reasonably fast specially in the Asian developing countries like China and India. The global human population is likely to reach 8.3 b and almost half of it will live in urban areas and demand foods with higher taste, nutritive value and satiety factor which only DA can meet. Since in South Asia a large population belongs to religions like Hinduism, Buddhism and Jainism which prohibit slaughter of animals and more particularly cattle which are considered religiously worth worshiping because of their role in providing food through milk and dairy products and providing draught animal power and organic manure and also meeting the fuel needs to burning of dung cakes or through conversion into biogas. They also contribute to country's GDP through their skins and hides and other products and by-products and services they provide to man. Further there is a growing realization that beef, kine (buffalo meat), mutton and chevon (goat meat), being red meats are injurious for health. There is therefore an increasing demand for meat from chicken, rabbits and pigs.

iii) The country has made large strides in DA development after attaining independence from the British rule in 1947. Although the livestock sector had received relatively lower public and private investment in research and development both of the central and state governments and further very little private investment, the progress in DA development has been impressive. Considering the population size, spread, their multiple functions, cattle have received a larger Research and Development (R&D) attention followed by sheep to meet the requirement of apparel wool for the large installed capacity in the worsted and hoisry of the woolen industry in the country. The other species, more particularly poultry, had received relatively lower R & D attention.

iv) After dairy production, poultry production has shown a tremendous progress in the country since 1970s. Earlier essentially a number of indigenous avian species were raised under extensive/ backyard management and primarily allowed to scavenge on natural resources both vegetable and insects in rural and peri-urban areas. Introduction of exotic breeds of both layer and broiler chicken started in 1950s, to be raised on government farms and breeding males were given to the poultry keepers for grading up indigenous birds. They were also advised to provide night shelters and some supplementary feed to the graded birds. There was thus some improvement in egg production and live weight gains of indigenous non-descript birds. Small scale intensive raising of layers and broilers was introduced in 1960s through the establishment of poultry estates by the State Animal Husbandry Departments where they built small sheds and rented them to poultry keepers and also provided them with the day old chicks, compounded feed and health cover and further arranged for marketing of eggs and broilers. The operational size of each unit and the whole estate was relatively small. At the same time large foreign franchisers had started establishing large poultry breeding farms to produce day old hybrid layer and broiler chickens and also advising the poultry farmers on feeding, health cover and management and providing them inputs and services for organized marketing.

v) In 1970s, the Government of India took a large initiative to import a large number of pure lines of layers and broilers and set up large regional research and development units, the former under the GOI, Department of Agriculture and Cooperation which is now a separate Department of Animal Husbandry, Dairying and Fisheries, which established Regional Central Poultry Breeding Farms in each of the four major regions of the country along with poultry training centers, random sample testing facilities on the performance of commercial layers and broilers produced by R&D organizations and private commercial poultry breeding farms and for feed ingredient analysis for nutrient content and quality specially the traces of mycotoxins. To avoid continuous import of grand-parent lines from large International Poultry Breeding Concerns and to make the country self sufficient in basic breeding stock, two All India Coordinated Research Projects (AICRPs) on Poultry for eggs and Poultry for meat with coordinating units at the Indian Veterinary Research Institute (IVRI), Izatnagar were started in 1971 with a number of research centers located in Central Avian Research Institute (CARI) and a number of State Agricultural Universities (SAUs). Subsequently, the Division of Poultry Science of IVRI was upgraded to a full-fledged central research institute, the Central Avian Research Institute, to undertake research on all aspects of poultry production for eggs and broilers and to coordinate the two AICRPs viz for egg and for meat. It was mandated to work on all domesticated avian species and in the process initiated work on quail and ducks for eggs and meat. Subsequently other species viz. guinea fowl, ducks, turkey, emu were also included in the research programme. Considering that the AICRPs took major funds, manpower and space of the institute as they were required to maintain a large number of layer and broiler pure lines, random bred control populations of layers and broilers and also undertake research on improving layers and broilers as a part of the two AICRPs which required performance recording on a number of sire progeny groups in different layer and broiler lines maintained as purebreds and their reciprocal crosses, and also provide random bred control populations to the cooperating centers as well as conduct central performance recording of the crosses produced by the cooperating center, it was decided to establish a separate Project Directorate on Poultry (PDP) at Hyderabad and transfer the pure lines, random bred control populations and coordination responsibilities and also initiate research on nutrition, physiology, housing and health of the pure lines.

vi) In addition to production, large research initiatives have also been taken on health, nutrition, housing and production and reproduction physiology, egg and meat quality assessment and processing and product technology and a large number of new value added products with long shelf life have been generated at the CARI. In 1970, decision was taken by the GOI to stop the import of grandparent and parent lines from the international and multinational poultry breeding concerns to reduce dependence on such imports for commercial poultry production in the country.

It imported pure lines of layers and broilers and initiated AICRPs on poultry on eggs and meat Layers and Broilers with coordinating unit at the Division of Poultry Science of the IVRI which was subsequently upgraded to an independent Central Avian Research Institute (CARI). It was expected that the research projects will generate sufficient superior germ plasm both of layers and broilers to be utilized by commercial poultry breeding concerns and by the State Animal Husbandry Departments to provide superior layer and broiler chickens to the commercial producers who were at that time dependent on the franchisers of the international poultry breeding concerns, however this did not succeed to the extent envisaged and under international and national pressure, the import of grandparent and parent lines was again allowed. In fact the GOI had expanded the facility of their large regional poultry breeding farm to multiply the lines generated under AICRPs and make breeding stocks available to state governments as well as private agencies for producing commercial layers and broiler chickens for use by the poultry industry.

vii) Intensive research both in the ICAR Institutes and State Agricultural / Veterinary Universities under the ICAR sponsored AICRPs and AP CESS funded projects and foreign assisted projects / bilateral research projects or on their own initiatives and a large R & D effort made by some private poultry breeding farms like Venkateswara Hatcheries and Kegg Farms which had led to be creation of high producing strains / lines which in crosses are producing eggs and meat with the same efficiency as in the rest of the world.

viii) Research on poultry diseases was carried out in the Indian Veterinary Research Institute under the Division of Avian Diseases and subsequently it is being carried out through the Center for Animal Disease Research and Diagnosis (CADRAD). The country is to a large extent self sufficient in commercial poultry genetic resources and can provide necessary management, feed and health inputs for commercial layer and broiler production.

ix) With the rethinking of allowing foreign collaboration in poultry breeding and free import of high producing commercial strains/ lines, there is a need to reconsider the large investment in commercial poultry breeding research in the public sector. It may be mentioned that in U.K. with privatization of seed production in most cereal and cash crops, the plant breeding research was left to be carried out by these companies, as there was patenting of the breeding approaches and of the commercial varities sold by them to the commercial poultry production concerns. The foreign companies allowed their franchisers to maintain the parent lines and create layer and broiler male and female parents to be supplied to other commercial farms for producing day old layer and broiler chicks for intensive egg and broiler production in the major eco-region with large feed and man power resource. The foreign companies are providing to their franchisers in India grandparent stocks/pure line to undertake their crossing to produce commercial layer and broiler chicks. Most of the foreign poultry breeding firms provided only the males of the male lines and females of the female lines to the commercial poultry breeding farms so that they could only produce commercial layer and broiler chicks and could not use the stocks provided to them for establishing pure lines and undertake selection for further improvement on the basis of the performance for purebred, crossbred or both.

x) The avian species, of which the chicken is the dominant species, have played an important role in meeting the economic, social and cultural needs and in providing high quality and balanced food through eggs and meat. With the growing apprehension of the role of red meat in human diseases, there is a growing tendency to consume chicken eggs and meat as a source of protein with essential amino acids and lower fat content. Chicken is further extremely efficient in converting feed nutrients into high quality human food in the form of eggs and meat and requires much smaller space and labor and can be raised under more intensive production conditions in urban and peri-urban areas which are the major centers of demand for eggs and broiler meat. Poultry production in India as in major part of the world, especially developing countries has emerged as a most dynamic component of DA sector with an average annual growth of 5% in layer and 10% in broiler components of this DA sub-sector during the last decade. The current contribution of poultry to the national GDP is Rs. 400 b comprising 0.05 percent of the Indian GDP and 10% of the GDP from the livestock sector. India has now attained the 3rd position in egg production with 61 b eggs produced per annum and 5th position in broiler production with 2.8 mmt of broiler meat which comprises relatively a smaller proportion of total meat produced in the country. Beef and kine are still dominant meat production in the country because of population size and distribution of cattle and buffaloes. However, their consumption is limited in case of socially and economically deprived classes in the country. Mutton and chevon have continued to be preferred meats. The population of sheep has remained almost static till 1980s when it showed a relatively a faster increase and essentially in the state of Andhra Pradesh. Unlike in greater part of the western world, the pig meat is becoming dominant but has a relatively lower importance in India because of large Muslim population considering pig an unclean animal because it lives on scavenging human waste and is a source of zoonotic diseases. Even high class Hindus and Sikhs prefer mutton and chevon and beef and now chicken is becoming important source of meet for these consumers.

xi) The poultry production has also a vital role in manpower employment, mostly self employment, in rural and peri-urban areas and mostly involving small and marginal farmers and landless laborers and other members of the economically, socially and culturally deprived classes. A large majority of people engaged in poultry production are women to whom poultry farming provides income to meet the essential family expenditure especially on food, education and health of their family members more particularly children. In addition it provides some eggs and occasionally meat for a family consumption. The poultry production is not only contributing to improvement in food and nutrition at household level but also health of the people through helping in education, employment and thus economic growth. The poultry sector has a large contribution of both the private and public sector. While the private sector provides major production inputs, public sector provides education, research and some services especially related to health. The major contribution in research leading to development of high producing strains and strain crosses of layers and broilers is from the ICAR through its Central Avian Research Institute (CARI), Project Directorate on Poultry (PDP), All India Coordinated Research Project (AICRP) centers located in different State Agricultural Univerties (SAUs)/ State Veterinary Universities (SVUs), Indian Veterinary Research Institute (IVRI) earlier through its Division on Avian Diseases, which now stands merged with Center for Animal Disease Research and Diagnosis (CADRAD) earlier through and support of various SAUs/SVUs in poultry disease research. Formerly the High Security Animal Disease Laboratory (HSADL) at Bhopal and now the National Institute of High Security Animal Diseases (NIHSAD) of Indian Council of

Agricultural Research which came into existence on 8th August 2014 contributed significantly by detecting many animal diseases of exotic origin and preventing them from entering our country look after the R&D needs of exotic emerging diseases that are likely to be introduced through international borders or import of breeding stocks from other countries. In addition, the National Bureau of Animal Genetic Resources (NBAGR) is working on description, evaluation, conservation and sustainable management of indigenous poultry genetic resources and aspects of their molecular genetics.

xii) The modern day chicken (*Gallus domesticus)* is known to have descended from the wild red jungle fowl (*Gallus galluse*) with five possible progenitor sub-species. While previous molecular studies suggest a single domestic origin in South East Asia (Thailand), at least six distinct maternal genetic lineages have now been identified corresponding to three distinct geographic centers of domestication. There is an agreement between genetic and archeological data which suggest that chicken was domesticated in Indus Valley some five thousand years ago and in Eastern China even earlier 7500 to 8000 years ago. Moreover, the species was probably domesticated independently in South East Asia in the Islands of modern day Indonesia.

xiii) Despite the phenomenal increase in egg and poultry meat production, the *per capita* annual consumption of eggs is 52 and broilers 2.3 kg against the world average of 102 eggs and 11 kg broiler meat. However the consumption in India is essentially confined to the urban population which comprises 32% of the total population of these countries and that too it is confined to rich and neo-rich families with better education, employment and incomes. There is a large regional disparity in production and consumption as the largest commercial egg and broiler farms are located in southern states, especially Tamil Nadu, Andhra Pradesh and also in Maharashtra, Punjab and Haryana. About 80% of the eggs are produced from hybrid layers in large commercial farms run in a similar manner and as efficiently as anywhere else in the world. The rest 20% are produced by indigenous birds or their grades with exotic layer breeds. Most commercial broilers are produced by large commercial broiler breeding farms located in urban and peri-urban areas and the contribution of the rural poultry production to commercial broiler is insignificant as most of dual type (egg and meat chicken of native type are used both for egg and broiler type).

xiv) Among the various avian species, the largest contribution is of the chicken which comprises 90% of the population of avian species followed by ducks (7%) and the rest all others avian species. Ducks are mostly reared in coastal areas. In addition, J&K and North Eastern region also has importance of rearing ducks. Commercial quail farming for meat and eggs is of comparatively recent origin and has run into problems due to the wild life laws of not raising wild life in captivity and more particularly for commercial purposes. There has been some relaxation after it has been explained that the quails that are raised for meat and eggs are of commercial varities and not the non-domesticated wild population, but it is disputed by GOI.

xv) In addition to chicken, other avian species have special importance in certain ecological niches such as with large water bodies where ducks can be raised with profit independently or through duck and fish culture/deep water paddy-fish-duck culture. Similarly, there are niches for other avian species or indigenous types of chickens such as Kadaknath which produces black meat with aphrodisiac value. Quails and ducks are becoming popular in a number of areas especially the quail eggs which are cheaper and can be pickled and preserved for a longer period. These may be included in child development, educational and poverty alleviation programmes. Guinea fowl is essentially a scavenger and can be maintained with least production inputs in rural areas under extensive management. Large flocks are maintained extensively and obtain their feed nutrients from insects and vegetable matter available from range land. They also do not compete with other DA species and rather help in control of liver fluke through consuming the snails which are intermediary host. Turkeys have more recently been introduced and can also be maintained under extensive management with limited supplementary feeding and health cover. Turkeys produce special kind of meat which has a religious significance for Christians and is religiously consumed on Thanks Giving and Christmas festivals. Further the breast meat in turkey has least fat and is liked by the meat consumers who are conscious of fat content of red meat. Ostrich and Emu are the latest entry into the family of domesticated avian species. Although they have a little importance for egg and meat production, but because of emu producing a large quantity of breast meat with fat which has medicinal value, its rearing is being increasingly taken up in some areas. Attention is however required for developing new products from eggs and meat from poultry which have longer shelf life without refrigeration and higher taste and market acceptability.

xvi) Other avian species have more regional importance and make relatively low economic contribution. In certain coastal areas like Assam, Bihar, Manipur, Kerala, Andhra Pradesh, Tamil Nadu, Odisha, Tripura and Jammu & Kashmir, duck farming has some importance. The Central Duck Breeding Farm of the Union Ministry of Agriculture at Hesaraghatta of Bangalore has been providing the germplasm and training facilities for duck farming. The Tamil Nadu Poultry Development Corporation Ltd. has also been popularizing raising quails. Other avian species have been given relatively lower importance by R&D authorities.

xvii) India is self reliant in poultry feed inspite it is allowing large quantities of oil cakes / meals and bran and polishes to be exported and diverting large quantity of molasses for industrial use. Nearly 2/3rd of about 14 mmt of poultry feed needed annually is manufactured in organized sector by companies which are members of Compounded Livestock Feed Manufacturers' Association (CLFMA) and the rest is essentially prepared by the farmers from the locally available feed ingredients. There are a number of feed analytical laboratories and disease diagnostic laboratories both in public and private sector.

xviii) The increasing feed cost and its relatively poor quality due to the purchase of cheaper feed ingredients such as spoiled grains and other agro-industrial processing byproducts which have larger crude fiber and some percentage of incriminating substances which have also a depressing effect on layer and broiler production. India exports a large quantity of oil cakes, bran and polishes to earn foreign exchange at the cost of the availability of quality feed for DA and more particularly poultry production in the country. Further, a large quantity of feed grains, are being diverted to bio-fuels which will make their availability difficult for DA and increase the feed cost. Molasses an important source of energy is not available in requisite quantity and at affordable cost for DA and poultry feed, because it is utilized for commercial alcohol production. Its availability at an affordable cost can improve the energy content of poultry and make it more affordable.

xix) Coarse cereals, oil cakes and cereal byproducts usually constitute the major part of the poultry feeds. The cereals and oil cakes almost comprise 50% of the feed. Coarse cereals such as pearl millet, grain sorghum, minor millets and ragi form the staple diet for millions of small and marginal farmers and landless laborers especially in arid and semi-arid regions with limited surface/ ground water irrigation resources. These coarse grains are nutritionally more important and most widely used in poultry rations throughout the world. Since they are grown in arid and semi-arid regions with highly erratic and low rain fall, there are serious risks of crop failure and since the seeding is to be done repeatedly if there is a intermittent drought and sometimes the crop does not yield even the quantity of grain used for seeding and reseeding. Coarse grains constitute about 22% of the total food grains produced and occupy about 38% of the total acreage under food grain production. The demand for coarse cereal is increasing at the rate of 4% per annum due to increasing human and DA population and demand for more DA products and services.

xx) The yield of maize per acre, which is the most important feed ingredient in poultry feeding, in India is just about 40% of the world average which is attributed to the limited availability of quality seeds, fertilizers and pesticides and irrigation facilities. The consumption is growing at 6% per annum and has outstripped production because of stagnation in area under maize production and yield per acre. Thus the consumption and production gaps will continue rising. Further, with the diversion of maize for production of ethanol, maize starch and high fructose corn syrup, the availability of maize for DA feeding is remaining below the desired level. Soybean is yet another important ingredient in poultry feed and an important protein source. Instability in production because of it being essentially a rain fed crop and indiscriminate export of soya meal is not allowing its fuller availability as poultry feed.

xxi) National Bank for Agriculture and Rural Development (NABARD) provides refinance to commercial/ cooperative/ regional rural banks for providing soft loans to poultry farmers and processers and traders in poultry inputs and products. NABARD has launched a large number of innovative schemes including the latest Poultry Venture Capital Fund Scheme to provide interest free loans to the extent of 50% of the cost of poultry production and processing schemes. The funds are provided by the Union Department of Animal Husbandry, Dairying and Fisheries, Ministry of Agriculture. The National Insurance Companies provide insurance to poultry farms and other poultry enterprises. The egg and poultry meat processing is at a nascent stage and most of the eggs are sold as table eggs and the broilers as live birds, largely dressed in the presence of the buyer and thus resulting in a large loss of slaughter by-products and offals. There is hardly any facility for freezing chicken meat and even letting the carcass set before it is sold for consumption as meat. There is further hardly any processing, value addition and products manufacture of poultry meat. There is a large market for indigenous chicken meat and eggs because of their taste. NECC and Broiler Marketing Cooperative Society (BROMARK) declare wholesale prices for eggs and broilers respectively but their operational area is limited. Poultry Farmers' Cooperative Societies and State Poultry Development Corporations developed for the purpose of helping in marketing of eggs and broilers have an extremely limited role. The export of eggs and broilers from India is highly limited and is primarily to Gulf, SAARC and South East Asian countries mostly as fresh frozen chicken and frozen egg products. The export from India constitutes only 0.6% of the world export. The major constraints of Indian poultry sector is characterized by a mixture of low input, low output; medium input-medium output and high input-and high output production units. While layer units are relatively widely spread, the commercial broiler units are concentrated in a few regions around urban and peri-urban areas where there is a large demand for broiler for meat. The problems of large poultry units are very different from the small non-commercial units.

xxii) Escalating prices of poultry feed has led to its shortage. The feed accounts for 60-65% of the cost of production of eggs and broilers. Further the export of oil cakes, meals, brans, polishes, and diversion of maize to starch and bio-fuel industry is resulting in escalation of feed prices and thus increases cost of poultry production in the country. The diversification of poultry production to rural areas, use of alternative avian species and alternative sources of feed are some of the areas which need immediate attention. Dietary interventions to produce designer eggs such as with omega-3 fatty acids, lower cholesterol content and improved egg shell quality to allow long distance transportation need attention.

xxiii) Rural poultry production has been seriously neglected by the poultry industry. The rural people are still dependent on supply of eggs and poultry meat from the indigenous, relatively low producing birds which are neither specialized as layers or broilers, nor are raised under proper housing, feeding and health management. Further, these stocks are highly broody and after laying a clutch of eggs would have a long pause and thus have relatively lower total number of egg laid. The eggs are also relatively smaller in size but have higher shell thickness and more dark yellow yolk and are preferred by Indian consumers because of better taste.

xxiv) Large efforts are now being made to create commercial layers and broilers involving crosses of relatively low producing exotic or exotic and indigenous breeds which have variable and brighter plumage color and shank length similar to the indigenous birds. A large number of layer and broiler strains have now been evolved from such crosses by CARI and PDP as well as some SAUs/SVUs. Kegg Farms, a commercial poultry breeding concern is also selling a commercial chicken which had been evolved by CARI through crossing relatively low producing exotic layer and broiler strains and is called Croiler and is suitable for raising under extensive / semi intensive production conditions in rural and peri-urban areas. The whole R&D for rural poultry production would require a serious re-planning especially in light of the larger ingress of the foreign poultry breeding concerns started after the liberalization of national economy under WTO in early 1990s. They are able to provide day old layer and broiler chicks with better productivity because of larger and long standing R&D inputs in a number of countries where they are located and are also able to support through cheaper and balanced feed, management and health inputs, and also help in marketing, primarily because of their size and spread in large part of the world. They may not venture into rural areas and may essentially continue their business operations in urban and peri-urban areas and the GOI and its various research and development agencies would have to consider ways to meet the needs of eggs and poultry meat of the large rural population which still constitutes 68.5% of the country's population and has so far been bypassed by urban poultry producers in production and consumption of eggs and chicken. It is therefore necessary to increase emphasis on rural poultry production and take initiatives for meeting the rural requirements of eggs and poultry meat. This can be met with through rural poultry production which can also contribute to the urban egg and broiler needs. The rural producers may be more competitive because of relatively lower space, feed and labour cost, and a large rural market, if eggs and broilers are provided at relatively affordable prices. In fact this will lead to large commercialization in production by small producers working together like in case of dairy cooperatives/producer companies. The present experience of rural dairy production reflects the possibility of success of similar other initiatives especially in case of poultry production which provides animal protein of high quality with essential amino acids, vitamins and minerals in the form of eggs which can be consumed even by vegetarian population being infertile. The availability of broilers in rural areas at reasonable prices and more readily will increase poultry meat consumption in the rural areas. This will also add to the rural employment and incomes and thus reduce the movement of rural people to urban areas seeking low level jobs and creating serious problems of housing and unemployment.

xxv) There are a large number of newer developments in Molecular Biology and Genetic Engineering which need proper attention in poultry production in the country, although some work had already been initiated both at CARI and PDP, particularly centres of AICRP. Heat stress will continue as an important factor impeding fuller expression of genetic potential of layers and broilers. Amelioration through proper housing and management, feed compounding such as replenishment of bicarbonates, ions and carbon-dioxide may help in alleviating physiological stresses due to physical environment. Further research on shelter management and evolving suitable semen dilution procedures are required. Poultry product processing is an area which has not received any serious attention. There are large regional imbalances in production and consumption and a cyclic boom and burst phenomena both in leading to over production and fallen prices and thus loss to poultry producers resulting in closure of a large number of farms or increase in prices resulting in poor consumption. This calls for a better development of infrastructure for storage, processing and transport. The Bureau of Indian Standards (BIS) and Agmark standards have been laid for poultry products but are not strictly followed due to lack of marketing intelligence and demand forecast. There are no serious efforts in assurance of quality. Except for NECC and the broiler cooperative, there is no serious effort in promoting consumption of eggs and broiler meat. Due to WTO obligations there is a possibility of large dumping of poultry products depressing internal production. There are raising environmental and ethical concerns resulting from intensive poultry production which need to be addressed immediately. Intensive poultry production especially in case of layers where more than one bird is housed in a cage with not sufficient space to move and have any social interaction leads to serious problems of picking on each other and result in serious injuries.

xxvi) The poultry sector in the world stands at $ 6.9 b which is expected to rise to $8.30 b by 2030. World's total production of poultry meat in 2010 was approximately 95 m mt comprising 85.6 % chicken, 6.8 % turkey, 4.6 % ducks and 2.6 % goose and guinea fowl. The quail makes a limited contribution and is only popular in a few countries like North Korea. Since quail is regarded by the wild life authorities as a wild avian species and is protected under Wild Life Act, 1972; the wild life authorities always raise objection to their farming in captivity. CARI has faced this problem and has not been able to extensively spread quail production for egg or meat inspite of its economic efficiency.

xxvii) The largest production of eggs and broiler has shifted from America and Europe to Asia and South America, especially Thailand and Brazil. The world *per capita* poultry meat availability was 13.8 kg per year. Global poultry meat production is likely to rise to 140 m mt by 2030. Global growth in egg production will continue to be unexceptionally high as is reflected from its increase from 20 m mt in 60's – 70's to around 40 m mt by 1990s and has reached 63 m mt by 2010. Of this 60 % is contributed by Asia alone. The global average *per capita* availability of eggs is about 9.1 kg/year and will reach 90 m mt by 2030 and about 55 % of this will be contributed by Asian countries.

Development in the US egg industry from 1960 to 2010 with respect to energy use and environmental impact, relative to other DA species and crop production showed that inspite of a 30% increase in output, use of life cycle assessment (LCA) developed by international organization for standardization (ISO 14044) which includes not only hen housed egg production but also factors involved in feed crop production and processing, energy use throughout the production cycle and transport of both inputs and outputs is lower than other DA species and crop production.

Enormous progress has been made in egg production in the last 50 years as reflected by decrease in lifetime mortality of layers from 15.8% to 6.7%, feed per kg eggs from 3.44 to 1.98 kg, rate of lay/ 100 hen days has increased from 59.2 to 75.3. Cumulative energy demand (CED), pollution due to green house gases (GHGs), acidifying emissions and other negative effects of commercial poultry production have shown a decline due to more appropriate management of layers and disposal of layer farm wastes. Layers have more favorably economic and environmental impacts than pork, beef and dairy production. Much of the improvements are the result of egg output and feed efficiency. Further there has been decrease or a complete ban, the latter in some countries like EU and India, of the use of animal byproducts in poultry feeds. These products have higher environmental impact compared to plant feeds and may also result in ill health in human beings.

Although crop yields have also increased during the last 50 years, the energy requirement and emissions of GHG associated with their production have also increased but there has been a little impact of the change in egg production indicating the egg industry to be more efficient and environmentally sustainable compared to other DA and crop production. Another benefit of egg and poultry meat production is not only CO_2 efficiency but also cost efficiency putting the poultry industry at the top as a source of animal protein without any major impact on environment. Although in India major economic growth and contribution to food and nutrition has been from milch animals particularly buffalo but the rate of growth has been higher in layer and broiler production.

xxviii) The number of undernourished people in the world has remained unacceptably high (0.93 b in 2010), although there has been a slight decline from 2009 (1.023 b). At present more than half of the world's protein-energy malnutrition problem is in South Asia, where a large percentage of people are vegetarian and depend on vegetable energy and protein or to some extent from milk and dairy products. The situation is however changing and there is an increasing consumption of eggs, being considered vegetarian because they are produced without being fertilized. The younger generation even among the ethnic groups like Hindus, Jains and Buddhist who earlier practiced vegetarianism, have now shed their religious taboo and have started consuming non-vegetarian food especially eggs, broiler meat and fish.

xxix) Poultry production has been the most dynamic sector of DA industry in recent times and is likely to continue expanding more particularly in the developing countries. China is rising as a major DA producer even when it is to import a large part of feed ingredients.

xxx) Feed International has estimated that out of a total of some 708 million metric ton compounded feed produced by commercial feed enterprises for all DA and avian species in the world in 2009, 290 m mt (41 %) was utilized for poultry feeding, making it a single largest segment of compounded feed industry in the world.

xxxi) Brazil, USA and Netherlands are the major chicken meat exporting countries together accounting for over 72 % of the world's chicken meat export, whereas; Russian Federation, Hongkong, China, Saudi Arabia and Japan are the major importer of broilers, accounting for 40 % of the total broilers imported in the world. Netherlands, Spain, Germany and China are the important exporters of chicken eggs and together account for 50 % of the world's hen egg export, whereas; USA, Germany and Spain are the major egg importers with a share of over 51 % of the world's egg imports.

xxxii) Among the DA enterprises, both extensive and intensive, poultry production occupies an important position and has enormous potential for expansion with relatively lower investment and can fulfill the world millennium goals of improving human food and nutrition with less effect on environment.

xxxiii) Currently poultry industry in India accounts for a total contribution to GDP of 0.7 % (Rs 400 b) and provides employment to over 5 m people, mostly in rural and peri-urban areas. The country has witnessed an annual growth of 7.3 % in poultry eggs and 10 % in broiler production compared to around 4 % in milk production and around 2 % in meat production from other animals. The high growth rate in poultry production has placed India at the 3rd position after China and USA in egg production with a production of 59.8 b eggs and 5th position after USA, China, Brazil and Mexico with a production of 2.6 m mt of chicken meat in 2009-10. Despite of such an impressive growth, the average *per capita* availability of eggs is 52 and of chicken meat 2.3 kg against the required level of 180 eggs and 11 kg broiler meat to meet the protein and energy requirement as laid down by Indian Council of Medical Research (ICMR). Since this availability, affordability and consumption is currently limited to 32% of the urban and extremely small and relatively rich rural population, the *per capita* consumption in rural areas will be almost of insignificance and they are to mostly depend on relatively costlier eggs and meat from local dual purpose chicken.

xxxiv) Ironically, India's 68.5 % of the human population, as mentioned earlier which lives in rural areas consumes hardly any commercially produced eggs and broiler meat. The large rural population neither contributes to the commercial poultry production significantly nor has any significant share in the consumption of intensively produced poultry eggs and meat and is primarily dependent on low producing chicken, a dual purpose bird, primarily raised under free range scavenging and producing 50-60 eggs per year and weighing around 1.5 kg at adult age. In addition, the indigenous chicken are late maturing, produce small sized eggs and thus small sized chicks which have low survival, slow growth and poor dressing percentage. However there is a great liking for the eggs and meat of the indigenous poultry because of their taste, which is essentially a myth. The meat of indigenous birds is extremely tough and takes a longer time to cook.

xxxv) The organized sector of poultry industry contributes nearly 70 % of eggs and most of broiler meat. The broiler industry is well established in southern states and accounts for 60-70 % of total output. In case of layer industry, Andhra Pradesh, Tamil Nadu and Maharashtra contribute 70 % of eggs produced in the country.

xxxvi) There is a large regional imbalance in the availability and consumption of egg and broiler meat. More than 60 % of the eggs are produced in Andhra Pradesh, Telangana, Haryana, Maharashtra, Punjab and Tamil Nadu and 60 % of poultry meat is produced in five states viz. Andhra Pradesh, Telangana, Karnataka, Maharashtra, Punjab and West Bengal. The other regions, more particularly the central and eastern region, have been bypassed both in production and consumption of commercial poultry eggs and meat and primarily depend on the indigenous chicken for eggs and meat.

xxxvii) The Hyderabad, Secunderabad region has the highest layer production in the country. It accounts for over $1/3^{rd}$ of the egg produced in theTelangana. The other pocket Bombay-Pune-Nashik, Sangli, Miraj in Maharashtra, Banglore-Mysore in Karnatka, Namakkal-Coimbtore in Tamil Nadu, Gurgaon-Yamunanagar in Haryana, Valsad-kheda in Gujarat and Ajmer in Rajasthan have developed a large layer industry which have also expanded around Punjab and Delhi. While marketing of eggs is relatively better organized due to the efforts of the National Egg Coordination Committee (NECC) which helps in gathering intelligence about availability and demand and also helps in regulating the prices, there are no such arrangements for broiler processing and marketing. Most broilers are sold locally alive and are slaughtered in the presence of the buyer. This results in large wastage of slaughter byproducts and creates serious pollution problems.

xxxviii) The egg consumption will increase with an increase in human population, change in age structure with more younger people, urbanization, increased education and employment and thus incomes, small nuclear families, larger funds to spare for food, desire for greater leisure, and all these factors combined will lead to higher consumption of ready to eat, tasty food with higher satiety factor and with an increasing non-vegetarianism and realization of ill effects of red meat, there is an increased consumption of chicken eggs and meat. Organization of egg production and distribution, realization of positive and negative effects of egg consumption, outbreaks of highly infectious avian diseases with zoonotic importance such as Avian influenza and other ethical consideration with respect to intensive raising of layer and broiler under confinement, are some of the factors influencing poultry production in the country negatively.

xxxix) There are some serious marketing problems of poultry eggs and broiler meat. Shell eggs are not traded over long distances because of their fragility and that they cannot be frozen. Therefore, most of the shell eggs are traded within confined markets. This is also true for liquid egg products but not however for egg powder which has still limited use in India. The broiler marketing has even more serious problems as most consumers of broiler meat demand that the chicken should be slaughtered and dressed in their presence as they consider the dressed frozen chicken as a dead chicken. In fact it is necessary that the carcasses after dressing must be maintained at a relatively cold temperature to set the meat through rigor mortis which allows the glucose to be converted to lactic acid which changes the composition of the meat and helps in increasing its shelf life.

xl) The future projection of the demand of eggs is difficult as in addition to eggs for human consumption, they are also used in hatching. However, there are other avian species which do contribute to egg production, though at present at a significantly lower level in India. Like duck eggs constitutes a relatively higher proportion of eggs consumed in some South East Asian countries and China.

xli) The biggest threat to poultry industry, as mentioned earlier, is from diseases with zoonotic importance such as Avian influenza caused by H5N1 strain. The outbreaks of this disease have devastated poultry industry in a number of states in India and a number of other countries.

xlii) In 2009, the total loss to poultry industry due to disease was Rs 2,200 crores. Further repeated outbreaks of Avian influenza have led to serious decline in egg and broiler production due to mandatory culling and destruction of layer stocks.

xliii) Avian diseases are a serious impediment in a sustainable avian egg and meat production and cause serious losses through mortality and morbidity and forcing large culling of birds due to their poor production after disease outbreak.

xliv) With large intensification in urban and peri-urban poultry production, the disposal of poultry wastes from production as well as processing units is becoming a serious problem and is causing serious environmental pollution problems. It is estimated that 22 m t of poultry waste annually is generated in urban intensive poultry production units and its disposal in a systematic manner so that it can be used as a valuable ruminant feed or organic manure and does not create environmental problems is a serious environmental pollution problem. Other than the poultry breeding farms, the dressing plants and hatcheries also generate poultry waste. Some of the alternative uses of poultry slaughter waste are as pet food, manure or bio-fertilizers such as through vermi-composting, biogas and generating electricity but is not fully utilized.

xlv) The major problems are however of disposal of dead birds and waste from slaughter house. There is a growing realization of the role of DA in causing global warming through methane production which contributes to GHG emissions and results in higher incidence of diseases and lower crop and DA production.

xlvi) Marketing of poultry products both eggs and broilers and more particularly the latter, causes major problems for the poultry industry both in serving the people as well as ensuring remunerative return to the producers. Lack of regulated markets like in case of agriculture produce especially cereals, vegetables and fruits and even to some extent in dairy sector, is also a serious limiting factor in expanding poultry production. Lack of adequate cold storage and ware housing facilities cause violent fluctuation in prices of both eggs and broilers, but more particularly in case of latter. Fragmented and remote rural markets also restrict reach of commercial poultry products to more difficult rural areas. In fact the marketing in poultry industry is a more serious problem than production. Elimination of a long chain of middle men through organizing poultry producers into cooperatives or rather producer companies which may take up in addition to production, collection, processing and marketing on a scale large enough that it will be able to compete with foreign multinationals having franchise hatchery. In addition to developing an organized marketing system, the processing, cold storage and proper transport arrangements for eggs, meat and their processed products will have to be created. The GOI, DAHD&F has already established a similar setup in poultry production like NDDB for dairy sector which with time and proper strengthening may help in removing the problems of poultry product marketing.

xlvii) There is a great potential for poultry industry to generate employment and incomes, especially in the rural and peri-urban areas and also improves nutrition and health of large rural population which has been bypassed both in production and consumption of poultry meat and eggs.

xlviii) In comparison to other DA farming, poultry farming requires relatively lesser investment, especially when raised in smaller units utilizing family labour and locally available feed resources. There is a relatively rapid return on investment as birds can be sold for meat at 6-8 weeks of age and the layers start laying between 120-150 days. The feed requirement both for egg and meat production is relatively low and the birds can be fed on a large quantity of coarse cereals and agro-industrial processing byproducts.

xlix) Compared to other DA species except fish, it has higher efficiency of feed conversion (4.6:1 in layers and 2:1 in case of broilers). In other DA species it ranges from 5 to 9. The water requirement in case of poultry is low. There is a more stable income compared to crops and other DA species. Poultry does not compete with human in feed except in high producing layers and broilers where 50% of the ration consists of maize and other coarse gains. Since poultry is a more efficient converter of feed into edible protein with essential amino-acids, vitamins and minerals, it provides better nutrition per unit of feed provided. Poultry farming can generate large employment opportunities for rural poor specially women as it requires only part time labour. Poultry droppings constitutes excellent organic fertilizer and being rich in nutrient can even be used as ruminant feed replacing costing, energy and protein component. Poultry manure contains 1.0-1.8% N and 1.4-1.8% P and 0.8-0.9% K and these are better balanced compared to the cattle dung, night soil and sheep and goat droppings. One ton of poultry litter is produced by 40 layers in a year and is equivalent to 140 kg of ammonium sulphate, 125 kg of super phosphate and 45 kg of potassium. This quantity of poultry manure is sufficient for 1 acre of paddy field and 1/2 acre of vegetable field. Birds under free range maintenance can spread their droppings more uniformly. Poultry feathers can be used as meal. They are also used as fillers for pillows, making fancy articles and making shuttle cocks for playing badminton. Poultry meat and eggs have high nutritive value especially essential amino acids, vitamins and minerals. In a country with large protein deficiency, egg which is considered as vegetarian and has high protein content and other essential nutrients, can meet the nutritional requirement at a relatively cheaper cost. Quail produces relatively larger number of smaller sized egg which can be easily pickled for long term preservation and can meet the protein need of school going children.

Summarizing the poultry R&D in India, following points needs to be considered:

1. The egg on an average comprises of 11% by weight of shell, 58% albumin and 31% of yolk. It consists of 65.5% water, 11.8% protein, 11.0% fat, and 11.7% ash. Albumin contains 88% water, 11% protein, 0.2% fat and 0.8% ash. The yolk contains 48% water, 17.5 % protein, 32.5% fat and 2% ash. The shell contains 96.0 % ash. One egg a day provides 90 Kcal of energy, 6.6 gm protein, 5.5 gm fat, 0.03 gm Calcium, 0.12 gm Phosphorus, 1.6 mg Iron, 600 IU vitamin A, 50 IU vitamin B, 0.095 mg vitamin B1, no vitamin C, 0.19 mg Riboflavin and 0.04 mg Niacin against the recommended daily requirement for a moderately active man of 3000, 70, 50, 570, 0.8, 0.9, 12, 5000, 400, 1.5, 75, 2.0 and 18 respectively. The beef, kine, mutton and chevon production have greater impact on soil and environment than poultry production for egg and broiler. Compared to lamb and pork, the broiler has higher protein (176g per kg meat and 177g per kg of edible DM of meat compared to 146, 354 of lamb and 166 and 225 of pork). The gross content of broiler meat is 65-85 % water, 16-22% protein, 1.5-13% fat, 0.65 to 1% ash and 0.5 to 1.5% carbohydrate. The poultry meat is an excellent source of minerals and vitamins and provides 190 mg Phosphorus, 1.5-1.8 mg Iron, 250-320 mg of Potassium for 100gm of edible meat. It is also a good source of Niacin and Riboflavin.

2. The country has impressive R&D facilities in all aspects of poultry production, health and product processing. But it is seriously lacking in ensuring their transfer to the industry due to relatively poor linkages and the poultry industry having developed their own R&D facilities and further depend on their parent companies and much less on government institutions/ departments. Further the limitations of feed both the quantity and quality and its ever increasing prices and relatively high disease incidence are impeding the growth of poultry production. India can be proud of a large research and educational infrastructure which inter-alia includes all aspects of poultry production, health and product technology. This will include breeding, nutrition, management, health, product processing and socio-economic aspects. The linkage between R&D facilities and the industry is still week and the industry does not depend on the R&D facilities available with the central and the state government organizations and have developed its own R&D and training facilities. There is need to have better linkage between the government efforts and the private sector R&D facilities.

3. Greater emphasis is required on R&D for rural poultry production. This should not be confined to low producing backyard poultry farming using currently mostly available indigenous or slightly improved indigenous chicken or other avian species utilizing local germ plasm but developing rural poultry production on the lines of cooperative dairy production through farmers' cooperatives or producer companies. The only difference between urban and rural poultry production may be that the urban units are large commercial units run by national and multinational companies, whereas; the rural poultry units may be small in size and may be linked for supply of inputs and services and processing and marketing of eggs and broilers. The size of the rural operations collectively could be large and competitive with the large national and multi-national commercial units. The layer and broiler lines developed by CARI, PDP and some units of AICRP which have similar plumage colour and shank length as in indigenous birds and relatively better adaptation to the rural production conditions can be applied in rural poultry production. The greater attention should be given to meeting the egg and chicken meat requirement of the rural and peri-urban people which still constitute 68% of the population in the country and are neither involved in production or consumption of poultry eggs and meat. In addition to the chicken for egg and meat, other avian species should also be propagated.

4. Dr. Wildhorst *et al.* at the Institute of the Spatial Analysis and Planning in areas of agriculture in the University of Vechta, Germany

has done a critical analysis of the present poultry development for egg production in the world in the last 10 years of the 20th century and projected the scenario till 2015. Changes in global environment especially its warming due to high green house gases (GHG) emissions arising from intensification of ruminant livestock production and industrialization and destruction of forest for increasing land under crop production and other civil uses such as construction of roads, markets, residential accommodations and establishment of new industrial units will lead to reduced availability of land for agriculture. There is already a serious depletion in availability of usable water both in quantity and quality and ingress of sea water in the coastal areas. Poultry production relatively makes less impact on environment compared to the ruminant DA and even pigs. The analysis of the current situation and predicting future egg production and their demand is extremely difficult over a relatively longer period. The lack of adequate data and a lack of clear definition of the commodity - egg from the large number of steering factor which decide about egg consumption and production. Even though the consumption of animal products is closely related to available income, a high income does not necessarily lead to higher egg consumption as the consumer may switch to other sources of food and nutrition especially in country like India with a large vegetarian population. The projected demand of 17.9 m mt will depend on some risk factors and political decisions. The biggest threat for the poultry industry in general is the disease outbreak especially H5N1-Avian Influenza virus which had a serious socio-economic impact in northern Italy. The Netherlands and several Asian Countries, resulting in a collapse of poultry industry in a few weeks it took a long period for it to recover. This has also resulted in serious import restrictions. Another factor impeding fast growth of poultry sector is the availability and cost of feed ingredients. The boom in bio-energy production in USA and some European countries, drought impacts in Australia, south eastern Europe and in increased in demand of cereals especially maize for food and feed grains in developing countries especially in China is leading to large increases in prices of poultry feed. This is expected to further increase and thus impact adversely poultry production. Far reaching impacts on the future of egg production and egg trade will be due to the imposition of restrictions on the sale and consumption of eggs produced under intensive system of production. Germany and Australia have already banned raising of layers in cages and similar action is expected in The Netherlands and UK. Welfare legislation will definitely increase production cost and reduce the competitiveness of egg production in the EU compared to Third World Countries. These three factors will definitely have considerable impact on the future development of egg production in the world and more particularly in the developed world which had enjoyed the large commercial egg production at the cheapest cost because of the import of cheaper feed ingredient and saving on labor through mechanization of production and handling of avian products. Several avian influenza outbreaks in important centers of egg production both in developed and developing countries and continuous rise in feed cost are likely to change the production patterns both in management and location.

5. The egg production in different regions of the world is currently projected based on population changes, change in age structure, development of GNP and allocation of family income for food, organization of egg production and distribution from backyard to intensive and from intensive to more extensive, increase in urbanization, education, employment and incomes resulting in a demand of food with taste and higher nutritional value and easy to cook and eat. The vertical integration of production and marketing and its becoming as a component of national agribusiness/ food chain, the health aspects of the food in terms of cholesterol content, outbreaks of highly infectious zoonotic poultry diseases and political decisions such as banning, raising chicken in cages are factors which will influence the development of the poultry production in future. It is difficult to predict the future situation for poultry production for eggs and more particularly broilers because of a large number of factors viz. human population growth, urbanization, education, employment and income and beliefs in consumption of eggs and poultry meat more particularly in rural areas where major human population in India still lives.

❑❑❑

CHAPTER-2

Domestication, Speciation and Diversification of Aves

i) In general, jungle fowl refers to the four species of birds under the genus *Gallus*, order *Galliformes* and family *Phasianidae*. These four species are Ceylon jungle fowl (*G. lafayetti),* Green jungle fowl (*G. varius),* Grey jungle fowl (*G. sonneratti) and* Red jungle fowl (*G. gallus).* The Ceylon jungle fowl inhabits exclusively the island of Ceylon (Sri Lanka), whereas Green jungle fowl is originally from Java, but is also found in Bali, Lombok, Komodo, Flores, Rinca and Island of Indonesia. Grey jungle fowl is indigenous to Southern and Western India, but extends into Gujarat, Madhya Pradesh and South Rajasthan. Red jungle fowl is most widely distributed from India in west to Bali in east.

ii) There are five subspecies of red jungle fowl. i. Cochin-Chinese red jungle fowl (*Gallus gallus*) which are found in Cambodia and Cochinchina and Annam now Vietnam, ii. Burmese red jungle fowl (*Gallus gallus spadiceus*) which is native of south-west Yunnan, Burma, Siam, with the exception of north-east Laos, the Malacca Peninsula and the area north of Sumatra. It is also found in north-eastern part of India while iii. Tonkinese red jungle fowl (*Gallus gallus jabouillei*) is native of Tonkin, south-east Yunnan (China) and northern Annam, iv. Javan red jungle fowl (*Gallus gallus bankiva*) inhabits the south of Sumatra and the islands of Java and Bali. It is likely to have been introduced in the Philippines, Tahiti and as far as Hawaii, v. Indian red jungle fowl (*Gallus gallus murghi*) is inhabitant of northern and central part of the India extending eastward to Odisha and West Bengal.

iii) There are two views about the origin of domestic fowl i.e. monophyletic and polyphyletic. Majority believe that the chicken has monophyletic origin and red jungle fowl is its sole ancestor based on high similarity between red jungle fowl and some of the early domesticated bird, free and successful mating between red jungle fowl and domestic fowl, better survival of crossbred progenies with good level of fertility on *inter-se* mating or mating with any of the parents and more close resemblance of the crow of the domestic cock with red jungle fowl in India as compared to other three jungle fowls. The early evidences against the monophyletic theory were the big difference between asiatic and mediterranean breeds, vertical long axis of the occipital foramen in Cochin breed against the horizontal in red jungle fowl, lack of sex-linked dominant silver gene in red jungle fowl, but its presence in grey jungle fowl as well as in some domestic chicken breeds and production of fertile offspring from the mating of grey jungle fowl and domestic fowl.

iv) Some molecular genetical evidences also support the polyphyletic origin of domestic fowl. The phylogenetic analysis of the entire mitochondrial DNA (mtDNA) genome and nuclear DNA (nucDNA) regions for four chicken repeat 1 (CR1) regions and OTC (ornithine carbamoyl transferase) strongly indicates of the free inter-species hybridizations between grey jungle fowl and red jungle fowl and between gray jungle fowl and **Ceylonese jungle fowl. Similarly domestic chickens have two skin color i.e. white and yellow.** A phylogenetic analysis has demonstrated that though the white skin allele originated from the red jungle fowl, the yellow skin allele originated from a different species, most likely the grey jungle fowl.

v) But there are several molecular genetics evidences, which strongly support the monophyletic origin of domestic fowl. It includes presence of two copies of a 60-bp-long unit containing the nearly invariant tetradecamer, AACTATGAATGGTT in red jungle fowl and domestic fowl, whereas other jungle fowls had 3 to 4 copies. Sequence homology comparison of 539 bases of mitochondrial DNA D-loop region revealed that the red jungle fowl in Thailand and its neighboring areas could be sufficed as the matriarchic ancestor of Chinese domestic fowls. More recent phylogenetic analysis based on microsatellite markers and mitochondrial D-loop sequences between Indian red jungle fowl, Indian domestic fowl, other three jungle fowls and other domestic fowls have provided a conclusive evidence regarding monophyletic origin of domestic fowl and Red jungle fowl as sole ancestor.

vi) The period and place of domestication of chicken is still debatable. Majority of earlier reviews, consider the Indus valley as the point of first domestication in 2500-2100 BC, however later, much earlier domestication of chicken in Chine than in Southeast Asia (~5000 BC) has been reported. In early reviews, the opinion of Peters (1913) did not get enough consideration as his statements lacked literary and/or archaeological evidences. Though, Darwin (1896) expressed a similar belief and lately West and Zhou (1988) have provided strong evidences in support of latter theory. However, the evidences of domestication of chicken at two different places in two different time periods are unquestionable and they are of Harappan culture.

vii) Several discoveries and supporting evidences of domestication of chicken in ancient China indicate that earliest domestic fowl was domesticated much earlier than the Indus valley culture i.e. as early as 5400 BC. From the archaeological site of Cishan, in Wu'an county of Hebei province, the chicken remains were found and most of them were tarsometatarsal bones (from males as well as females). Among other bones (Clavicle, humerus, femur, radius and ulna specimens were also found. These chicken bones were in abundance in the animal remains and the much larger in size in comparison to those of red jungle fowl which gives a positive evidence for domestication.

viii) West and Zhou (1988) had reviewed several evidences and found that 16 Neolithic sites in Northern China have now yielded evidence of domestic fowl, all of them predating Mohenjo-Daro by many centuries. At 13 sites in Europe and western Asia, chicken bones older than those of Mohenjo-Daro have also been discovered. Eight other sites in China, Turkey, Syria, Spain, Romania, and the Ukraine have yielded osteological evidence that is contemporary with that of Mohenjo-Daro. Further, using information from Ho (1977) and from other sources, West and Zhou (1988) stated that the semi-arid climates at the 16 Neolithic sites during at least past 10000 years, was the normal climate for jungle fowl, hence they proposed the domestication point of chicken somewhere in southeast Asia and its subsequent travel to Northern China by about 6000 BC. These evidences put the question mark on the Indus valley as the first domestication centre.

ix) Using archaeological evidence for chicken domestication from China, Asia and Europe, as well as palaeo-climatic evidence from China, it is concluded that chickens were first domesticated from the red jungle fowl (*Gallus gallusmurgi*) in Southeast Asia well before the sixth millennium BC and taken north to become established in China by 6000 BC, when they were later introduced to Japan via Korea during the Yayoi Period (300 BC-300 AD). Domestication occurred in India much later than that in China (~2000 BC), either independently or as a diffusion from Southeast Asia. Although the Iron Age was the main period for dispersion of chickens throughout

Europe, they were already present in some areas during the late Neolithic and early Bronze Age. It is proposed that the earliest European material may be derived from China via Russia.

x) The storage of grains and the conservation of live meat in the form of domesticated birds and animals is a major achievement of the man in the Neolithic agricultural revolution. Plants capture the radiant energy of the sun through their green coloring material-chlorophyll and re-organize and store it in their leaves, roots and seeds which the man consumes as food directly or as feed for his DA and avian species and uses them for food, work, fuel and a number of other industrial and non-industrial purposes. This had led to food and nutritional security for man and hence, an increase in human population which also resulted in an increased area under crop and DA production and consequently an increase in DA population. This also resulted in a large spread of human population spatially and increase in its reproduction rate leading to Malthusian predicament of an imminent danger of large scale famine and human misery.

However, man with his ingenuity of improving crops, DAs and fish production, has been able to avoid large scale hunger and starvation, although spatially and temporally there have been regular human devastation due to serious food shortages and consequent starvation, disease and mortality.

xi) It was only after the man became free from the worry of getting food through hunting and gathering, he started cognition and developed better intelligence which led to higher things in life and development of science, art and culture.

xii) It is believed that inspite the fowl originated in India around 2300 BC, it took long time for India to breed fowl for eggs and meat and it was primarily maintained for sport. This led to development of a large number of types with different shape of comb varying in shape and size and feather and their color. The birds were primarily kept for cock fighting which is still a common sport in some rural areas using indigenous birds. In addition to its use in sport, chicken was kept as a fancy pet animal and the beauty of its plumage had given rise to a large number of breeds / type including the famous Aseel and Kadaknath. The former has black skin and has not only a better adaptability to hot and humid climatic conditions but also produces meat with higher taste and aphrodisiac value.

❑❑❑

CHAPTER-3

Poultry Breeding Research and Development in India - Historical Perspective

Systematic research and development in poultry improvement in India started in 1932 with a grant of Rs 32,000 from Royal Commission on Agriculture to Mission Farm in Etah for breeding experiments. Initially major emphasis was on improving indigenous chicken for egg production through selection and crossing them with exotic layer and broiler breeds and among the exotic breeds. Although the Central and State Governments started breeding exotic stocks and distributing day old chicks of exotics or their crosses with indigenous non-descript chicken. Major research and education in poultry science started in 1960s with the assistance of Technical Cooperation Mission (TCM) of US Government later named as United States Assistance for Development (USAID) and the FAO. A number of exotic layer and broiler breeds were imported and experimented with for studying their performances under Indian environmental and managemental conditions. Two projects for studying the purebred performance of important indigenous poultry types and their crosses with exotic layer breeds were undertaken under PL-480, a project supported by US Government. It involved studies on performance of indigenous birds and their crosses with exotic and layer breeds with respect to their body weight gains, efficiency of feed conversion, carcass yield and quality and egg production and egg quality, survival and disease resistance. The day old chicks of indigenous and exotic breeds and their reciprocal crosses were raised under disease free condition and a representative sample of each of the genetic group was exposed to Ranikhet and Spirochaetosis to determine the percent mortality and morbidity. It was seen that the crosses involving indigenous males and exotic females had higher disease resistance. There was also some improvement in body weight gains, efficiency of feed conversion, sexual maturity, egg production and egg weight. Another PL-480 funded project was implemented by Venketeshra Hatcheries, Pune and involved studying genetics of efficiency of feed conversion in broilers and studied its inheritance and genetic relationship with live weight gains and carcass yield and quality.

A major leap towards in-house research and development programme was start of All India Coordinated Research Programme (AICRP) on poultry for egg and poultry for meat in 1970-71. Extensive research on improving layer and broiler production was undertaken under AICRP on Poultry for egg and AICRP on Poultry for meat. A large number of superior performing layer and broiler pure lines were imported and placed at a number of centers of AICRP to study their purebred performance and performance of their reciprocal crosses. The lines were to be selected on the basis of an index combining age at first egg, short duration egg production and egg weight in layers and body weight at 12 weeks, and efficiency of feed conversion in broilers. These lines were regularly crossed to observe the crossbred performance in reciprocal crosses. Since the same lines were maintained at more than one location, it allowed testing of the same line and sire progeny group within line at a number of locations to study the genetic, environmental and genotype x environment interaction. The sire progeny groups were to be selected within each line based on their purebred and reciprocal crossbred performance with data pooled over the centers where same lines were maintained. Considering the size of breeding operations, the number of lines maintained, were gradually reduced and their reciprocal crossbred performance was tested only after longer intervals. The project did provide information on genetic aspects on egg and broiler production and effectiveness of selection and mating programmes in improving egg and broiler production and led to development of a number of commercially viable layers and broiler strain crosses.

At Central Avian Research Institute high producing layer strain cross ILI-80 and now called CARI-Priya has been evolved which has age at first egg 17-18 weeks, 50% egg production at 150 days, peak production 26-28 weeks, growing survival 96%, layer survival 94%, egg production peak 92%, hen housed to 72 weeks egg production, 298, hen day to 72 weeks, 301 eggs feed consumption per dozen eggs 1.77 kg and per kg mass 2.57 kg, average egg weight 57 g with an excellent internal quality, the bird is easy to handle and performs well under variable management conditions, is an efficient converter of feed in to eggs and has low laying house mortality.

Biotechnology Research

Chicken can be used as a model bio-reactor to produce proteins of medicinal importance through transgenesis. The multi cellular stage of embryo in freshly laid eggs, breaking of egg shell to get access to embryo and the presence of large quantity of yolk create hurdles in development of transgenic chicks. However sperm mediated gene transfer method is used in developing transgenic chicken through developing transgenic spermatozoa. Integrating foreign DNA in spermatozoa genome which includes separation of spermatozoa through centrifugation and their washing with a buffer and subsequent dilution in fixed concentration in a buffer and addition of foreign DNA plus liposome mixture is prepared and incubated at room temperature. Similarly, a restriction enzyme (Ncol) and liposome mixture is prepared by mixing both in a fixed concentration and incubation at room temperature. Subsequently both the mixtures are combined and incubated for a fixed duration at room temperature and used for inseminating a hen.

Estimating parental genomic properties using micro-satellite markers: The basic protocol includes identification of polymorphic micro-satellite markers, isolation of genomic DNA from the parents and offspring to make a panel of genomic DNAs. PCR amplification using this panel of genomic DNA for each micro-satellite marker, resolution on metaphor agarose, sizing of alleles and estimation of the proportion of the common alleles at each marker as well as cumulative on all markers. The cumulative proportion of common bands will show the genetic similarities between the parents and offspring and ranges from 0-1. Higher the proportion, higher will be the parental genomic proportion.

Multiplex PCR has been used for sexing guinea fowl. A common band of both the sexes is amplified and female specific band, only in female simultaneously is used to overcome the sexing problem, a set of primers such as USP-1 and USP-3 specific to w-chromosome-0.6 kb EcoRi fragment specific to females and another set of primers i.e. DS-1 and DS-2 specific to partial 16S rRNA gene, hence common in both sexes, a multiplex PCR has been developed. The female shows 2 bands i.e. 370 bp female specific and 590 bp common band while male show 590 bp band. The method can be used at birth, since sexual bi-morphism is poorly defined in guinea fowl.

PCR RFLP in identifying meat of different species: DNA based methods for identification of species from which the meat has originated is based on mitochondrial DNA sequencing. The basic protocol includes isolation of genomic DNA from meat samples, amplification of the common bands and its subsequently digestion with all the identified species specific restriction enzymes. The species is identified on the basis of restriction enzyme profile.

Selection criteria for enhancing immuno-competence: Immuno-competence improves disease resistance through selection without compromising the production. Both humoral and cell mediated response parameters are increased in successive generation without any loss of body weight in broiler chickens.

Recombinant cytokines production and their use as an adjuvant in growth promotion: Cytokines offer a class of protein substances that can be used in a recombinant form as a naturally occurring immuno-adjuvant, immuno-modulator and growth promoter. Avian cytokines viz. IFN-ã led to higher humoral and cell mediated immune responses to New Castle Disease Vaccine as well as higher body weight in broiler chickens.

Molecular markers for immune responses against NDV: Molecular markers for enhancing protection against specific diseases have been pursued in poultry genetics. The SNP (A318G) in IFN-ã promoter region has been located which is associated with immune response with NDV. A simple procedure applicable in commercial breeding programme has been developed to improve the NDV response.

Silencing of myostatin gene in cultured chicken embryo fibroblast: It is used in overcoming physiological barriers for increasing muscle development. The application of RNAi for silencing myostatin gene is a step in this direction. siRNAs for myostatin designated and procedures were developed for silencing myostatin gene in cultured embryo fibroblast.

□□□

CHAPTER-4

Poultry Genetics and Breeding - Basic Principles and Their Applications

Primary aim of a genetic study is to identify inherited variations which may be discrete or continuous in nature. Qualitative genetics is the study of traits showing discontinuous variation i.e. they can be grouped as discrete classes. These traits are relatively less influenced by environment and are generally governed by a single or a few genes under simple Mendelian inheritance. The examples of qualitative traits include simple phenotypic differences in plumage colour, skin colour, shank colour, feather development, comb type as well as immunologically or biochemically polymorphic characters.

The quantitative genetics can be defined as the study of inheritance of traits, which show continuous variation and are governed by a number of genes located on the same chromosome or on different chromosomes. These traits are called as "quantitative traits" as they can be quantified through weight or measurements. Some of them are called metric traits as they are measurable on some metric scale e.g. body weight in gram (g) and shank length in centimeter (cm). Some traits are measured in terms of numbers such as number of eggs laid during some specified period. Quanlitative traits come in "all or none" class and have only two values i.e. either present or absent. Such traits are fertility, hatchability and mortality. Inspite these traits are recorded in percentages but can be converted into a continuous distribution by different statistical procedures. The basic inheritance of all the quantitative traits is complex as they are governed by a number of genes with different relationship with each other viz. additive/ dominance/ epistatic and these genes may interact with other genes located on the same or different chromosome. The genes affecting the same trait and located on the same chromosome but at different loci are linked and depending up on the distance they may continue go together or segregate often. The size of linkage disequilibrium would depend upon the distance between the two linked loci and they may continue to create disequilibrium in the gene sequence for a longer time and may thus cause a correlation between the linked traits for a longer / shorter period. Further the phenotypic expression of these traits is influenced to a varying degree by environment. The environment is both internal i.e. interaction with other gene and production environment in which the gene are to express their effects. This involves nutrition, physical environment determined by ambient temperature (maximum and minimum), relative humidity, solar radiation and wind velocity and health environment. Most of these environmental factors are either controlled by determining needs of different production types and providing them with the requisite feed with nutrient contents, providing shelters to protect from inclement weather and protecting the birds from infectious and non-infectious diseases.

In chicken, the important quantitative traits are growth rate, egg production, feed efficiency, carcass yield and quantity (dressing percentage and bone: meat: fat ratio). Meat and egg quality traits as well as reproductive and fitness traits are important in determining the economics of poultry production for meat/ eggs. Though most of the economic traits are quantitative in nature, however; some traits such as plumage color, feathering rate show qualitative inheritance.

4.1 Qualitative Economic Traits

4.1.1 Plumage color

There is a large variation in plumage color which helps in discriminating among different breeds and varieties within a breed and sexing of day old chicks. It has also been used as a model for study of gene action at the cellular level. Plumage color has economic importance not only in layer but also for broiler production. The tinted eggs from colored germplasm get an extra price in market. Similarly colored broiler is preferred over white one. Hence, it is important to know different plumage types and their inheritance. The solid plumage colors are white, black, red and blue. A number of other plumage colors are also encountered and are inherited in a simple Mendelian system.

a) ***White plumage***: White plumage is breed characteristic of White Leghorn and White Plymouth Rock. In White Leghorn it is dominant, whereas; in Rock it is recessive. The epistatic gene I in White Leghorn prevents the expression of color gene leading to white plumage, whereas; in White Plymouth Rock, the epistatic gene I is absent. The epistatic gene I is also present in strains of Rhode

Island Whites, White Minorcas, White Wyandottes and White Plymouth Rocks.

b) ***Black plumage***: Black plumage is a characteristic of Jersey Black Giants, Black Sumatra, Black Hamburgs, Black Leghorn and Black Minorca. It is recessive to white in White Leghorn but dominant in other breeds and varieties.

c) ***Red plumage***: Red plumage is a characteristic of Red Leghorn and is also seen in Rod Island Red (RIR), New Hampshire and Red Sussex. The intensity of red color varies greatly in different breeds suggesting a control of a number of genes and influence of the environment.

d) ***Blue plumage***: It is found in Blue Andalusian. It is due to heterozygous condition of gene BL.

e) ***Buff plumage***: It is found in Buff Brahmas, Buff Cochin, Buff Leghorn and Buff Orpingtons. It is dominant to recessive white but is recessive to black. It is autosomal.

f) ***Columbian plumage***: It is a characteristic of Columbian Leghorn, Columbian Plymouth Rocks and Light Sussex. It is due to dominant sex linked gene S and a non sex-linked gene which restricts the spread of black to the neck, wings and tail. It is located on sex chromosome.

g) ***Sex linked barring***: The barring gene which produces barred plumage is sex linked and expresses at the time of hatching. When males of RIR / New Hampshire are mated with females of Barred Plymouth Rocks all the male chicks have bright yellow shanks and spot marking on head and the females are solid black without head spots but with black or very dark shanks. The difference in the color pattern in the two sexes helps in sexing chicks at the time of hatching.

4.1.2 Skin color

Yellow and white are predominant skin colors. Yellow skin is characteristic of most American breeds and white of European breeds. A single pair of genes W and w represents white and yellow colors respectively. White color is dominant. The gene is autosomal and causes a deposition of carotenoid pigment xanthophyll. W gene prevents the transfer of Xanthophyll pigment to skin, beak and shank causing them to be white.

4.1.3 Ear lobe color

Color of ear lobes is inherited and helps in identification of the breed of the chicken. White ear lobe is a characteristic of Mediterranean breeds and all the breeds with white earlobes lay white shelled eggs. Breeds with red ear lobe lay brown shelled eggs.

4.1.4 Slow and fast feathering

Mediterranean breeds have early growth feathers relative to Asiatic, English and American breeds and a fast growth of feathers. The slow feathering (K) is dominant to fast feathering (k). The gene is located on sex chromosome and is used for sexing chick at hatching.

4.1.5 Plumage pattern

The rate of development of feathers, their distribution and texture result in large variation in plumage pattern in chicks. The classical example is of naked neck where the feathers are absent on the neck region and dominant Na gene is responsible for the condition. Frizzle plumage is not completely dominant to normal plumage. The genotype FF produces complete frizzle plumage, whereas; those with Ff are semi frizzle. The gene is autosomal.

4.1.6 Comb type

Six types of combs have been reported in chicken which include single, rose, pea, walnut, duplex and breda. Both rose and pea comb are dominant to single comb and are incompletely dominant among themselves. Duplex comb is seen in polish, sultan and La Fleche breeds. The duplex comb is inherited differently from the previous four comb types. Two different alleles (Dv and Dc) have been identified and are incompletely dominant. Breda is found in ducks Breda breed. The bd is recessive to Bd and those with the gene have duplex comb.

4.2 Quantitative Economic Traits

The different domesticated avian species especially chicken is reared primarily for economic purposes viz. for egg/ meat production and the aim is to get maximum meat of desired quality and eggs with optimum size and good internal quality. There are some breeds where both eggs and meat are important economic traits such as in indigenous breeds of chicken. While the meat is produced both from males and females and in the case of broilers both the males and females are raised and marketed for meat. In case of layers, the chickens are sexed at one day of age and males are generally destroyed or may be occasionally raised for meat production in rural areas as they are cheaper than broiler chicken but take much longer to reach the marketable weight. There are a number of factors which influence the meat and egg production from chicken. It is known that the meat and egg production is genetically controlled to different levels being higher in meat production and relatively lower in egg production. Both these characters are also influenced by genetic and environment as well as the interaction/ correlation between genetic and environment. It is also known that for meat and egg production, a large variation exists between populations as well as within a populations, but this variation is continuous in nature i.e. no distinct phenotypes exists for these traits (like plumage colour), rather the individual performance is distributed in a range from minimum to maximum (such as in case of body weight at any specific age say day old may range from 28 g to 38 g in chicken. The traits showing continuous variation are called quantitative (metric) traits. These traits are measurable in term of a quantity such as in grams. The body weight of a chick at day old age averages 31.5 g or a bird produces 300 eggs in a year. The quantitative traits are polygenetic in nature, which means that these traits are influenced by a large number of genes, generally with small effects and with a large environmental variation. There may be some genes with major effects and have a larger control on the variation in that trait. These genes may interact in an additive or non-additive or both manners with each other. In addition, there may be epistatic interactions with other genes located on the same or other chromosomes. Further, as stated above these traits are influenced by environment and the interaction between genetic and environmental effects. Hence the inheritance of quantitative traits is complex and difficult to measure at a gene level or even accurately at the level of the influence of all genes contributing to the variation in quantitative characters. These characters may also be correlated with each other and this correlation may be positive, as between body weight and egg weight (means heavier eggs from heavier birds) or negative, as between egg production and egg weight (means birds producing more eggs generally have low egg weight). This co-relationship between the traits is also controlled by genes and is also influenced by production environment. Since the part of the variations existing in the traits and co-variations existing between the traits is controlled by genotype is inherited, therefore it is essential to measure it. The measures of estimating the genetic variance and co-variance and are hertibility, repatability and genetic corelation.

4.3 Heritability

The heritability estimates the proportion of the total phenotypic variation that is due to heredity. More precisely, it is the proportion of the differences for that trait in a population that are due to additive effects of genes. For example if, a trait has a heritability of 0.5, it means that 50 % is due to environmental effects of the total phenotypic variation observed for that trait is due to genetic differences governing the trait, while remaining 50 % is due to the environment. Therefore in general, heritability (h^2) is defined as the ratio of genotypic variance and phenotypic variance i.e. V_G/V_P. This is the definition of heritability in broader sense. In narrow sense, heritability is the ratio of variance due to additive genetis effects and total phenotypic variance i.e. V_A/V_P. The heritability can also be defined in terms of regression coefficient.

4.4 Genetic and Phenotypic Correlations

The relationship between two traits in statistical term is expressed by correlation (phenotypic, genetic and environment). Genetic correlation between two traits is defined as the correlation between genetic effects that influences the two traits (Falconer, 1960). As the phenotype is considered to be a function of both the genotype and environment; therefore, the observable or phenotypic correlation between two traits will arise due to correlations between genetic and environmental effects that influence the two traits in a similar or different manner which will result in a positive or a negative genetic correlation. Genetic correlation between two traits may arise due to pleiotropy or linkage between genes affecting the two traits (Falconer, 1960). Pleiotropy is an expression of a gene/genes whereby it affects two or more traits, so that when the gene/genes segregate results in simultaneous variation in the two characters. The degree of correlation arising from pleiotropy expresses the extent to which two characters are influenced by same genes. But as the correlation resulting from pleiotropy is the overall or net effects of all the segregating genes, some gene/genes may have positive effects on both the characters while in another case a relationship may be negative and an increase in one trait may result in a decrease in the other correlated traits. Genetic correlation may also be caused by linkage disequilibrium, which is transient in nature. Genetic correlations may also be caused by different breeding goals within a population (Pirchner, 1983). Genetic correlation, like heritability can be estimated from pair of traits using variances in and covariance components between the two traits (Snedecor, 1940). This may be calculated from the regression of one trait in offspring and another trait in parents or vice versa (Hazel, 943). Becker (1986) has outlined the procedure of estimating the genetic correlations using analysis of variance and covariance, analogous to estimation of heritability.

4.5 Traits Important for Meat Production

4.5.1 Body weight

Fast growth is the foremost desirable characteristic for meat production. Most simple measure of growth is body weight at a specific age. It measures the cumulative growth up to the age at which body weight is taken, however; it does not measure the rate of growth between two ages. Body weight gain, either absolute or relative between two points of time in the age of an individual reflects the rate of growth. In view of high positive correlation between body weights and weight gain, the body weight at a specified age is a reliable and simple criterion of growth in chicken. Body weight at early ages i.e. 4 to 6 weeks of age have extensively used as selection criterion to improve early growth rate in meat type lines/ breeds. Juvenile body weight is highly heritable trait and highly positively correlated with subsequent body weights as well as weight gains.

4.5.2 Voluntary feed intake (Appetite and efficieny of feed conversion, Feed conversion ratio/ FCR)

Feed conversion is amount of feed consumed to gain a specified weight at a specific age or feed consumed to gain one kg body weight, whereas; feed efficiency may also be defined as weight gain in a specified quantity of feed e.g. weight gain per kg feed. Both the parameters may be for a period between two points of age or may be cumulative up to a specific age. The term FCR is quite commonly used and understood term and may be calculated as amount feed consumed in kg to gain one kg body weight up to market age i.e. up to 4 weeks or 5 weeks of age. Lower the estimate, better the feed conversion efficiency of the bird.

4.5.3 Body (skeletal confirmation traits)

For meat production, it is not only the amount of meat, but the appearance of carcass is also important. Hence some skeletal and conformation traits received attention of the breeders. These traits may include keel length, breast length, shank length, leg length, leg circumference, body depth, breast angle etc. at market age. Among these three traits are more commonly measured and used. The shank length is measured as distance from hock joint to carpal joint, whereas keel length is the distance between the point of ischium (anterior end of keel bone) and the point of keel (posterior end of keel bone). Both the measures are measured with the help of Vernier Calipers and expressed in centimeter. The breast angle is measured in degrees at a point about 1 inch posterior to the anterior end of the keel bone, using Virginia type breastometer.

4.5.4 Carcass traits

For broiler production, carcass traits are essentially important. Carcass traits include the yields from different edible body parts and the losses in the form of inedible body parts. More yield and lesser losses are desirable for profitable broiler production. Different carcass traits usually measured are given below.

i) ***Shrinkage loss***: Loss in body weight due to withdrawal of feed and water before 24 hours and 12 hours respectively, before intended slaughter is taken as shrinkage loss. Percent shrinkage loss is calculated as ratio of shrinkage loss and pre-slaughtering body weight, multiplied by hundred.

ii) ***Bleeding loss***: Birds are bled in a bleeding cone. Difference in pre-bleeding body weight and post-bleeding carcass weight is a measure of blood loss. Percent bleeding loss is calculated as ratio of bleeding loss and pre-bleeding body weight, multiplied by hundred.

iii) ***Feathering loss***: Carcass are de-feathered mechanically/ manually. The loss in pre and post de-feathered carcass weight is taken as de-feathering loss. Percent feathering loss is calculated by dividing the feathering loss by pre-slaughter body weight and then multiplying the product with hundred.

iv) ***Offal loss:*** The head, shank, feet and viscera except heart, liver and gizzard are considered as offal. Percent offal loss is the weight of offals divided by pre-slaughter body weight and then multiplied by hundred.

v) ***Evisceration yield***: It includes the carcass excluding offal and giblets. Percent evisceration yield is the ratio of eviscerated carcass weight and pre-slaughter body weight, multiplied by hundred.

vi) ***Giblet yield***: Giblets includes edible visceral organs i.e. heart, liver and de-skinned gizzard. Percent giblet yield is calculated by dividing the weight of giblets by pre-slaughter body weight and multiplying the product by hundred.

vii) ***Cut up part yield***: The eviscerated carcass is cut into standard cuts including breast, neck, wings, back, thigh and drumstick as per BIS standards. The percent yield of different cut-up parts may be calculated by dividing weight of cut-up part by eviscerated carcass weight and multiplying the product by hundred.

viii) ***Abdominal fat weight***: Abdominal fat consists of both leaf fat and gizzard fat. Leaf fat is removed from around the cloaca and under the viscera. Gizzard fat is removed to the point between pro-ventriculus and gizzard and at the attachment of duodenum. Percent abdominal fat is calculated as ratio of weight of abdominal fat and pre-slaughter body weight, multiplying by hundred.

4.5.5 Livability

Good livability is extremely important for profitable layer and broiler production and is measured in most simple terms i.e. percent mortality up to market age/ and of layer.

4.6 Selection for Economic Traits

Selection can be defined in terms of its observable consequences as the 'non-random differential reproduction of genotype' and may be either natural or artificial (human endeavoured). The purpose of artificial selection for a metric character is to modify its mean or its variation or to extend its range in one or the other direction. The change in a population mean resulting from selection is brought through changes of gene frequencies at the loci that influence the character and are under selection. The change produced by selection that is of interest to breeder is the change of population mean and may be referred as response to selection. Basically, response to selection is the function of additive genetic variation and intensity of selection, but some other factors such as effect of natural selection, inbreeding etc. also influence the response to selection.

Selection for metric characters in DAs including poultry is being done largely for improving the traits of economic importance. Since majority of the traits are related to production such as growth rate, egg production, have positive contribution to returns from sale hence the selection is on positive side i.e. the individuals having higher estimates for these traits are to be selected. In very few cases such as abdominal fat in poultry, individuals having lower estimates are selected. Therefore, either on higher or lower side; the individuals are selected on their individual performance for the trait. This is most simple way of selection and is called as mass selection or individual selection. The effectiveness of this selection depends upon the degree of reliability of the measurements of phenotype of an individual to be a measure of the genotype of that individual for the trait being selected. This reliability depends upon the extent of influence of the environment on that trait as we know that the phenotype of an individual (P) is equal to the genotype (G) plus environmental influence (E) i.e. P = G + E. In case, where environmental influence is less, P may be a good indicator of G, but in the traits under large environmental influence, P may not be good indicator of G. Therefore, to improve the prediction of G from the P; the information from different sources such as ancestors, collaterls (sibs or progenies may be considered after giving proportional weightage depending upon the relationship of the individual used for predicting the breeding value of other individual. Hence the selection may be classified in the following methods depending upon the source of information used.

4.6.1 Individual selection

In this method, the individual is selected on the basis of its own performance. It is also called mass selection.

4.6.2 Pedigree selection

In this method, the individual is selected on the basis of the parents/ grandparents.

4.6.3 Progeny selection

In this method, the individual is selected on the basis of its performance of progenies.

4.6.4 Selection based on the performance of the collateral relatives

In this method, the individual is selected on the basis of its collateral relatives such as full sibs or half sibs.

The selection may be done for one, two or more than two traits at a time. Depending upon the number of traits under selection, the selection methods may be classified as follows:

Tandom selection: In this method, one trait is selected at a time. After improving one trait, another trait is taken up for improvement.

Independent culling level: In this method two traits are improved simultaneously by fixing the minimum culling levels for both the traits.

Selection index method: In this method two or more traits are selected simultaneously through an index, in which due weightage is assigned to each trait. The weightage may be simple with a difference of an individual from the population being or based on heritability of gentic and phenotypic corelations among traits of interest and their relative economic value.

4.7 Breeding Programmes for Improving Productivity

a) Egg/Meat production

The primary objective of any DA breeding programme is to increase the production efficiency/productivity which is a function of reproduction, survival and actual production of economic products/services. The basis of selection, as mentioned earlier, can be individual's own performance or of relatives viz. parents, collaterals (full and half sibs) and progeny. The relationship with full sibs is similar to that with progeny but the limitation is the number of full sibs available relative to the progeny and since the subsequent progeny of selected parents is to perform in the same production environment as the earlier progeny on which genetic merit of the parents has been determined, the accuracy of selection can be very high. Further, the intensity of selection can relatively be higher in progeny especially in layers and broilers where large number of chicks from each parent can be tested in a large number of locations, thus, reducing the effect of genotype x environment interaction/correlation. Genotype-environment correlation should also be avoided by ensuring that all birds irrespective of their level of performance are provided free choice, *ad lib* feed to exploit differences in their appetite / voluntary feed intake which also has a large genetic variation and determines not only the performance but also economic efficiency of production.

b) Survival

Survival is the most important economic trait as higher susceptibility to disease and environmental stresses lead to serious problem of morbidity and mortality and economic losses in any commercial DA production. Although survival or susceptibility to disease has a discontinuous distribution at phenotypic level calling a few categories and the underlying genetic variation, however; is normally distributed. There are large variations among breeds, strains within breeds and sire progeny groups within a strain with respect to disease susceptibility / resistance. The diseases investigated for genetic resistance in poultry include Marek's disease, Leucosis, Blue Comb, Coccidiosis, Nematode worm infestation, Rhanikhet disease, Aspergillosis, uric acid nephritis and various respiratory infections. The number of genes controlling susceptibility/ resistance to a disease is not clearly known. Possibly, the resistance is polygenic with a large number of genes with small effects and spread over a large part of the genotype. However, there are some major genes related to Major Histo-compatibility Complexes (MHC). Research is now in progress for identifying micro-satellites related to production and disease resistance in DA as well as other major and minor genes which may help in identifying more resistant animals/birds and improving genetic resistance to microbial and parasitic diseases. It is known that indigenous DA species are more adapted to tropical environment and diseases and have been used for introducing disease resistance in high producing layers and broilers. Although major efforts in controlling mortality and morbidity have been through disease surveillance and monitoring and taking strategic control and eradication methods but still the economic losses due to various diseases which are currently endemic is very large. The pathogenic agents often mutate resulting in failure of immunity caused through vaccination and if there exists resistance to diseases in general, the losses resulting from disease will be relatively less. Testing of stocks against Pullorum and Mycoplasma infections, vaccination against infections like RD, Fowl Pox, Marek's, Bronchitis, Infectious Bursal Disease (IBD) and medication to prevent and cure has been the usual procedures for reducing economic losses due to mortality and morbidity in poultry. Perpetual applications of chemotherapeutic agents results in drug resistance. Similarly, the mutation of disease causing organisms leads to breakdown of immunity resulting from protective vaccination, it is therefore necessary that genetic resistance to disease should be increased through selection or introducing inheritance from resistance stocks. The need for breeding for disease resistance is therefore large as the number of diseases in poultry could not be controlled through conventional approaches.

4.8 Role and Present Status of Biotechnology (Molecular Biology and Genetic Engineering) in Augmenting Poultry Productivity for Eggs and Meat

Till more recently, major genetic progress in economic traits related to egg/meat production viz. egg production, egg size/weight, egg quality and efficiency of feed conversion in case of layers, live weight gains, efficiency of feed conversion, carcass yield and quality in case of broilers, have been made on the basis of the phenotypic expression or estimates of breeding value derived from the phenotypic measurements without indepth knowledge of genetic basis (gene/ genes controlling these traits). This has led to selection based on multiple traits using selection indices combining different economic traits weighed according to their genetic variances and co-variances and relative economic value, with some emphasis on generation interval. This had also led to complex breeding schemes such as reciprocal selection with a constant texture, reciprocal recurrent selection and inbreeding and hybridization, the latter requiring development of a large number of inbred lines with a large inbreeding coefficient and testing different lines in largest possible combinations and identifying lines with superior performance in different traits and their combining ability with other lines either for the traits not selected for or utilizing non-additive variance/covariance primarily due to dominance and over dominance.

The conventional breeding approaches although have led to a large progress in poultry production for egg and meat production, the approach has certain limitations like relatively slow progress, requiring continuous measurement of phenotypic variance and maintenance of a large, well structured population with proper feeding, management and health cover, incurring large expenditure on housing, management and technical manpower. The selection results in a large culling of genetically inferior birds at various stages of life when their performance can be recorded and thus results in large economic losses incurred on their production through feeding, health cover and management. This is truer in case of layers where the expression of the economic traits related later age. Further characters like disease resistance would require exposure of animal to the disease and selecting survivors or with higher immunological responses. Similarly in carcass traits the birds need to be slaughtered and in such cases only related animals can be selected.

The recent advances in biotechnology related to molecular biology and genetic engineering have provided opportunities to understand the molecular architecture of the individual bird and select them early in life for traits expressed late in life and requiring knowledge of pedigree, collaterals. These approaches can further strengthen the conventional breeding schemes through knowing the genetic architecture related to the traits of economic importance and thus an increase in accuracy and intensity of selection for the desirable economic traits as well as reducing unnecessary expenditure on raising animals for traits of economic importance.

4.8.1 Genetic profiling

Chicken was the first non-mammalian domestic animal species known to have been domesticated in south China some 10,000 years back based on DNA studies on conserved bones. It is also first known mammalian species sequenced for the whole genome. Chicken genome comprises 18 pairs of autosomes and 01pair of sex chromosome (2n=78). The females are heterogametic (ZW) and males homogametic (ZZ), unlike in mammals where male is heterozygous (XY) and the female homozygous (XX). Autosomes in chicken are classified in to five large macro-chromosomes, five intermediate chromosomes and 28 micro-chromosomes. Chicken genome is estimated to be 1.2 x 10^9 base pair and ~ 4,000 Cm (Centi morgan) in length. It comprises of 20,000 – 23,000 genes. Chicken genome contains ~ 2.8 million of Single Nucleotide Polymorphisms (SNPs) with one potential biomarker at every 374 base pair along the genome.

4.8.2 Marker assisted selection (MAS)

During the second half of the 20th century imperial selection based on physical characteristics viz. size and shape of comb, plumage colour and intensity and height of flightiness and aggressiveness and fighting ability, as chicken was used mostly for sports. It is only later that biometrical approaches strengthened the foundation of Quantitative Genetics in most animal improvement programmes but it was poultry which adopted the utilization of both additive and non-additive components of genetic variances in and co-variances between different economic traits and using more complex breeding schemes such as reciprocal selection, recurrent reciprocal selection/ inbreeding hybridization.

In the last two decades there has been an emergence, though slowly of biotechnology which has made us know more of the "black box genetics". The current understanding that each phenotype is controlled by a gene or a group of genes has led to the use of Marker Assisted Selection (MAS). MAS involve the selection of individual based on genetic markers associated with economic trait of interest. In 1970s traits related to blood groups, protein and enzyme polymorphism and cytogenetics were studied with respective to their variances and possible relationship with economic traits. Except for some relationship with congenital abnormalities or some specific disease problems, variation in them and their relationship with most economically important traits was low and they could not be used for selection of individuals with superior genotypes for economic traits.

As mentioned earlier, MAS involves selection on the basis of genetic markers associated with economic traits. Genetic markers used for MAS are candidate gene markers either based on SNP's of anonymous markers such as DNA finger prints/microsatellites. Accurate understanding of the genes controlling a trait *per se*, estimation of environmental variation in gene expression and development of sophisticated statistical techniques are now being employed in MAS. MAS may enhance rapid genetic gain due to higher precision in estimating genetic merit (breeding value) of an individual. This is more true in sex limited traits, expressed in one sex, while the genetic merit for the genetic trait in other sex although carrying genetic variance does not express in the phenotype. DNA based selection is highly accurate as it is not based on physical expression and thus selection can be made directly in both sexes and can lead to higher genetic gain per unit time. Similarly some traits, as mentioned earlier, are expressed late in life at a later age for which the breeders have to wait to select the animals till expression of the trait. This unnecessarly increases the expenses on maintenance of birds which may subsequently not be selected to contribute to the next generation. This is more true in case of layers where only a few males are selected and the use of AI has further resulted in the retention of even fewer males. To minimize the economic loss due to retention of birds which are not going to be used for breeding, DNA based selection can be performed at an early age even before the trait is expressed. This is even more true for traits requiring slaughter of the animals or their exposure to a disease in case of carcass yield and meat quality or susceptibility to a disease. In such cases individual selection is not possible and only family selection is resorted to. In case of family selection, the relationship of the individual with the family member on the basis of whose phenotypic/genetic merit individual will be selected and its effect on generation interval will determine the rate of genetic gain per unit time. Gene based selection can be followed without the above mentioned limitations on the basis of DNA or marker assisted selection.

With the advancement in biotechnology, a number of genetic markers such as Amplified Fragment Length Polymorphism (AFLP), Restricted Fragment Length Polymorphism (RFLP), Random Amplified Polymorphism (RAP), DNA, Microsatellite, Quantitative Traits Loci (QTLs) and Single Nuclotide Polymorphism (SNP) have become available and not only help in predicting the genetic merit of an individual with higher accuracy but at an early age and at shorter life span. This can further help in understanding population structure and development of genetic approaches for improving DA population are economic production purpose. Molecular markers are helpful in identifying the genetic merit of an individual at an early age and in both sexes. MAS has a number of advantages in most DA improvement programmes as they:

i) Do not need a large structured population for implementing selection programmes for animal improvement,

ii) The process can be applied at birth or before the expression of desired trait.

iii) It reduces the cost of maintenance till the expression of the trait.

iv) The rate of genetic improvement is higher than conventional selection because of higher accuracy and intensity and reducing generation interval such as milk yield/egg production

v) The cost of genotyping is not very high and is around Rs 60 per sample.

4.8.3 Quantitative Trait Loci (QTL)

Majority of economic traits in domestic animals (DAs) are polymorphic and polygeneic in nature and are controlled by several genes located on the same or different chromosomes, each contributing only to a small component variation in a trait. Such loci/genes are called QTLs. With the genetic markers, QTLs controlling a specific economic trait are identified and these QTLs are then mapped to determine the linkage status with other markers. The closely linked marker for QTL is most desirable for accurate determination of genetic variation and thus a higher genetic gain through selection.

In poultry, several QTLs have been mapped on different chromosomes and are being used in selection of traits such as live weight, egg production and disease resistance. The QTL for live weight at 48 days of age in broilers and voluntary feed intake have been mapped on chromosomes 16 and 17 and Marek's disease on chromosomes 2,4,7 and 8.

Beijing You Chicken has been genotyped at five SNPs by using PCR and associated with growth and reproduction traits. The T 50639403C (T808C) SNP of the Insulin Growth Factor binding protein 1 gene has been associated with body weight of 10 weeks of age and C56072547T (C968T) SNP of insulin like growth factor binding protein 3 gene is associated with body weight at 8 and 10 weeks of age respectively. The C4535156T (C1591T), G4533815A (G250A) and G4533675C (G110C) SNP of the STAT 5B gene are associated with age at first egg ranging from 0.0088 to 0.0143. The SNPs have a significant association with early gain in body weight or sexual maturity or both and may be used as potential markers for MAS.

QTLs affecting resistance to Marek's disease have been identified by a panel of 15 SNPs and 217 microsatellite markers. 21 QTL regions affecting post challenge survival have been identified and all distributed on 11th chromosome (GGA1,2,3,4,5,8,9,15,18,26) and Z.

Salmonella infected poultry products are a major source of zoonotic infection and need alternative approaches. A high density marker set of 1255 SNPs covering the whole genome to identify QTL responsible for salmonella colonization has been identified. Four QTLs on chromosomes 2, 3, 12, and 25 have been identified. These include one genome wide significant QTL on chromose 2 and 3 additional QTLs on chromosomes 3,12 and 25 at 96, 15 and 1MB respectively which are significant at the chromosome wide level.

4.8.4 Restriction fragment length polymorphisms (RFLPs)

Restriction enzyme can break DNA at a particular nucleotide and in different patterns. The variation in sequence fragment length is used as a measure of variation in a population. The technique has limitation in predicting variation due to site specificity of restriction enzyme. Molecular markers for high humoral immune response in

Kadaknath breed of indigenous chicken have been identified. M x i interferon induced gene brings prolification of single stranded RNA virus including influenza viruses. SNP Mx I gene has been reported to be associated with influenza virus leading to the study of partial intron 13 and partial Axon 14 of Mxi gene using PCR-RFLP to explore polymorphism in Aseel breed.

4.8.5 Microsatellite

Microsatellites are pallandrome repeats of 3-4 bp DNA sequence randomly distributed across the genome. They are highly polymorphic, codominant in nature and can allow study of variation in a genome with a relative ease. For polygenetic and conservation studies, this marker has extensively been used. Further for the genome mapping, genetic diversity study, monitoring population dynamics and parentage determination, this marker has also been used. Association has been found between body weight at different intervals with microsatellite markers specially ADL 212 and LEI 147 on chromosome 2 with weight at hatching and at 12 weeks.

The microsatellite ADL 023 is significantly associated with egg production upto 64 and 72 weeks. Association with egg weight at 28 weeks has also been reported. There are similar other reports of association of microsatellite with body weight at different ages. Evidence of 8 QTL regions associated with a total of eight egg traits with specific gravity, albumin height, Haugh score, shell shape, total number of eggs, terminal body weight, live weight gain and efficiency of feed conversion has been observed.

4.8.6 Single nucleotide polymorphism (SNP)

Advancement in the genomic tools like high throughput gene sequence had provided to reveal gene sequence units of genome-nucleotide. Single Nucleotide Polymorphism (SNP) can be present all over the genome (promoter, axon). Those in the axonix regions are classified synonymous (change does not result an amino acid substitution) types. In chicken more than 2.8 million SNPs have so far been reported. One potential biomarker is present at every 470bp along the total genome. Out of the total SNPs studies in chicken, at least 70% are common SNPs for broiler and layer. Focusing on linkage mapping of genes, association studies using candidate gene approaches, and evolutionary analysis, are the areas of importance to study SNPs in chicken. The most common approach has been comparative analysis of the DNA sequence of a breed. This has been facilitated by PCR.

Comparative analysis of DNA sequences across the breeds has used SNPs. An alternative approach for SNP is expressed sequence tag (EST) data mining. SNPs of pit-1gene and its association with growth traits has been studied and indicates an association. Similarly SNPs in the promoter regions of Prolactin genes have significant association with egg production in layers.

4.8.7 Genome wide selection (GWS)

GWS is also known as Whole Genome Selection. Genome Wide Selection has used a large panel of SNP markers which can increase the accuracy of predicting breeding value at an early age. This approach was first applied in dairy cattle. In an animal model, a multistep evaluation is done through extraction of pseudo-observation and estimation of genomic effects for genotyped animals. This assumes equal contribution of each marker to variance in a trait. This is equivalent to BLUP.

The concept of GWS is gaining global importance in predicting breeding value of parent stocks in poultry with high accuracy and in shorter time. SNPs and other genetic markers on a single or a few candidate genes are either gene specific or base pair specific and hence incapable of estimating genetic variation across the whole genome and at one time. GWS determines genes flow and segregation in whole genome at a time. It requires very high density location of the SNPs and vast array of genotypes to determine association with the economic traits. However traits with low heritability or those which are sex limited or sex influenced, expressed late in life or requiring slaughter or exposure to infection can be measured. It can be used in a non-pedigree population and can thus avoid maintenance of identification and performance record on pedigree. This is more relevant to the situation where small numbers of birds are maintained under more extensive management and not identified and their parentage is not known. Comparison between genomic and phenotypic information for estimation of accuracy of selection indicates that inclusion of genetic information increases the accuracy of selection for 6 week body weight and breast meet content.

4.8.8 Sex determination

In case of layers where only few selected breeding males are required for breeding and even in broilers where there are differences in meat production related traits between the two sexes, the determination of sex at hatching may be important. In past, phenotypic methods such as plumage pattern and vent sexing have been used. The latter needs lot of experience and skill and adversely affects the health and production of bird. Several genes have been mapped on Z chromosomes, mainly housekeeping genes and a few more specialized functions. DMRD1 is among those genes mapped on the Z chromosomes which can be used for sex determination. The smaller W chromosome is analogous to the mammalian Y chromosome. Several genes like ATP5A, CHD and ASW are specifically located on W chromosome. A novel gene FET1, a probable ovary determinant is unique to the W chromosome and is a potential candidate gene for sex determination. The molecular methods for sex determination have the advantage of a use (i) at an early age ranging from a day old to adult age requiring small quantity of tissue. (ii) applicable in all avian species with female with heterozygous, (iii) is not age or sex specific, (iv) requires less time after collection of a feather follicle, (v) is simple and rapid and does not require similar expertise and accuracy as in vent sexing or in feather sexing where the genes connected with pattern of feather characterization needs to be introduced may be from lower performing breed and this adversely affects productivity.

4.8.9 Microarray techniques to express the function of multiple genes affecting traits

A group of genes can be up-regulated or down regulated for a particular condition through microarray analysis. It involves collection of a group of genes on microchips which can be used to study the global expression as well as to identify SNPs in the whole genome. The development of high throughput microarrays has made the study of gene expression possible by including thousand of genes on a silicon chip. It is an important tool to explore gene networks and to identify highly conserved genetic pathways. These have been used to study gene expression differences among a range of broiler chicken and to investigate activities of T cells responsible for inducing immune response against pathogens. The technique has also been used in other avian species such as turkeys and quails.

4.8.10 Gene sequencing

It is emerging as the most effective tool in biological research to study gene function. It can be done at the transcriptional or post transcriptional stage. At the transcriptional stage, the silencing is done by homologus recombination by manipulating gene sequence through inserting mutation into a specific region of the gene, producing a modified or non-functional protein. Another approach is to genetically modify organism through null mutation in the genome. Post-transcriptional gene silencing involves the down regulation of gene expression through specific mRNA degradation. It is achieved by using antisense oligo-deoxy-ribonucleac acid, ribosome and small interference RNAs. The transitional silencing of myostatin in chicken embryo fibroblast using 5 different small hair pin RNA expression constructs have been reported. Upto 68% of mRNA in transiently transferred fibroblast could be achieved. Its use in growth regulating genes in chicken can help in enhancing growth in indigenous growth relatively poor growing chickens. There are a number of genes like Myostatin, limiting muscular growth at different stages and the expression of genes negatively regulating muscle growth, if blocked can increase body weight by 20-30% at an early age.

4.8.11 Transgenic technologies

The introgression of a foreign gene into an organism leads to a transgenic organism. In the last two decades a better understanding of molecular basis of growth and development in living organism has been achieved. The technique has potential in accelerating traditional poultry breeding for further improvement in production traits in layer and broiler stocks. Most avian species have short reproductive cycle and are ideal for introgressing gene of interest for creating transgenic birds to be used as bioreactors for the production of pharmaceuticals and industrial proteins. The serious protein energy malnutrition can be overcome through producing transgenic chicken with higher level of protein through eggs and meet. The transgenics can also be produced for higher disease resistance and better product quality for example low cholesterol content of eggs and meat.

4.9 Role of Biotechnology in Avian Reproduction

There is a large importance of body mass and egg number in poultry production for meat or eggs. This has resulted in a serious decline in most economic traits specially those with low genetic diversity/ hertability. The large germplasm resources of Indian avian species, which though less productive for eggs and / meat have unique properties of withstanding extremes of environmental stresses and has a higher disease resistance. The understanding of the unique characters of these breeds through biotechnological tool and assisted reproductive techniques can help in sustainable management specially meeting for livelihood and nutritional security of economically and socially deprived people in rural and peri-urban areas who have chicken under low production. Because of extremely small number of birds with a family and maintained with little and no production and health inputs have made them low producers but not inefficient producers. The use of genetic diversity and better production inputs can improve their productivity.

Further the techniques of cryopreservation of semen, cryopreservation of blastodermal cells or primordial germ cells may offer the preservation of entire genome. The low efficiency and high cost involved are currently impeding the progress in their use. Cryopreservation of avian semen is the only approach for efficient sustainable management and conservation of avian genetic resources other than *in situ / ex situ* the live bird conservation.

The use of chicken embryos to produce transgenics which can be used as bio-factories for higher production of proteins and pharmaceuticals such as vaccines and immunoglobulins are areas needing priority research. Use of semen or sperms of avian species as the medium for transfer of exogenous genes in to poultry eggs can be an alternative for producing transgenic chicken.

Avian species especially chicken raised for eggs/meat have a tremendous potential for increasing employment and incomes in urban, peri-urban and rural areas. Unfortunately the modern approach to poultry production for eggs and meat has been confined to urban and peri-urban areas which have not only by-passed the large rural population in production but also in consumption of high protein rich foods viz. eggs and meat of avian origin.

The vast avian genetic resources available in the country in terms of species, production type and breeds witin production types needs an urgent research and development for their sustainable use and conservation urgently so that they can serve as an important genetic resource for adaptation to adverse climatic conditions and poor production inputs and wide variety of diseases.

4.10 Selection for Behavior

Animal welfare is becoming an important issue in consumer perception as a component of product quality. The main welfare issues in poultry production especially in layers are related to limited space and the restriction on the natural behavior which could be expressed in conventional large cages. The production cost is likely to increase both in terms of space and labour. The change from non-cage management system would require effective control on feather picking, pecking and Cannibalism, for both of which there are differences among and within breeds. Breeders are selecting against these two behavioural problems which are more difficult to control in floor management where larger groups of birds are maintained than in cages where the birds are maintained in small groups. Feather picking and cannibalism are undesirable behavior and must be reduced if not, completely avoided. There may be genetic differences as reflected by production type (broilers and layers, breeds and strains within the production sites. Hence selection of birds with no or relatively low aggressive behavior may reduces the losses. Recently QTL, involved in gentle and severe feather picking have been indentified on chicken chromosome and they may play important role in reducing feather picking and cannabilism in Cannibalism layers through MAS.

4.11 Selection against Metabolic Disorders

Increase in production performance has also resulted in higher incidence of metabolic disorders. These are :

i) ***Ascites***- which is a growth related disorder of broilers. This results in high hypertrophy of the smooth muscles of pulmonary arterioles, right ventricle to total ventricular ratio, lung capacity, (lung length and width), electro-cardiography changes, pulmonary arterial pressure, pulse oxymetry, heamatocrit and packed cell volume. These traits have moderate heritability and their incidence could be reduced through selection.

ii) ***Skeletal problems***- These are major economic welfare concerns in broilers. These involve tibial dyschcondropalasia, epiphyseal ischaemic necrosis, epiphyseal separation, skeletal fractures, Valugs-Varus deformity spondylolisthesis and gastrocnenimus tendon rupture. Genetic studies on leg disorder have revealed large differences among commercial lines crosses and traits were classified as these traits have medium heritability. Selection produces favorable results through reducing leg disorders have been eliminated at the level of pedigree by *ad libitum* feeding so that weakness can be detected and incorporated in family selection. Genetic improvement is the most effective method of preventing non infectious skeletal disorders and has made a major impact in reducing incidence of disorder such as tibial dyschondropalsia. The main skeletal problems in layer hens are osteomalacia and osteoporosis which are associated with the loss of bone minerals during the laying period. There are large individual differences in the bone characteristics of hens at the end of the laying period which are un- related to egg production in a flock of high producing hens. This suggests that osteoporosis may be alleviated through selection without serious loss in egg productivity.

4.12 Reducing Environmental Stress

Several major differences are present in a tropical raised avian species compared to temperate/sub-temperate climate. The naked neck gene (Na) is responsible for reduction of feathers over the body surface and particularly complete loss in the neck region which helps in alleviating heat stress. The heterozygous naked neck layers have significant higher egg production, egg weight, egg mass and body weight under continuous heat stress. Similarly frizzle gene (F) also has a favorable effect on chicken productivity but less pronounced than the naked neck gene. The dwarf gene reduces body size and thereby causes a reduction in egg number and egg size but has a significant lowered depression due to heat stress. This may not be uniform in all genotypes which indicate genotype x environment interaction.

4.13 Application of Genomics in Poultry Breeding

There is a significant expansion in SNP panel development, high throughput genotyping and sequencing platforms. In addition, there has been a significant improvement in genetic merit in layers and broilers through conventional breeding approaches and biotechnology.

□□□

CHAPTER-5

Chicken Genetic Resources- Exotic and Indian Breeds and Those Evolved Through Various Genetic Approaches (Selection and Mating Systems)

Breed refers to a group of DAs within a species with a common ancestry, preferably registered with a breed association and conforming to a breed type in terms of physical conformation and production traits and following a set of breeding programme with performance recording and using the same in selection of parents for the next generation. There are large differences in definition of a breed given by different geneticists.

The genetic progress through selection in poultry has resulted from utilizing both the additive and non-additive genetic (dominance and epistatic) variation through selecting within pure lines for different characters such as in one line for egg production and the other line for body weight gains/fertility and hatchability and crossing the grandparent lines to create parent lines with specific characters related to either the male or female parents and crossing specific pure lines for producing commercial chicks which have higher general and more particulary higher combining ability, thus utilizing not only additive but also non-additive genetic variation which would not have been possible through selection in a single population (intra population selection) because of possibly negative relationship among different characters and different levels of genetic variation due to the influence of environmental factors leading to confounding of genetic and environmental effects or a correlation between genotype and environment. Like in case of corn, complicated breeding plans involving different selection procedures in male and female parents and using inbreeding and hybridization through crossing of inbred lines or using recurrent reciprocal selection for in producing commercial layer/ broiler stocks. This would require maintenance of a large number of pure (inbred) lines which meet the market requirement, provided it will involve their continuous selection and testing as purebreds and in all possible reciprocal crosses and identifying pure lines which will meet the requirement of a combination of desired economic characters in parents and ultimately in commercial chickens.

Industrial system of poultry production, in which environmental stresses are largely reduced by maintaining birds under intensive housing with environmental controls and intensive use of health inputs have allowed a greater focus on production efficiency in terms of maximizing profit per bird and ensuring more efficient utilization of production inputs and/product quality. There has however been a lower emphasis on adaptation to local production environment especially the changes that are fast occurring due to global warming and disease incidence arising from international trades and too frequent movement of people throughout the world.

Climate change, as mentioned earlier, will have a large impact on production environment and will require changes in the production system, both the types of DAs and production environment in which they are performing. Although there is a large diversity between and within strains/ lines which can be used for selecting birds for adaptaion in addition to production. The increase in temperature alonwith humidity will impair reproduction and increase the incidence of vector borne diseases.

The consumer demands will have to be kept in view with larger consideration on health, environment, ethics and animal welfare issues. There is a growing demand for free range and organically produced meat and eggs with no use of hormones or chemicals used for increasing live weight/ egg production from ranged and confined birds in sheds. The meat produced by indigenous bird though less soft and lower fat but has a higher taste especially for rural people who are accustomed to eat indigenous bird. The eggs produced by ingenious birds have higher yellowness of yolk even though small in size.

5.1 Exotic Chicken Breeds

The exotic chicken breeds are classified based on their place of origin and have four major classes i.e. i. American breeds, ii. Mediterranean breeds, iii. English breeds and iv. Asiatic breeds. While the most eggs production by commercial layers use American and

Mediterranean breeds, English and Asiatic breeds are used to develop most of commercial broilers.

5.1.1 American breeds

The most popular American breeds have been Plymouth Rock, New Hampshire, Rhode Island Red and Wyandotte. Most of these breeds are characterized by yellow skin, yellow shank with no feathers and red ear lobes. Eggs are mostly brown shelled. Plymouth Rock is used both for eggs and meat and is known for its egg size and meat characteristics. Barred and White Plymouth Rocks are very popular. Varieties like Buff, Silvered, Penciled, Columbian and Blue are also recognized by their genes for barring. Rhode Island Red is a dual purpose breed developed by the poultry farmers of Rhode Island and is a mixture of Malay Game, Red Shanghai, Brown Leg Horn, Cornish and Wyandotte's breeds. Some strains are single combed. They produce brown shelled eggs. Standard weight is 3.8 kg in cock, 2.9 kg in hen, 3.4 kg in cockerel and 2.5 kg in pullet. New Hampshire was developed from RIR by New Hampshire poultry farmers for early maturity, rapid feathering, large egg size and good quality meat. Some strains are used for broiler production and the others for brown shelled eggs.

5.1.2 Mediterranean breeds

These are mostly of Italian origin and are Leghorn, Minorca, Andalusian, Spanish and Ancona. They are light bodied and developed for high egg production. Leghorn is a most popular layer breed with compact light body, uniform blending, pretty carriage, long shanks, and small head with well set rose or single comb. Popular varieties are white, brown and black. Standard weights are 2.6 kg for cock, 2.0 kg for hen, 2.2 kg for cockerel and 1.8 kg for pullet. Minorca is also known as red faced Spanish. It has probably originated from Spanish. Single comb, black rose comb, white single comb, white rose comb and single comb buff are five varieties in the breed. Comb is erect with six evenly and deeply serrated points.

5.1.3 English breeds

These are known for their fleshiness and with the exception of Cornish, all the English breeds have a white skin and red earlobes. Except Dorking and Red Cap, all other breeds lay brown shelled eggs. They were earlier most broody but the character has been removed through selection. Major breeds are Cornish and Australorp. Cornish had originated in England in the 19th century through breeding Aseel, the Malay and English game birds. It has close and compact feathers and heavy flesh. The breed is very deep and broad giving the shoulders great width. The breed is pea combed. There are dark and white varieties. The cock weighs 4.5 kg, hen 3.4 kg, cockerel 3.6 kg and pullet 2.7 kg in dark variety and 3.6 kg, 2.7 kg, 3.1 kg and 2.2 kg in white laced red variety. Australop was developed in Australia. It is more upstanding and less massive and is primarily a layer. The plumage is lustrous, greenish black in all parts of the body.

5.1.4 Asiatic breeds

Brahma, Cochin and Langshan are the three recognized Asiatic breeds which are virtually extinct now and were characterized by a large body size, heavy bones, feathered shanks, red ear lobes and yellow skin. They were broody and poor layers. They have however made a significant contribution to the development of American breeds.

5.2 Indian Breeds

The most common breed raised as rural chicken is desi or non-descript and is considered as the best mother for hatching of eggs being broody and looks after the hatched chicks very well. It is smaller in size and poor layer with long pause within each cluch. It is also very well adapted to extensive free range management with a limited supplementary feed mostly household kitchen waste and protection from inclement weather. Several names have been given to the local birds available in different regions such as Tenis, Naked Neck, Punjab Brown, Ghagus, Lotab, Kashmir Faberella, Titri, Bursa, Tellicherry, Denki, Nicobari and Kalahasti. Only four breeds Chittagong, Aseel, Kadaknath and Bursa can be considered as breeds in the strict sense. A large number of fowls of different sizes, shapes and colours and mostly resembling jungle fowl are found throughout India and have been named as independent breeds mostly on the basis of their home tract or some distinct physical conformation traits. Most of these breeds are highly variable in physical conformational traits and production of eggs and meat.

There is a large intentional and un-intentional intermixing of breeds/ types located in a region or even across regions. In fact there may be hardly any indigenous breeds / types still available as over the last 50 years there has been distribution of cocks of exotic breeds for improving poultry production in rural areas. Except in highly interior tribal areas where such development programs were not taken up or made a little impact. Some indigenous avian genetic resources both of chicken and other avian species may still be available.

5.3 Description and Evaluation of Indian Chicken Breeds

As mentioned earlier, majority of indigenous chicken are non-descript with a large variations in size, plumage colour, morphology and production in terms of body weight gains, efficiency of feed conversion, carcass yield and quality, egg production, egg size and both external and internal egg quality traits especially shell thickness and shell colour. A number of breeds have been described by different investigators with similar or different conformation and production. Most of these descriptions are based on smaller population size maintained mostly under extensive/semi- intensive management. Of the breeds described, important breeds are Ankaleshwar, Aseel, Busra, Chittagong, Danki, Daothigir, Ghagus, Haringhata Black, Kadaknath, Kaalasthi, Kashmir Faverolla, Miri, Nicobari, Punjab Brown, Tellichery and Red Jungle Fowl. In addition, the most common bird, as mentioned earlier, is non-descript or Desi with highly variable size, comb shape and size, body weight, growth rate, survival, egg production, egg weight, egg size and quality. Some studies on the non-descript Desi fowls as purebreds and in crosses with exotic layer and broiler breeds have been carried out under various external (PL-480) and internal (supported by the ICAR, Ministry of Agriculture, Government of India, Department of Agriculture / Department of Animal Husbandry, Dairying and Fisheries). Most of these research and development programmes have been of short duration and based on relatively smaller populations and did not yield any concrete information which can be used for sustainable use and conservation of these breeds. More recently, the National Bureau of Animal Genetic Resources (NBAGR) has conducted field surveys through a network project involving a number of State Agricultural / Veterinary Sciences Universities. Based on these studies, some information about the description and production performances and molecular genetics characterization is now available.

5.3.1 Ankaleshwar

It is a hardy and tropically adapted breed, associated with the tribal (vanbasi) culture. It is also referred as Desi, has low egg production, slow growth, late sexual maturity, broodiness, small egg size and deep yellow yolk colour. The breed is essentially raised in free range conditions. The breed known to be distributed as a backyard poultry production system in tribal areas. Little information on breed characterization either of physical conformation, adaptation and production characteristics is available. A recent detailed survey carried out at Anand Agriculture University (AAU) has given morphological characterization and has also studied management practices and product attributes. The microsatellite studies for molecular characterization have been done by NBAGR.

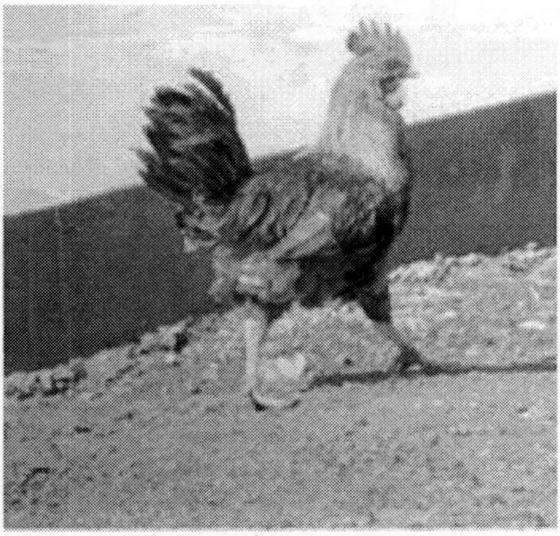

Fig. 5.1 Ankaleshwar
(*Source:* http://sapplpp.org)

The breed is distributed in Bhrauch and Narmada districts of Gujarat, mostly Ankaleshwar, Jambusar, Zagadia, Bharuch, Hansor and Vailia talukats, whereas; in Narmada district it is found in Dedipada, Rajpipla, Tilakwada and Nandod talukas. The breed is most probably named after Ankaleshwar in Bharuch district. The breed is kept primarily for meat, although eggs are also consumed in addition to being hatched for raising chicken for meat. The birds are raised under free range system in the backyard and some shelter is provided at night to avoid predation. The flock size ranges between five and ten. In addition to scavenging, some household kitchen waste and coarse grains are also provided. Incubation and hatching is carried out by the broody hens throughout the year. No prophylactic and curative treatment against diseases is provided except more recently vaccination against Ranikhet and Fowl pox is being done in areas where these diseases prevail.

Plumage colour has wide variations and is generally white with light grey to brown and golden admixture. The plumage pattern is generally striped or spotted with golden yellow feathers having black tips. Golden yellow plumage colour is predominant in males and black golden in females. Comb is red and single or rose type. Beak is small and yellow in colour. The skin is yellow or pinkish. Ear lobes are white and large in cocks and small in hens. Shank is yellow in colour. Eyes are black with yellow reddish ring. Feathers are also observed on legs, cap and beard (Fig.5.1).

The average day old weight of chick is 28.9±1.0 g. The average weight of males and females is 551.0 ± 3.0 g and 458.0 ±2.0 g respectively at 8 weeks and 830.0 ± 4.0 and 750.0 ± 4.0 g respectively at 12 weeks of age. The average weight at slaughter is 1.76 and 1.49 kg around 72 week. The average age at first egg is 180 days and annual egg production averages 79. The hatchability percent is 84. Mean egg weight is 35 g. Egg shell colour varies from cream brown to white. The shell is strong and thick. The egg has thick albumin and deep yellow yolk. Albumin index, yolk index and haugh index average 0.09, 0.36 and 83.7, respectively. The dressing percentage averages 62.

Genetic characterization: The average number of alleles is 9.88 using 25 nucleotide microsatellite loci. The number of alleles with frequency higher than 5% are 5.4. The effective number of alleles is 4.6. The alleles present in Ankaleshwar are not available in any other indigenous breed of chicken and belong to LEI155, LEI174 and HUJ003. The frequency of three alleles is 0.013, 0.038 and 0.013 respectively. Mean observed heterozygosity is 0.62 against the expected of 0.74 pointing to certain degree of inbreeding due to small effective population size as the number of male used for breeding are small which was found to be 0.162 with 4 loci showing a negative value. Ten loci had significantly different allelic frequency than expected under Hardy-Weinberg equilibrium principle, whereas; 11 loci were in equilibrium. Non-random (selective) mating appears to be responsible for the deviation. The quantitative and qualitative tests did not reveal any recent genetic bottleneck or any event resulting in such genetic differences.

5.3.2 Aseel

Aseel is an Arabic word meaning pure or thoroughbred. It is a breed of game fowl, which may have been domesticated some 3500 years back essentially for sport such as cock fighting which is also mentioned in Indian religious scriptures-Manu Srimiti. The breed has probably descended from the Indian Red Jungle fowl, the progenitor of the current day chicken breeds in the world, created through generations of selection for egg/meat production and removal of broodiness which is usually found in most indigenous fowl types/ breeds. Aseel is also known Malay fowl and may have given rise to most European breeds of layers and broilers. It is an important breed for cock fighting and sports. It produces delicious meat and has excellent heat and disease tolerance. These characteristics have resulted from long term human and natural selection. It is included in the FAO list of breeds needing conservation. The breed predominates in North Bastar and South Bastar of Chattishgarh and Khammam district of Andhra Pradesh. The farmers maintaining these birds are small and marginal and maintain a small flock. The former king of Vijayanagram state is known to have patronised the breed and helped in its conservation and sustainable use for meat and sport. Although flock size is usually less than 10, however; larger flocks as large as 20 are also observed. The breed is still not commercially farmed. The birds of the breed can thrive under extensive range management, essentially scavenging on natural plant and insect resources. Some kitchen waste and coarse grains are also provided as supplemental feed. Adequate drinking water is also provided.

The breed is known for its endurance and fighting power. There is large variation in physical conformation and plumage colour which ranges from brownish red to reddish brown and black. Some birds with white and golden plumage colour are also present. The colour is generally patchy but solid and stripped pattern are also observed. The skin colour is mostly yellow, shank colour is also yellow. Ear lobes are red. Comb varies from single pea to rose, of which pea comb is more common. Eye colour is brown, although black colour is also observed (Fig. 5.2).

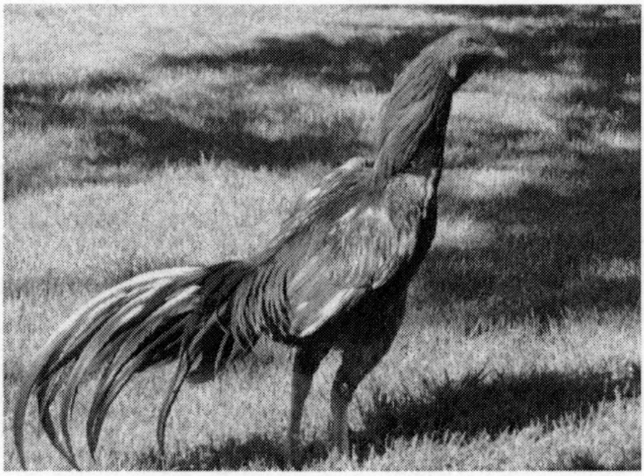

Fig. 5.2 Aseel
(*Source:* indianfarm.com)

Body weights average 29, 234, 934 and 1964 g at 0, 8, 20 and 40 weeks. Feed conversion efficiency in terms kg of feed/kg body weight gain ranges from 2.45 to 5.29 upto 10th week and decreases after 10th week. Age at first egg ranges from 27 to 29 weeks. The period of lay at a time ranges from 15 to 20 days, when the hen broods on the eggs laid to hatch and then starts again laying. Generally in three laying cycles 30 to 36 eggs per year are produced. The predominant egg shell colour is brown. There is no fixed age at slaughter, however the birds are slaughtered/sold at 28 to 32 weeks of age. Dressing percentage averages 75. The breed is highly fertile with 74% hatchability on egg set and 85% on fertile egg basis.

The most predominant diseases affecting the breed are Ranikhet, Fowl Pox and Bacillary White Diarrhoea, Ascariasis is also common. Among external parasites, ticks and lice are commonly prevalent. The mortality averages 13% in adults and 40% in chicks.

Genetic characterization: Based on DNA extracted from random blood samples, microsatellite studies were carried out on dinucleotide repeats and it was seen that they undergo higher rate of mutation. It was further observed that the microsatellite loci were in the public domain, are not in linkage disequilibrium and follow Mendalian laws of inheritance. Microsatellite alleles ranged from 2 to 9 with an average of 4.2. Heterozygosity estimates based on a set of microsatellite loci showed higher values. The selected loci are highly polymorphic and thus suitable for genetic diversity analysis.

5.3.3 Bursa

The breed is reared by tribals in area bordering Maharashtra and Gujarat comprising Peint and Surgana talukas of Nasik, Sakri taluk of Dhule and Navapur, Taloda and Dhedgaon talukas of Nandurpur districts of Maharashtra and Uchchal, Songath Nizer taluks of Surat and Ahawad of Daang districts of Gujarat. These birds are known as Busra, possibly because of their predominance in Busrawal village in Sakri taluka of Dhule district or the name given in Marathi. These birds are maintained under free range management in small numbers by rural households and primarily sold for meat. Birds are maintained under free range system in a flock size varying from 2 to 25, with an average of 9. 48% of the birds are chicks, 39% hens and 13% cocks. Only bamboo baskets are used to provide protection from weather and predators, that too at night as during day they are allowed on natural graizing.

The birds of this breed are relatively smaller in size, have wide variations in plumage colour, which is generally white mixed with black feathers on neck, back, tail and reddish brown feathers on shoulders and wings. Some solid white birds or with mixed brown and black or black and golden colour or solid black plumage are also available. Skin is pinkish in colour. Comb is red. Ear lobes are white or brown. Beak is yellow; wattles are red and small to medium in size. Shank is yellow. Beak, eye rings and shank are blackish grey or black (Fig. 5.3).

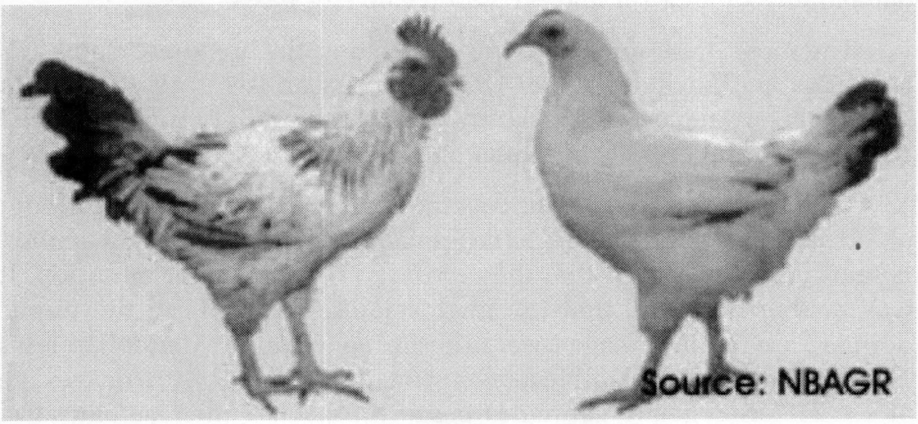

Fig. 5.3 Bursa
(*Source:* http://sapplpp.org)

The weight of the adult male ranges from 0.85 to 1.25 kg with an average of 1.11 kg. The weight of hen ranges from 0.8 to 1.2 kg with an average of 0.9 kg. The age at first egg ranges from 5 to 7 months. The hen lays 12-13 eggs in a clutch of 2 weeks, when it goes in brooding to hatch the eggs and then starts laying again. Annual egg production ranges 40-55. Hatchability ranges between 60-85, dressing percentage between 65-70. Eggs are small in size and on an average weigh 32 g with a range form 28-38 g. Shell colour ranges from light brown to dark brown, although some creamish white eggs are also laid. Egg shell is strong. Albumin is thick and yolk colour is mostly dark yellow.

Genetic characterization: The mean number of alleles observed is 10.6 with a range from 6 to 17. The number of alleles observed is significantly lower than the effective number of alleles. The expected heterozygosity is more than the observed heterozygosity for all the loci (0.535). The mutation drift equilibrium using three mutation models showed to be in mutation drift equilibrium. The breed is not experiencing any significant population reduction.

5.3.4 Danki

The breed is distributed in Vijayanagaram district with some presence in adjoining districts of Srikakulam and Visakhapatnam of Andhra Pradesh. This breed is also known as Dinki. It is a game bird and is used for cock fighting. The birds can fight for one to one and half hour. The chicks are sold at Rs. 50 to 150 at 3 days, Rs. 300 to 500 at 4 months and Rs. 600 to 1000 at 1 year of age. These birds are sold for cock fighting and meat. Danki differs from Aseel being larger in size, grows faster and have shorter and stronger neck, strong body, broader wings, longer spur and sharp eyes. The birds are generally managed on free range and are kept in open. Cocks are more ferocious and are normally restrained under a bamboo basket or tied with a long thin rope, which is secured to one of the leg and the other end to a wooden pole.

The birds are essentially maintained on free range scavenging and very rarely some supplemental grains such as ragi, oats, jowar, broken rice, rice bran are given in small quantities. The cocks are forced to run at least 2 km before fighting to exercise. Sometimes, almonds, resins, egg, milk etc. are also given to fighting cocks. The flock size averages 17 with range from 6-42 with 56% chicks, 17% hens and 27% cocks. Mortality ranges from 20-30% upto 2 months of age. It is higher in winter than in summer. The birds are not generally vaccinated but larger relatively better managed flocks are vaccinated against Fowl Pox and Ranikhet. Brooding is done in bamboo basket hung from the roof. Hatchability ranges from 70 to 85% and can go to as low as 50% during summer and as high as 100% during winter.

Predominant plumage colour is brown followed by black. Some birds with red white or golden yellow colour are also observed. The males have shining bluish black feathers on wings, breast, tail and thighs. Neck is slightly darker in shade than the rest of body. The hens generally have brown feathers mixed with black or white feathers. The birds have white or pinkish white skin with large patches of rose red colour on breast, thighs and wings. Ear lobes are red in colour. Eye colour is mostly black and eye ring is generally red. Comb is large and red in colour. It is relatively smaller in hens than in cocks. Pie comb is most common. Beak is generally shorter and yellow in colour. Upper part is slightly broader and curved and extends beyond the lower part in downward direction. Spur is long and sharp in cocks making it difficult to walk. Shank is yellow in colour but greyish or black coloured shanks are also observed (Fig 5.4).

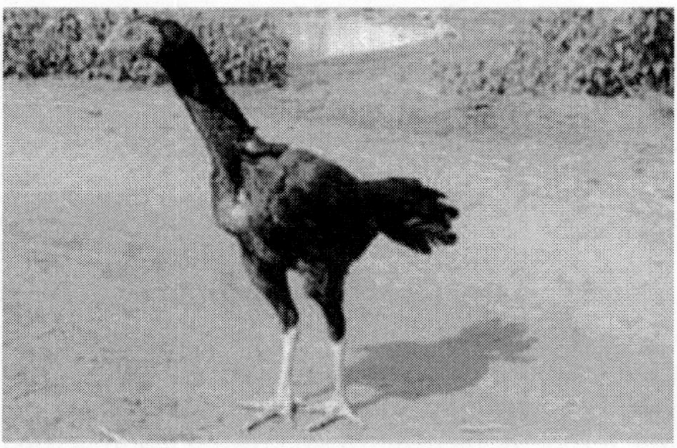

Fig. 5.4 Danki
(*Source:* http://sapplpp.org)

The average body weight is 3.12±0.09 kg and 2.22±0.06 kg in adult males and females. The age at first egg is around 6-8 months. The clutch size is 8-12 in 15-20 days. After hatching the eggs, the hen looks after the chicks from 2.5 to 3 months. The egg production ranges from 25-35 eggs in a year. Egg weight ranges from 37 to 54 g. Egg yolk is deep yellow in colour.

Genetic characterization: Multi locus genotyping indicates that the 25 microsatellite loci have a large number of alleles (243) with 50% of the loci having low allelic frequency with an effective number of alleles averaging 4.64±1.77. The observed heterozygosity is high (0.74) and close to the expected (0.76). The within population variation, a measure of inbreeding was 0.03 and was significant.

5.3.5 Daothigir

The breed is distributed in Bodoland region of Assam with breeding tract mainly in Kokrajhar district and in some parts of Dhubri, Bongay Gaon, Barpeta and Nalbari districts located on north bank of river Brahmaputra. It is generally reared by Bodo community for meeting domestic requirement for meat and eggs. The estimated population is 14,000. The birds thrive on thigir (*Dillinia indica*). The plant bears flowers of different colour similar to plumage colour of the breed. The shape of the flowers also resemble the shape of comb.

Flock size ranges from 10-60 with an average of 23. The birds of the breed are raised mixed with non-descript/desi birds. The flocks are maintained without any shelter and mostly kept on scavenging natural vegetation and insects. Some owners provide supplementary paddy grains. Males are caponized at 2-4 months of age for fattening, which gives them better growth and meat quality. The incidence of the disease is also low in capanised birds and they fetch better price. Eggs are generally hatched through broody hens. The mortality is low. Coccidiosis and Ranikhet are common diseases and birds are generally vaccinated against Ranikhet and Fowl pox.

The birds are small in size with a compact body but long and heavy legs. Plumage colour is generally black interspersed with white feathers. Striped pattern is also seen. Wings and tail feathers are black and brownish. Neck and back has golden yellow or brownish feathers. Skin is creamish in colour. Ear ring is red and ear lobes are also mostly red but sometimes white or white mixed with red are also observed. Wattles are medium to large in size and are red in colour. Comb is red, single and erect and relatively large in size. Beak and shank are yellow in colour. Tail is short and almost at level with the beak (Fig 5.5).

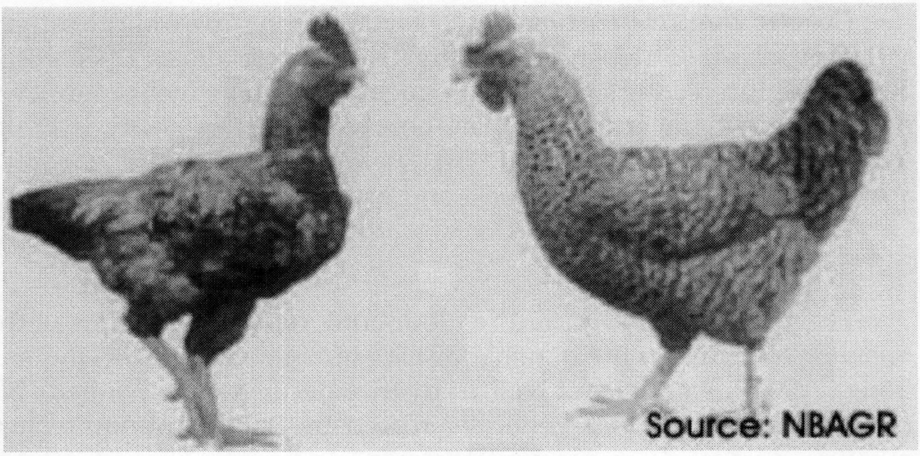

Fig. 5.5 Daothigir
(*Source:* sapplpp.org)

The adult males on an average weigh 1.79±0.1 kg and females 1.63±0.13 kg. Age at first egg ranges from 5-8 months with an average of 6 months. The clutch size is 20 and annual egg production is between 60-70 eggs. The hatchability is 80-85%. Egg weight ranges from 42-48 g. Shell colour is mostly light brown. Shell is strong and thick. Albumin is generally very thick. Yolk is mostly deep yellow in colour.

Genetic characterization: A total of 237 alleles were observed at 25 loci with high polymorphism and with dinucleotide repeats. The value of effective number of alleles was significantly lower than expected according to Hardy-Weinverg equilibrium and could be due to a large number of alleles at very low frequency. The effective number of alleles was 5.18 and was significantly less than expected. The mean observed heterozygosity was 0.78 indicating variable population structure. The polymorphic content estimated on the basis of allelic frequency was 0.77. The mean value of F was 0.081, which was significant. The breed is under mutation drift equilibrium and has not gone through any genetic bottleneck.

5.3.6 Ghagus

The breed is distributed in Kollar district and adjoining areas in Banglore district of Karnataka and Chittoor and Anantpur districts of AP. The birds are locally known as Desi/ Chigu and generally maintained for meat and recreation/game. A large number of Giriraja, a cross between exotic and indigenous chicken breeds is also available in the region. The birds are mostly reared by Kukarni community and on average a bird cost Rs. 200 to 500. The birds are reared under free range system in the backyards. The average flock size is 27 with a range from 10-60. Little housing is provided. The cocks are tied with a thin rope to a pole to avoid fighting. Some supplementary feed in the form of kitchen waste, ragi, broken wheat and rice are also given. The birds have good growth rate and are generally vaccinated against fowl pox and Ranikhet diseases. Broody hens are used for hatching of eggs.

The predominant plumage colour is brown followed by black. The males have shining bluish black feathers on breast, tail and thighs. Neck is covered with golden feathers. The throat is some time loose and hanging. Wattles are small and red in colour. Comb is red and pie or single type (Fig. 5.6). Hens are generally brown and black. The newly hatched chicks are light in colour. The breed looks like a mixture of Aseel, Danki and Kalasthi, but produces more eggs than the other breeds mentioned.

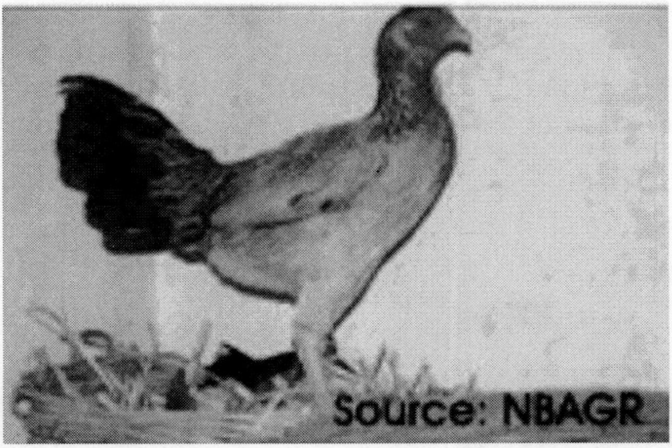

Fig. 5.6 Ghagus
(*Source:* sapplpp.org)

The adult weight averages 2.16±0.25 kg in males and 1.43±0.81 kg in females. Age at first egg ranges from 5-8 months. The clutch size averages 15-20 in a cycle of 25-30 days. Brooding period averages 2-3 months. Before entering in to broodiness, average number of eggs produced range between 45-60 days annually. The mortality is high during summer. Average egg weight is 40±2 g. Egg yolk is deep yellow in colour.

Genetic characterization: A total of 257 alleles with a mean number and effective number as 10.3±3 and 4.8±1.8 respectively. A large number of loci have a low frequency. Heterozygosity is quite high- 0.70, on an average observed against 0.77 expected. 13 loci were not in equilibrium. The test for the mutation drift equilibrium shows severe reduction in population size in recent past, which is supported by a normal L shaped curve.

5.3.7 Miri

Local name of breed is Porog, however, Miri has been derived from the name of the tribe, Miri or Mising. The birds are essentially scavengers and a little feed, health and management inputs are provided for their survival and production. They play an important role in the daily life of tribal people and are an integral part of their social, religious and cultural life. They provide primarily meat, which is highly delicious and forms an important source of protein for the local people. There is no commercialization of production/sale of chicken in the region. The population is large and widely distributed and does not face any threat of genetic bottleneck /extinction. The breed is distributed in Dhimaji North Lakhimpur, Siv Sagar and adjoining districts of Dibrugarh and Majauli island in upper Assam.

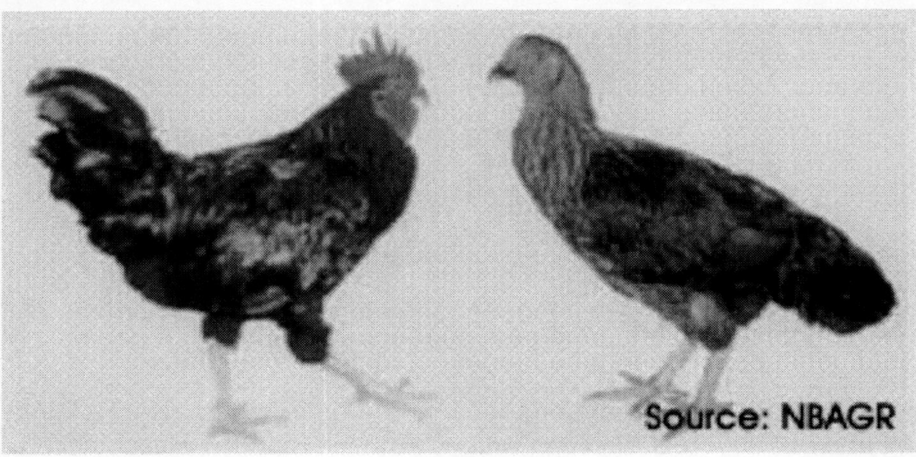

Fig. 5.7 Miri
(*Source:* sapplpp.org)

The average flock size is 25 with 11 males and 14 females both adults and chicks. Most of birds are housed in bamboo houses with thatched roof with flooring 5 feet above the ground level. Birds are also kept in the backyard and housed during night, generally in cane/ bamboo cages. In the cages, paddy straw bedding is provided. The egg production is 15-25 in a laying cycle before the birds become broody and starts laying after the eggs have been hatched and the chicks are able to look after themselves. The mortality reported is around 11% in the first four weeks. No vaccination or deworming is provided.

There is no standard plumage colour and majority of birds are white, with some percentage brown/black. Birds of mixed colour are also present. The colour is normally solid but spotted/stripped birds also exist. The skin colour ranges from white to yellow. Ear lobes are red. Comb is single and red in colour (Fig.5.7). The eyes are mostly brown.

It is essentially a meat breed and the birds are slaughtered during social and religious functions. Dressing percentage is between 65 and 74. Eggs weigh around 42 g. The average weight at 6 month is 1.06±0.04 kg and at 12 months 1.52±0.05 kg. Age at first egg, average is 212 days, clutch size 4-5, average annual egg production 62 with hatchability of 79%. Mortality upto 1 month ranges from 12-15%. Shell colour is light brown but brown and dark brown eggs also occur. Egg weight averages 42 g.

Genetic characterization: Microsatellite loci gave average number of alleles and average effective number of alleles as 4.24 and 2.93, respectively. The average expected and observed heterozygosity was 0.59 and 0.57, respectively, which points to little loss of genetic variability due to natural/artificial selection. The normal "L shaped" curve showed that the population has not gone through any genetic bottleneck in the last few generations.

5.3.8 Nicobari

The breed is found in Andaman and Nicobar islands in Bay of Bengal on eastern side of India and maintained under semi-intensive system. Naked neck and frizzle fowl are also available and can withstand high humidity. The local chickens have continuously been improved through grading with high producing layer and broiler breeds both indigenous and exotic. The breed has originated in Nicobar group of Islands and is maintained by tribals since a long time under a free range management.

The birds are mostly kept without any confinement and are not provided any shelter but are provided some supplementary feed. The birds are left in the morning in search of feed and return their home stad in the evening. They meet nutritional requirements especially of proteins of their keepers. In addition to free range rearing scavenging some supplementary feed comprising of broken grains, kitchen waste and coconut gratings are also provided to the birds during night. Small low cost houses are made up of bamboo or simply bamboo baskets are used to protect the birds from predators at night. The birds are resistant to most of infectious diseases of chicken and no vaccination is normally done.

The birds are brownish matty in colour and are hardy (Fig. 5.8). Black and white coloured birds are also seen. The plumage colour is generally solid. The birds are medium sized with short legs and compact body. The comb is single and red in colour. Wattles and ear lobes are pinkish. The shank and body skin is pinkish white. The neck is short and thick with black plumage tipped with brown shade. Breast is prominent, tail is of medium size. The birds are highly tolerant to hot and humid conditions with temperature varying from 23.3 to 30.5 °C and humidity varying from 74-90%. The mortality is generally low. The breed is used for egg production under free range management with some supplementary feedings.

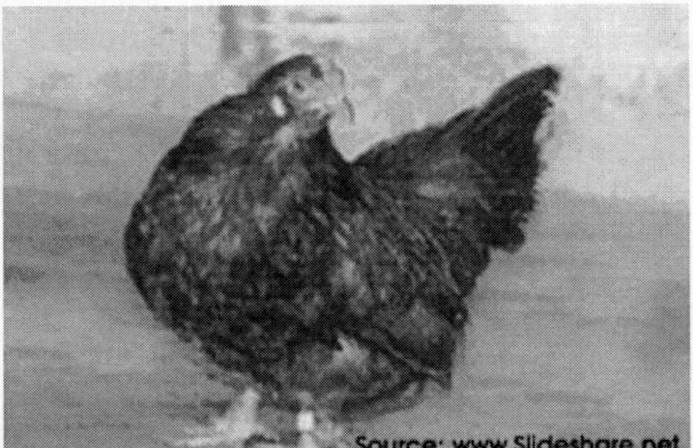

Fig. 5.8 Nicobari
(*Source:* http://sapplpp.org)

In addition to the 8 breeds studied by NBAGR for their description and evaluation for physical conformation and production characteristics and some molecular characterization, there are other breeds which have been studied by the Central Avian Research Institute, PD Poultry and some cooperating units.

5.3.9 Chittagong (Malay)

Chittagong (Malay) is found in the North Eastern states of India bordering Bangladesh. Average weight of cock is 3.5–4.5 kg and hen 3.0 – 4.0 kg. It is a large bird, very strong and hardy with a fighting nature. It possesses all the characteristics of a good game bird such as colouring (primarily bay, chestnut, gray, roan, palomino, black, etc.), large eyes, long mane and tail, strong, yet refined legs, high headset and and low tail set when in action, (Fig 5.9).

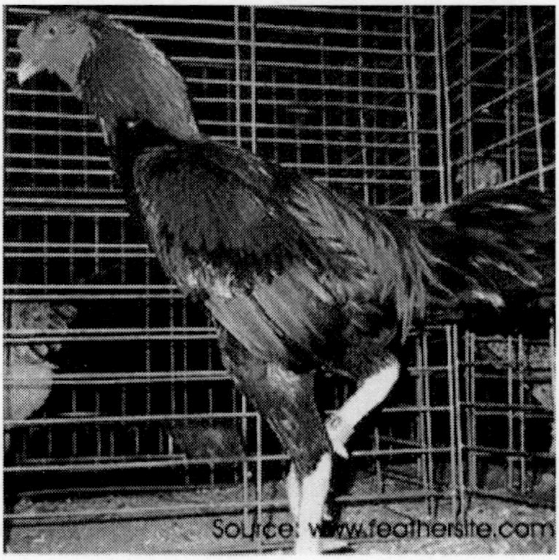

Fig. 5.9 Chittagong (Malay)
(*Source:* sapplpp.org)

5.3.10 Harringhata black

Harringhata black is reared throughout West Bengal. The core-breeding tract comprises the northern part of North 24 Parganas and the southern part of Nadia, West Bengal. It is Jet black in colour with red comb and wattles while the shanks are white in colour. The average weight of cock is 1.5 kg and hen 1.2 kg. Annual average egg production is 130. It is a small bodied black bird with typical features of a layer (Fig. 5.10). The breed is very alert, highly mobile, and capable of escaping predator attack while scavenging. Farmers maintain the birds on scavenging with negligible supplementation of grains, crop byproducts and kitchen waste. The breed is highly broody and has a good mothering ability is used by farmers to hatch and brood eggs of other fowls and even ducks. The breed demonstrates effective tolerance to common diseases.

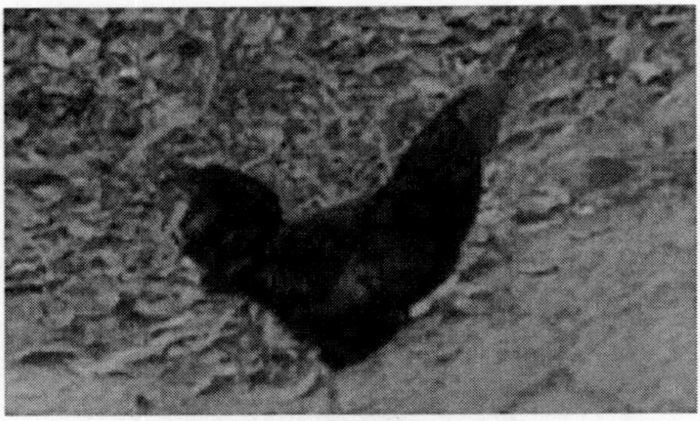

Fig. 5.10 Harringhata Black
(*Source:* sapplpp.org)

5.3.11 Kadaknath

The native tract of Kadaknath is in the Jhabua and Dhar Districts of Western Madhya Pradesh. A day-old chicks are bluish to black with irregular dark stripes over the back. Adult plumage varies from silver and gold- sprinkled with bluish-black and without any spankling. The skin, beak, shanks, toes and soles of feet are slate like in colour (Fig. 5.11). The comb, wattles and tongue are purple. Most of the internal organs show intense black colouration, which is pronounced in trachea, thoracic and abdominal air-sacs, gonads and at the base of the heart and mesentery. The blood is darker than normal. The black pigment is the result of melanin deposition.The average adult weight in males is 1.5 kg and hen 1.0 kg. Annual egg production is 80 in numbers. The eggs are light brown in colour. The average egg weight is 46.8 g. The original name of the breed is Kalamasi, meaning a fowl with black flesh, which, though not very appealing to the eye, is very tasty. The bird is resistant to diseases in its natural habitat under free range management but is more susceptible to Marek's disease under intensive rearing conditions. Kadaknath chicken is said to be rich in a number of amino acids and vitamins and are a powerful source of protein.The meat is known to have affordable value.

5.3.12 Kalasthi

The breed is native to the Chittoor district and adjoining regions of Nellore district in Andhra Pradesh. The common plumage colour is bluish black but brown birds are also seen. The colour pattern is generally patchy in males and spotted in females. The cocks possess shining golden

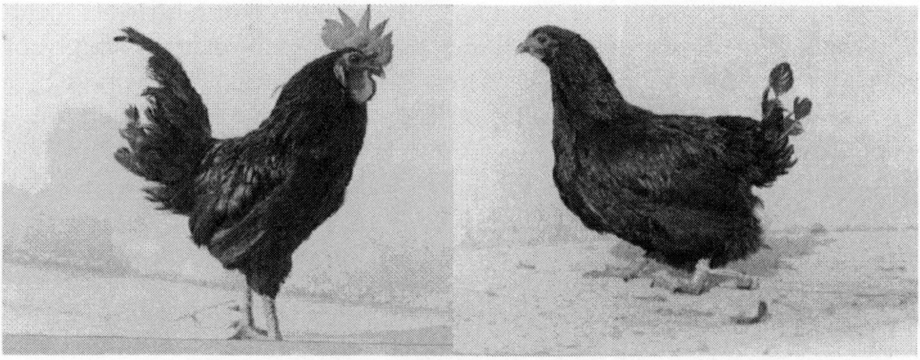

Fig. 5.11 Kadaknath
(*Source:* http://www.slideshare.net/

feathers on the neck and wings (Fig.5.12). Legs are proportionately longer. Wings are dorsally set revealing thighs enveloped with smooth feathers. Wattles are absent. Comb is red, pea type and compressed. Spur is smaller in size. Average adult weight of cock is 2.48±0.13 kg and that of hen 1.85 ± 0.10 kg. The average age at first laying cycle is 6-8 months. Number of eggs laid in one egg laying cycle of 15-25 days is 9-14. Annual egg production is 30-40. Average egg weight is 42.91 ± 1.94 g. These birds are reared in the backyard farming system primarily for meat.

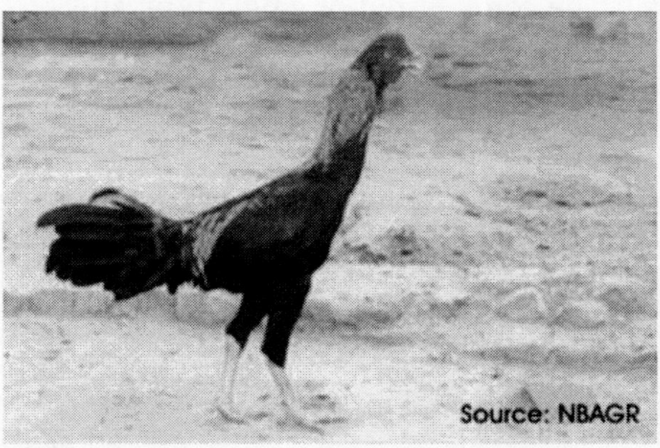

Fig. 5.12 Kalasthi
(*Source:* sapplpp.org)

5.3.13 Kashmir Favorolla

This is the indigenous chicken of Kashmir and thrives at an altitude of 1,500 to 2,000 meters above mean sea level (MSL). They are small sized birds with small single combs and wattles. Their feathered comb is the peculiarity of this breed (Fig.5.13). The average adult weight of cock is 1.72 ± 0.04 kg and that of hen 1.25 ± 0.02 kg. The average egg weight is 46.06 ± 0.48 g. This breed is most suitable for cold climates and mountainous terrains.

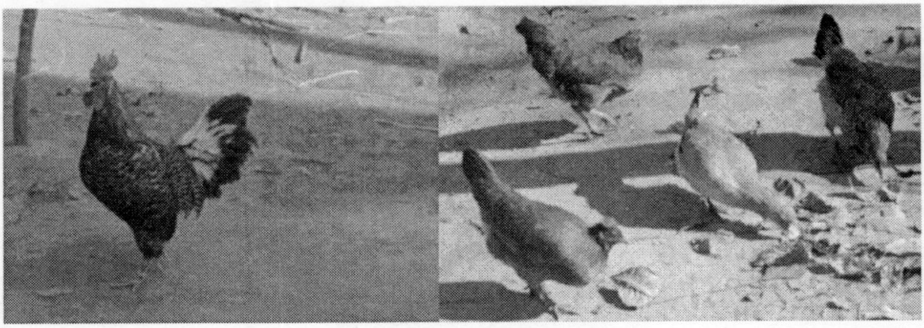

Fig.5.13 Kashmir Favorolla
(*Source:* http://image.slidesharecdn.com/

5.3.14 Punjab brown

This breed is found in rural areas of Gurdaspur in Punjab and in Ambala and Yamunanagar in Haryana. The plumage colour is mostly brown and the pattern is usually solid but is sometimes spotted or striped. The males in particular have black spots/stripes on their neck, wings and tail. The comb is red of single type and erect in position (Fig 5.14). The average flock size is 9 birds. Average weight of cock is 2.15±0.94 kg and that of hen is 1.57±0.04 kg. The average age at first laying cycle is 5-6 months. Annual egg production is 60 - 80. Average egg weight is 46.0±1.91 g. Egg shell colour is mostly light brown. It is a multi-purpose breed, yielding good quality meat and eggs. Birds are reared in the backyard and shelter is provided only at night in the form of small enclosures mostly made up of mud and wood.

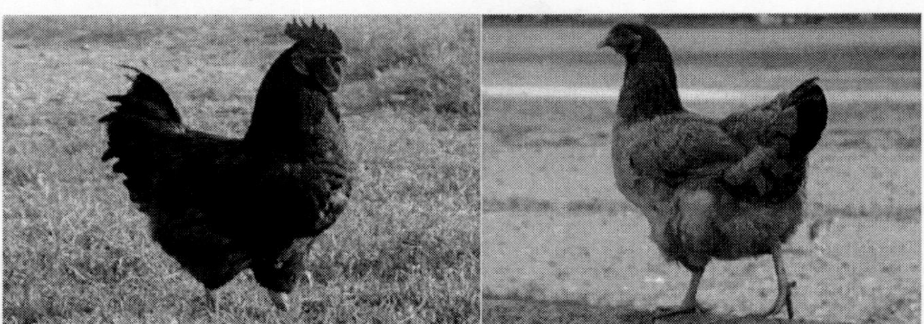

Fig.5.14 Punjab Brown
(*Source:* http://image.slidesharecdn.com)

5.3.15 Tellicherry

This breed is found mainly in the Calicut district but also in the surrounding areas in Kannur and Malappuram districts of Kerala and the adjoining Mahe region of Puducherry. Plumage color is black with a shining bluish tinge on hackle, back and tail feathers. Comb is red, single and large in size (Fig.5.15). Average weight of cock is 1.62±0.16 kg and that of hen 1.24±0.10 kg. The eggs are tinted. Annual egg production is 60–80. Average egg weight is 40.02 ± 0.94 g.

In addition to the 15 breeds described above, there are other breeds of less known description and importance viz. Phulbani, Kalahandi, Dumasil, Vezaguda, Gujuri and Hansli, which are relatively less known and are described below.

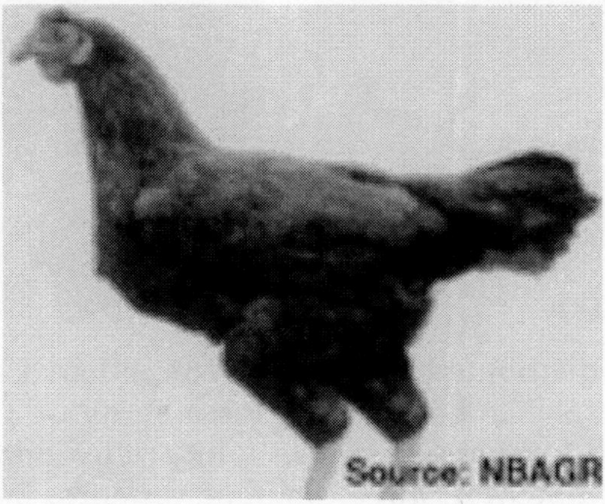

Fig. 5.15 Tellicherry
(*Source:* http://sapplpp.org/)

5.3.16 Phulbani

This breed is mostly found in the districts of Phulbani and Boudh in Orissa. The birds of both sexes are alert and active and small to medium in size. Length of the bird varies from 42 to 71 cm. Plumage colour is varied, predominantly being black, with various shades of brown and white (Fig.5.16). Based on comb, types two varieties are recognized - rose comb and single comb. Combs are fairly large in males. Wattle is poorly developed. The weight of cock varies from 2.0 to 2.5 kg and the weight of hen varies 1.0 to 1.2 kg. The age of first egg is 6 to 7 month. Egg production is 8-12 per clutch with an average of 3 - 4 clutches in a year. The average annual egg production is 40 eggs.

Egg shell colour is White. This breed is used both for eggs and meat production. Females are broody hence used for hatching and rearing of chicks. Cocks are rarely used for fighting. The birds are reared in the smallholder production system and are well adapted to their environment. Flock size varies from 4 to 30 birds.

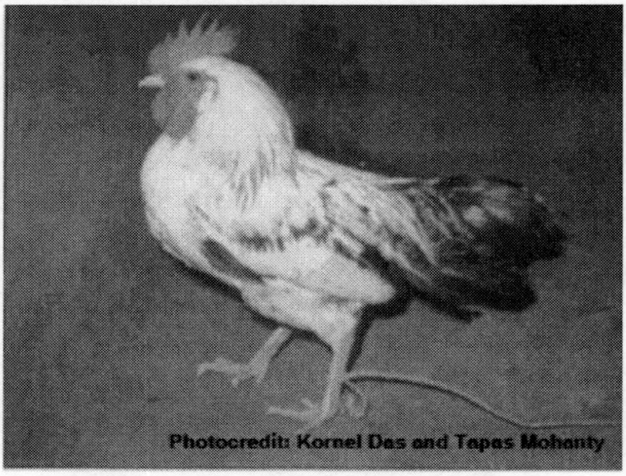

Fig. 5.16 Phulbani
(*Source:* http://sapplpp.org)

5.3.17 Kalahandi

It is widely distributed in Bhawanipatna, Khariar and Nawapara subdivisions of Kalahandi district of Orissa. Birds are alert, active and vary from small to medium in size with well-proportioned body. Plumage colour differs in three different varieties. Brown or Khairi Black or Kabri Barred or Chitri. The average body length in males is 70 cm and in females 55cm. The height of male is 69 to78 cm and that of female 51 to 64 cm. Single comb with five serrations is most common. Wattles are fairly large and well-rounded and red in colour (Fig.5.17). The head is small to medium in size. Eyes are medium sized, usually gray or black in colour. The weight of cock is 2-3 kg and that of hen 1.3 - 1.7 kg. Egg laying starts at the age 5 to 6 months. Average annual egg production is 100 to 150. Egg shell colour is white. The birds are raised in the backyard in the smallholder production system. Flock size varies from 8 to 100 birds. It is a dual purpose breed and is used for production of both eggs and meat. About 50% of the eggs are consumed and the remaining are used for hatching. The birds are well adapted to their environment and capable of protecting themselves from predators.

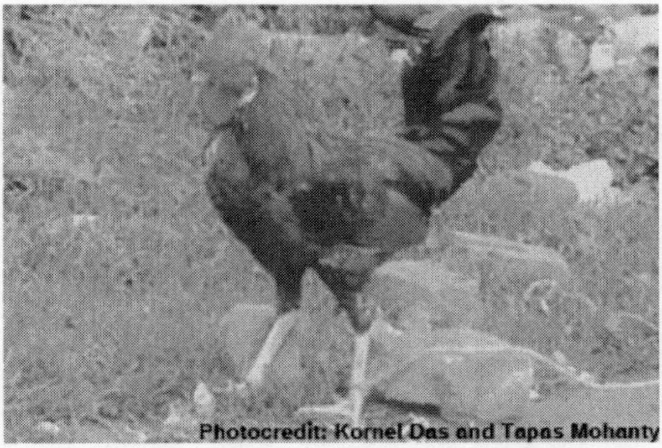

Fig. 5.17 Kalahandi
(*Source:* http://sapplpp.org)

5.3.18 Dumasil

The breed is mostly found in Karaya and Jashipur blocks of Mayurbhanj district in Orissa. Birds of both sexes are active and alert and fairly large in size with 80 cm in length and 70 cm in height. There are two recognized varieties - black and brown as far as plumage colour is concerned. In the black variety, the plumage colour of entire body including wings is black with a greenish sheen. In the brown variety the plumage colour is uniformly lustrous dark brown from head to tail. Pea comb is common. Wattles are red in colour and are of moderate in size in males , moderately sized in males, rounded at the bottom and free from wrinkles. Eyes are compact and small. Eye lids are light red in colour (Fig. 5.18). The weight of cock is 3 to 3.6 kg and that of hen, is 2 to 2.5 kg. The laying age is 6 months. Average annual egg production is 100 to 150. Egg shell colour is light to medium brown. It is a dual purpose bird used for both egg and meat production. The males, though used for cock fighting, are less aggressive. The birds are reared in the smallholder production system in a family flock size ranging from 4 to 7. The hens are less broody compared to other indigenous domestic fowl. The eggs are hatched through use of broody hens of other indigenous breeds. The birds of the breed possess the ability to survive and perform in a low production input system and in harsh physical environments.

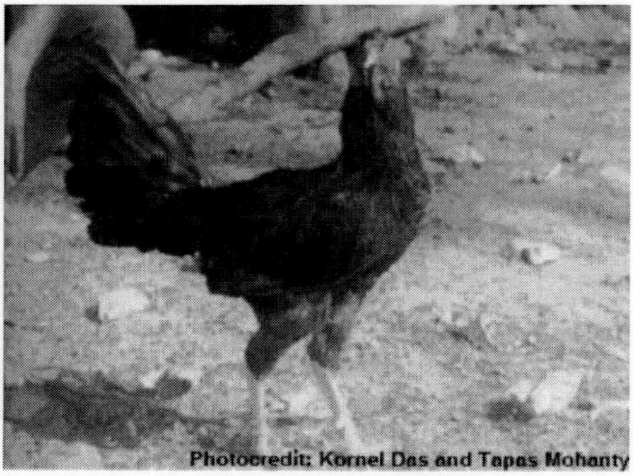

Fig. 5.18 Dumasil
(*Source:* http://sapplpp.org)

5.3.19 Vezaguda

It is widely distributed in rural particularly in tribal areas and even small towns of Malkangiri district and Jeypore subdivision of Koraput district of Odisha and even adjoining areas of the state of Andhra Pradesh. Adult cocks are fairly large with majestic gait and high stamina. Predominant plumage colours are black, brown and white. Comb, wattles, face and ear lobes are red in colour, head is light red and beak yellow. Pea comb is common, fairly large in size and firmly set. Eyes are compact (Fig.5.19). Body length in males is 70 to 91cm and in females 52 to 70 cm. The height of males is 67 to77cm and that of females 47 to56 cm. The weight of cock is 2.5 to 3.5 kg and of hen 1.6 to 2.5 kg. Age at first egg is 7 to 8 months. Egg production is 8-15 per clutch; an average of 3-4 clutches in a year. Average annual egg production ranges from 50 to 60 eggs. Egg shell colour is light brown. Most of the eggs produced are used for hatching the chicks as they fetch a higher price than eggs. Eggs are consumed only when it is absolutely necessary (ceremonies or during severe summer when hatchability is poor). Males are mainly used for cock fighting and are sold for a very high price. All the birds are maintained under smallholder production system with a flock size varying from 5 to 40. The breed is well adapted to the environment and is capable of protecting itself from predators.

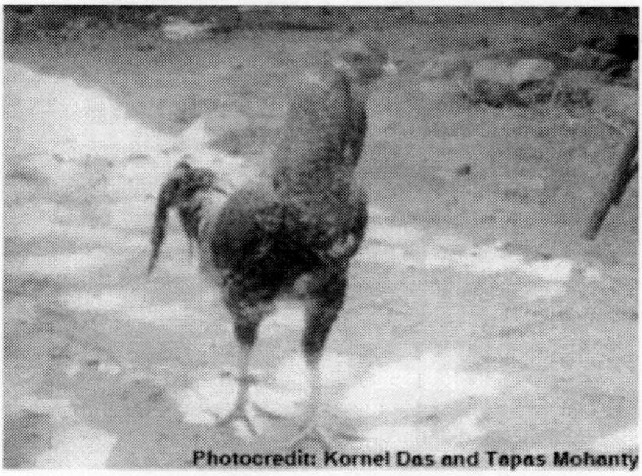

Fig. 5.19 Vezaguda
(*Source:* http://sapplpp.org)

5.3.20 Gujuri

This breed is widely distributed in Baripada and Khunta blocks of Mayurbhanj district in Orissa. Birds of both sexes are active and alert with a well-proportioned body. Plumage colour varies from dark brown to maroon all over the body. Buttercup comb is very common which is big in size and well developed in both sexes. Wattles are bright red in colour, well rounded but smaller in size. Eyes are small, round and brown in colour (Fig.5.20). The length of body in males is 66 cm and in females 53cm. The height of male is 57cm and of female 54 cm. The weight of cock is 2.5 kg and that of hen 1.5 kg. The egg laying age is 6 months. The egg production is 15-20 per clutch with an average of 3-4 clutches in a year. Average annual egg production is 80 to 100 eggs. The egg shell colour is light to medium brown. Locally it is also known as Thusuri, Kadamkhadia, Khairi, Kalua and Bansabania. It is a dual purpose bird and used for both production of eggs and meat. Males are good fighters and hence used for cock fighting. Most of the eggs produced are hatched since chicks fetch a better price than eggs. The birds show an excellent adaptability to their native environment and are tolerant to heat and cold.

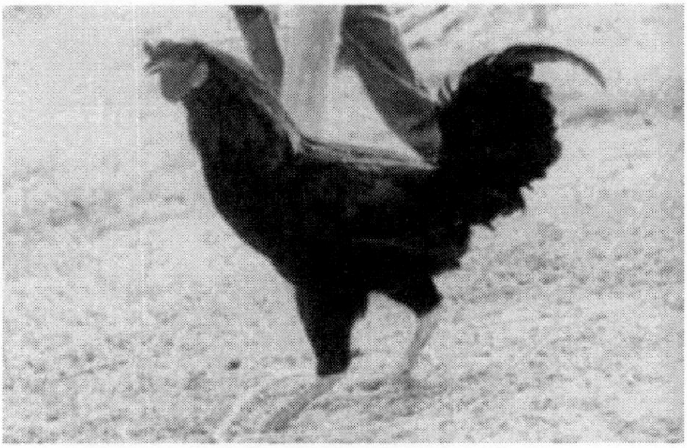

Fig. 5.20 Gujuri
(*Source:* http://sapplpp.org)

5.3.21 Hansli

It is widely distributed in Udala and Kaptipada blocks of Mayurbhanj district in Odisha. Also found in varying numbers in other blocks of the same district as well as the adjacent district of Keonjhar. Birds of both sexes are fairly long. The length of body of male is 71 to 74 cm and that in female 48 to 57 cm. The height of male is 61 to75 cm and that of female is 45 to 63 cm. The comb, wattles, face and earlobes are red. The birds of the breed are characterized by pea comb. The beak and head are light yellow and eyes are light gray (Fig. 5.21). The weight of cock is 2.5 to 3.0 kg and that of hen 1.75 to1.85 kg, cockerels 1.5 to 2.0 kg and pullets 1.2 to 1.4 kg. Age at first egg is six months. Egg production is 10-20 per clutch with an average of 3-4 clutches in a year. Average annual egg production is 50 to 60 eggs. Egg shell colour is light brown. The males of the breed are very aggressive with high stamina and dogged fighting qualities and are used for cock fighting which is a popular sport in the region. All the eggs produced are hatched and rarely used for human consumption, unless the weather conditions are adverse for a good hatch. Meat fetches a good price in the market since it is considered tastier than that of farm-bred chicken. Fighting cocks are sold at exorbitant prices, usually 3 to 4 times higher than when they are sold for meat purposes.

In addition to the domesticated indigenous breeds described above Red Jungle Fowl, which is the progenitor of the modern day chicken is also found in wild in north eastern region. Efforts to domesticate or kept these birds in captivity or cross them with the domestic indigenous or exotic breeds have not been very successful.

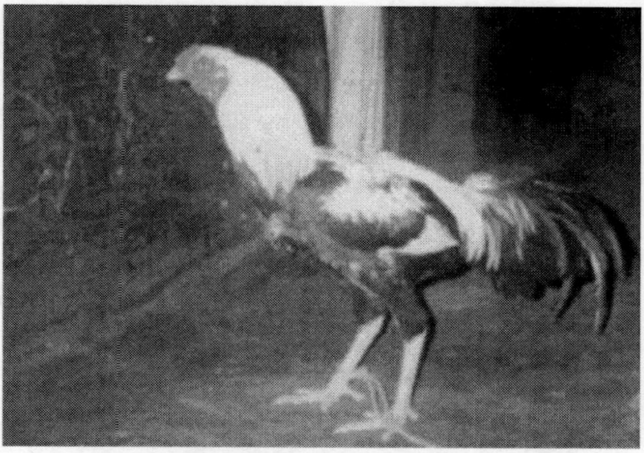

Fig. 5.21 Hansli
(Source: sapplpp.org)

5.3.22 Red Jungle fowl

It is native to southern and Southeast Asia and in India. It is found in India in east Arunachal Pradesh, Odisha and the forests of Chhattisgarh. The red jungle fowl inhabits tropical and subtropical habitats throughout its extensive range, including mangroves, scrubland and plantations, although it seems to prefer flat or gently sloping terrain, forest edges and secondary forest. It is also found in the foothills of the Himalayas. The length of cock ranges 65-75 cm and that of hen 42–46 cm. Average weight of cock ranges 672–1,450 g and that of hen 485-1,050 g. The vibrant male has a long, golden-orange to deep-red crown and neck feathers, and a dark metallic-green tail with a white tuft at the base. The under parts are dull black while the upper parts are a combination of glossy blue-green, rich dark red, maroon-red, fiery orange and blackish brown. The colourful cock also has vivid scarlet-red facial skin, throat, two lappets and a heavily dented fleshy crest (comb), and red or white ear patches on the sides of the head. The female is a dull brown-gold colour with a partly naked, pale red face and throat (Fig. 5.22). Hens produce four to seven eggs per clutch, which are incubated for 18 to 20 days by the hen. At twelve weeks of age, the young are chased out of the social group by their mother, and go off to join another group or form their own. A tropical member of the pheasant family and is widely believed to be a direct ancestor of the domestic chicken. It was first raised in captivity at least several thousand years ago in the Indian subcontinent and the domesticated form has been used around the world as a productive food source both for meat and eggs. The red jungle fowl lives in small mixed flocks during the non-breeding season. These have a hierarchical social system in which there is a 'pecking order' for both males and females. In the spring, at the onset of the breeding season, each of the stronger cock maintains a territory with three to five hens. Meanwhile, young cocks live isolated in twos and threes. Red jungle fowl forages on the ground for seeds, fruits and insects, using their feet to scratch away leaf-litter in search of food. Jungle fowl have been extensively used in medical research benefiting mankind.

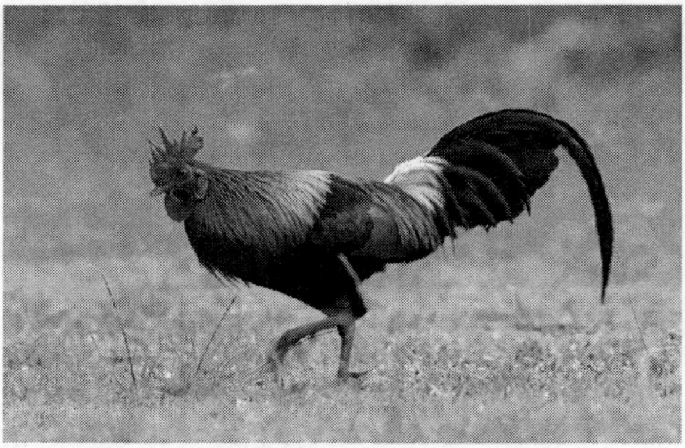

Fig. 5.22 Red Jungle fowl
(*Source:* sapplpp.org)

5.4 Indigenously Developed Chicken Germplasm Through Crossbreeding

A large number of new breeds have been evolved through crossing various exotic layer and broiler breeds or their strains/inbred lines with indigenous descript/non-descript breeds and with an emphasis on expanding rural poultry production and generating breeds/types of chicken similar to the indigenous breeds in plumage colour and adaptation to extensive rural poultry production. Similarly a large number of new layer and broiler breeds have been evolved through selection in relatively low producing exotic layer and broiler breed/strain crosses with long shank length and plumage color similar to the indigenous breeds. These breeds have been tested under extensive management in rural areas in a number of agro-ecologies and have performed better than the indigenous breeds both in egg and meat production and product quality. The breeds/strains of layers and broilers are described below-

5.4.1 Germplasm from Central Avian Research Institute, Izatnager, Bareilly

5.4.1.1 Egg type germplasm for commercial farming

5.4.1.1.1 CARI Priya Layer

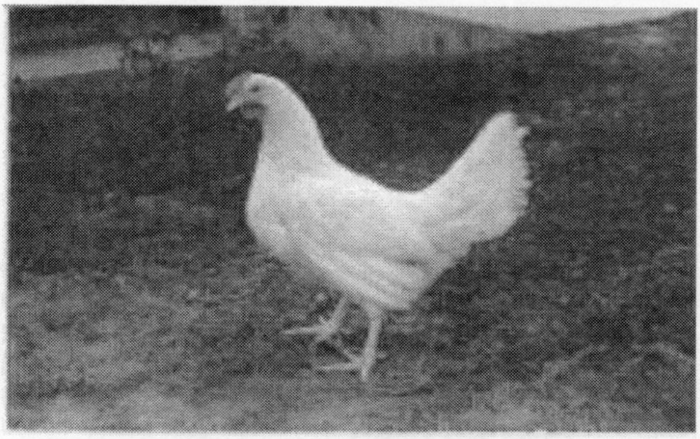

Fig. 5.23 CARI Priya Layer
(*Source:* www.icar.org.in /cari/varieties_deve.php)

CARl Priya was developed by crossing superior male and female strains of White Leghorn. Their performance has been studied and indicated age of first egg at 17 to 18 weeks, 50% production at 150 days, peak production at 26 to 28 weeks, liveability of grower (96%) and layer (94%). Egg production at peak 92%. Hen housed to 72 week more than 298 eggs. Egg weight averages 57 g (Fig. 5.23).

5.4.1.1.2 CARI Sonali Layer (Golden-92)

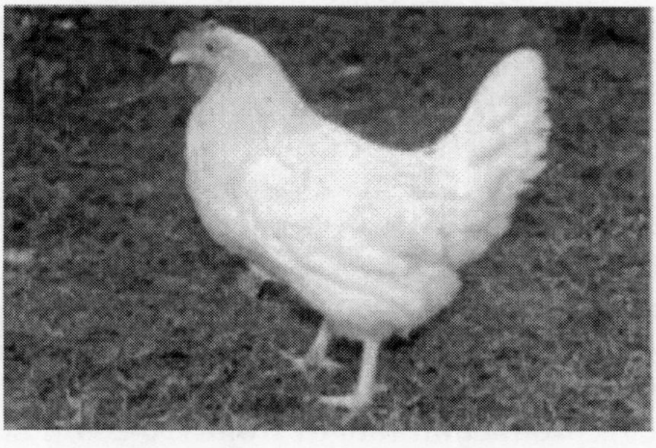

Fig. 5.24 CARI Sonali Layer (Golden-92)
(*Source:* www.icar.org.in /cari/varieties_deve.php)

To cater to the needs and high demand of the consumers of the golden brown egges, Sonali layer was evolved and released for its commercial exploitation in the year 1992 using White Leghorn as male line and Rhode Island Red as female line. The performance study indicates age at first egg at 18 to 19 weeks. 50% production at 155 days. Peak production at 27 to 29 weeks, livability of grower 96% and layer 94%, egg production at peak 90%, and hen housed to 72 week more than 280 eggs. Egg weight average 54 g (Fig. 5.24).

5.4.1.1.3 CARI-Devendra

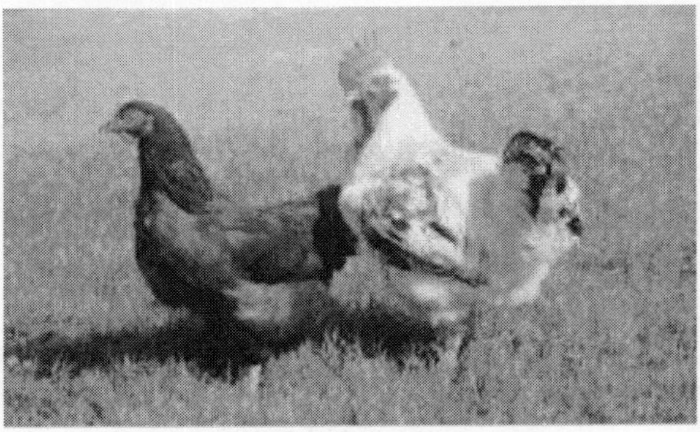

Fig. 5.25 CARI-Devendra
(*Source:* www.icar.org.in /cari/varieties_deve.php)

CARI Devendra is a medium-sized dual-purpose bird, produced by crossing coloured synthetic broiler line as male line and Rhode Island Red as female line. It is the most suitable bird for Indian poultry farmers due to its attractive bright plumage colour. The bird achieves moderate body weight at eight weeks of age with a relatively economic feed conversion ratio. The meat has lower carcass and abdominal fat than broiler meat, which makes it a consumer's preference. CARI Devendra is also a suitable bird for rural poultry production because of its better survivability and moderate egg production ability and being medium sized and dual purpose bird, efficient feed conversion and giving high positive return over feed cost. It is superior to similarly stocks with low laying house mortality. Body weight at 8 weeks averages 1100-1200 grams, at 10 weeks 1400-1500 grams, and at 12 weeks 1700-1800 grams. Age at sexual maturity ranges from 155-160 days. Annual egg production ranges from 190-200 (Fig. 5.25).

5.4.1.2 Meat type germplasm for commercial farming

5.4.1.2.1 CARI BRO -VISHAL (CARIBRO-91)

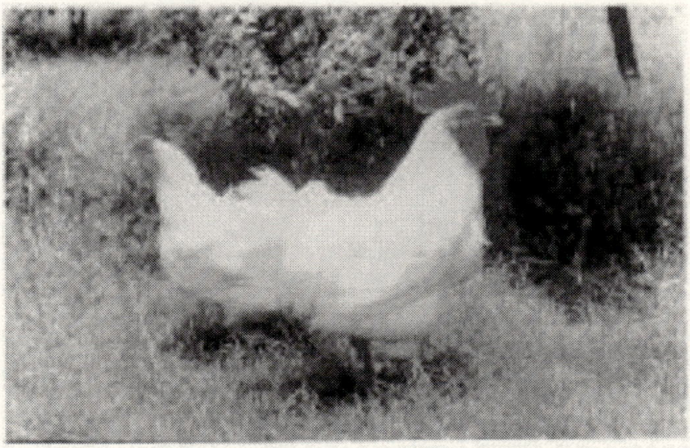

Fig. 5.26 CARI BRO -VISHAL (CARIBRO-91)
(*Source:* www.icar.org.in /cari/varieties_deve.php)

Weight of chickem at hatching at day old 43g. Weight at 6 weeks averages 1700g and at 7 weeks 2000 to 2150g. Dressing percentage ranges from 75-80%. Livability percentage ranges from 97-98%. Feed conversion ratio at 6 weeks is 1.85 (Fig. 5.26).

5.4.1.2.2 CARI-RAINBRO (B-77)

Weight at day old 41g. Weight at 6 weeks 1300 g. Weight at 7 weeks 1600 g. Native tract native to Southern and Southeast Asia and in India it is found in east Arunachal Pradesh, Odisha and the forests of Chhattisgarh. The red jungle fowl inhabits tropical and subtropical habitats throughout its extensive range, including mangroves, scrubland and plantations, although it seems to prefer flat or gently sloping terrain, forest edges and secondary forest. It is also found in the foothills of the Himalayas. Livability percentage 98-99%. Feed conversion ratio at 6 weeks 2.3.

5.4.1.2.3 CARIBRO-DHANRAJA (Multi-Coloured)

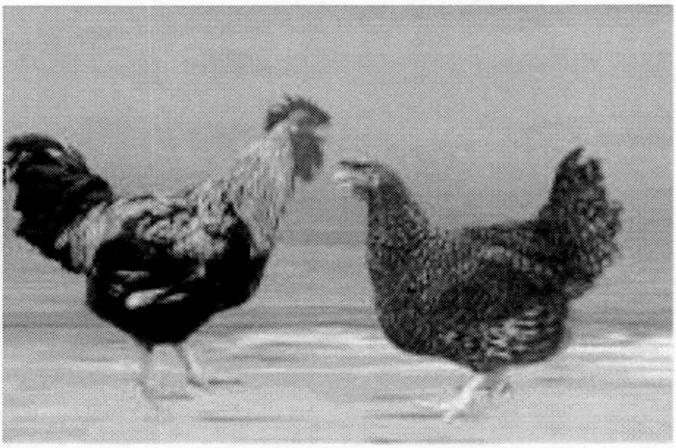

Fig. 5.27 CARIBRO-DHANRAJA (Multi-Coloured)
(*Source:* www.icar.org.in /cari/varieties_deve.php)

CARIBRO Dhanraja is the most preferred bird among farmers because of its multicoloured plumage and high economic returns. CARIBRO Dhanraja produced by coloured synthetic male and female lines. This stock is characterized by its bright plumage colour with single comb. It is also less susceptible to adverse environmental conditions. Average weight at one day 46g, weight at 6 weeks 1500 to 1700g, at 7 weeks 2000 to 2150g. Dressing percentage ranges from 73-75%, livability percentage 96-98%, feed conversion ratio at 6 weeks 1.90 (Fig.5.27).

5.4.1.2.4 CARIBRO-MRITUNJAI (CARI Naked Neck)

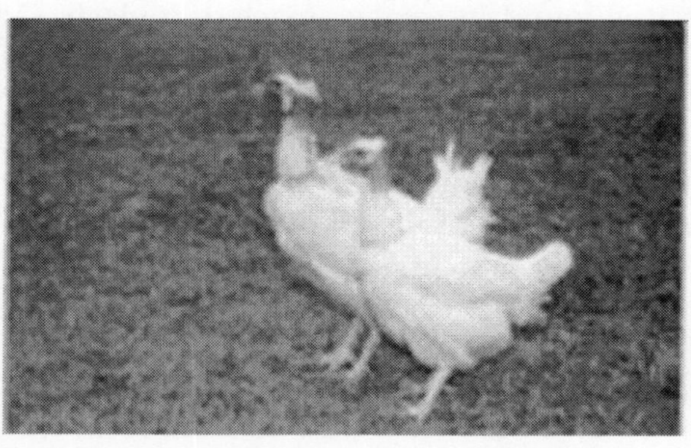

Fig. 5.28 CARIBRO-MRITUNJAI (CARI Naked Neck)
(*Source:* www.icar.org.in /cari/varieties_deve.php)

CARIBRO Mrityunjay is a commercial cross produced through introgression of naked neck gene into coloured and white synthetic broiler lines by repeated backcrossing. Both coloured and white plumage stocks of CARIBRO Mrityunjay are available. The stock is characterized by its adaptability to high ambient temperature, which make it the ideal bird for tropical environment. Weights at day old ranges from 38-42 g, at 6 weeks 1400 to 1500g, at 7 weeks 1800 to 2000g, dressing percentage 75 - 77%, livability percentage 97-98%, feed conversion ratio at 6 weeks 1.95 (Fig. 5.28)

5.5 Germplasm for Rural Poultry Production

5.5.1 UPCARI (Frizzle Cross)

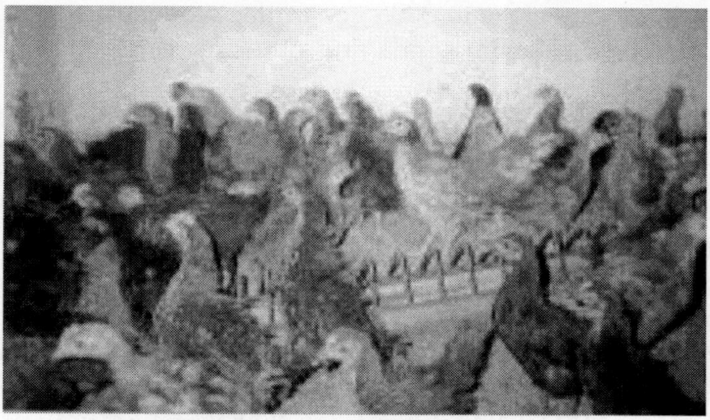

Fig. 5.29 UPCARI (Frizzle Cross)
Source: www.icar.org.in /cari/varieties_deve.php)

Indian native chicken with Frizzle plumage has been crossed with CARI Red for development of UPCARI birds. Unique scavenging type birds, having typical desi fowl look, better tropical adaptability and disease resistance, exceptional growth and production performance. Best suited for backyard system of poultry production. Four varieties of UPCARI birds suitable for different agro-climatic conditions are available and have been evolved through crossing different breeds as given below:

1. Kadakanath x Dehlam Red
2. Aseel x Dehlam Red
3. Naked Neck x Dehlam Red
4. Frizzle x Dehlam Red

Body weight at 20 weeks in males is 1688g and female 1285g. Age at sexual maturity 165 days. Annual egg production 220 eggs. Egg weight at 40 weeks is 60 g. Fertility 90%. Hatchability (FES) 84%.

5.5.2 Krishi Layer

It is a commercial layer variety, evolved utilizing IWH and IWI lines for the benefit of the farmers. The variety has the potential to lay about 280 eggs/year on hen housed basis.

5.5.3 Swethapriya

It is egg type variety developed for small scale intensive and rural poultry. The bird has white plumage with brown/black spots and has potential to lay close to 200 eggs under scavenging conditions. It is particularly popular in Kerala and other regions.

5.5.4 Krishibro -meat type germplasm for commercial farming

Developed by the Project Directorate on Poultry (PDP of ICAR), Hydereabad. Multi-colored commercial broiler chicks. Attain body weight by 6 weeks of age with less than 2.2 feed conversion ratio. The survivability of this bird upto 6 weeks of age is around 97%. These birds have attractive colour plumage and are well adapted to tropical weather conditions. The commercial Krishibro has highly resistance against the common poultry diseases like Ranikhet and Infectious Bursal Disease (IBD). Advantages are that it is hardy, well adapted and better survivability

5.6 Germplasm for Rural Poultry Production at Project Directorate on Poultry (PDP)

5.6.1 Vanaraja

Suitable bird for backyard farming in rural and tribal areas developed by Project Directorate on Poultry (PDP), Hyderabad. It is a multi-coloured dual purpose bird with attractive plumage. It has better immune status against common poultry diseases and is adaptable to the free range rearing. Vanaraja males attain moderate body weight at 8 weeks of age under regular feeding system. The hen lays 160-180 eggs in a laying cycle. Due to their relatively light weight and long shanks, these birds are capable to protect themselves from predators which are otherwise a major problem observed in birds reared in backyards.

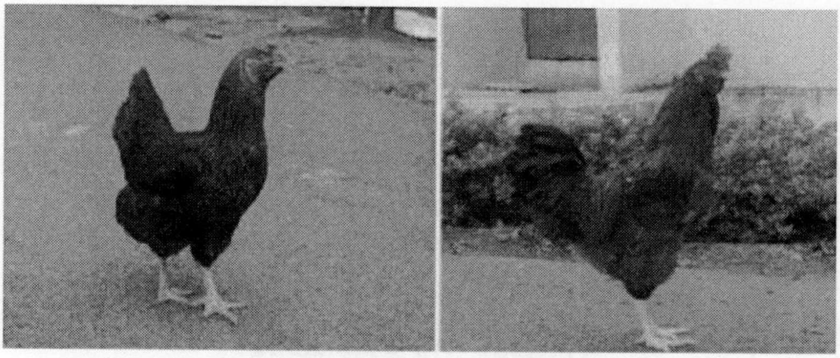

Fig. 5.30 Vanaraja
(*Source:* www.icar.org.in)

5.6.2 Grampriya

It is a multi-colored bird layer variety, developed by PDP for free range farming in rural and tribal areas. It is with moderate body weight and longer shank, which make it less prone to predator attack, which is a desirable characteristic under free range system. Average body weight at six weeks ranges from 400-500 g, whereas the weight at sexual maturity is 1600-1800 g. The males weigh around 1.2 to 1.5 kg at 15 wks of age and suitable for *tandoori* preparations. The bird has the production potential of 230-240 eggs in a year and can lay 160-180 eggs in free-range conditions with minimum supplementary feeding. The bird lays brown eggs weighing 57-59g. It is hardy and livability is high. The rural and tribal farmers of many states are being profitted by this variety.

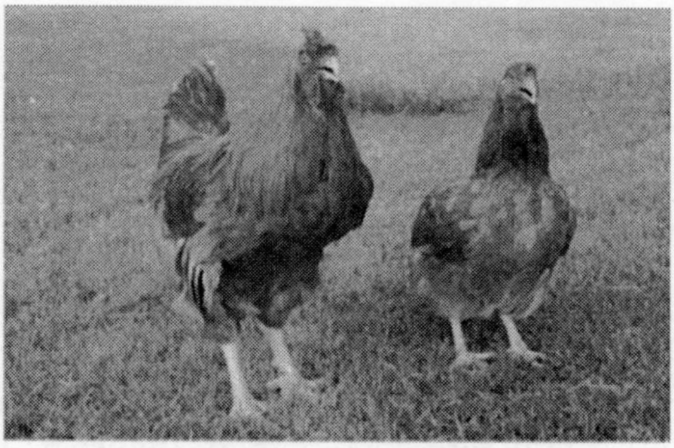

Fig. 5.31 Grampriya
(*Source:* icar.org.in)

5.6.3 Srinidhi

It has been developed by PDP and has multi-colored plumage and longer shanks. It's weighs ~ 650 g at 6 weeks of age, while males have body weight of more than 2.3 kg at 15 weeks of age. It is an early maturing bird. The egg production upto 40 weeks of age is 90 eggs and the annual egg production is 228 eggs under intensive system of rearing. The survivability is more than 95%. Under field conditions, it gives a body weight of 500-550 g at 6 weeks of age and has potential to lay 140-150 eggs per year. Eggs are brown in color and are big in size (53-55 g) (Fig. 5.32).

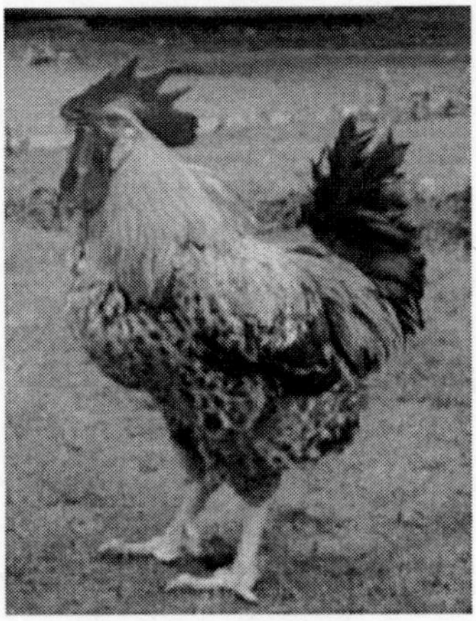

Fig. 5.32 Srinidhi
(*Source:* icar.org.in)

5.7 Germplasm Developed At SAUs/ SVUs

5.7.1 Giriraja

Giriraja is a suitable bird for small scale farmers and tribals, developed at the Karnataka Veterinary, Animal and Fishery Science University, Bangalore. It has resemblance with local birds in color and appearance. Giriraja are sturdy and less prone to common diseases and can acclimatizes to any region and weather. It is well adaptable to scavenging conditions. Giriraja attains a body weihgt of 1600-1700 g at 8 weeks of age under scavenging system and can lay 140-150 eggs in a year. Eggs are bigger in size (55-65 g) and have colored egg shell. Adult male birds weigh 4500-5500 g, whereas; female weighes 3500-4000 g (Fig. 5.33).

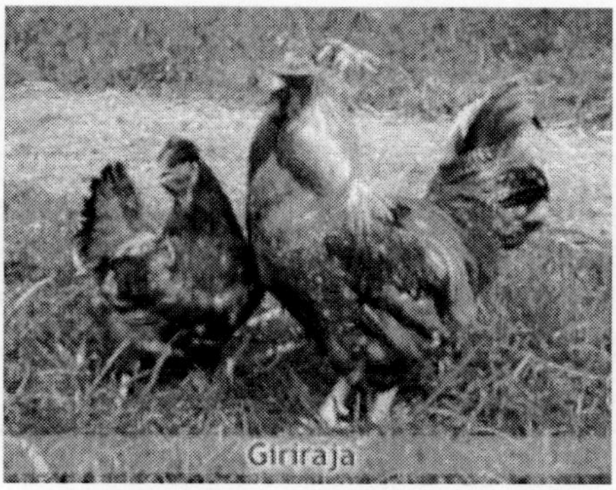

Fig. 5.33 Giriraja
(*Source:* toppoultrymarket.blogs)

5.7.2 Sawarandhara

This breed yields 15-20 eggs in a year, more than Giriraja breed and was released by the Karnataka Veterinary, Animal and Fishery Sciences University, Bangalore in 2005. Swarnadhara chicken has a high egg production potential along with better growth compared to other local varieties and are suited for mixed and backyard farming. Compared to Giriraja breed, Swarnadhara breed are smaller in size with a lighter body weight, which makes them easier to escape attacks from predators such as jungle cats and foxes. The bird can be reared for its eggs and meat. It attains maturity from the 22-23rd week after hatching. Hens attain a body weight of about 3 kg and the cocks about 4 kg. Swarnadhara hens lay about 180-190 eggs in a year (Fig. 5.34).

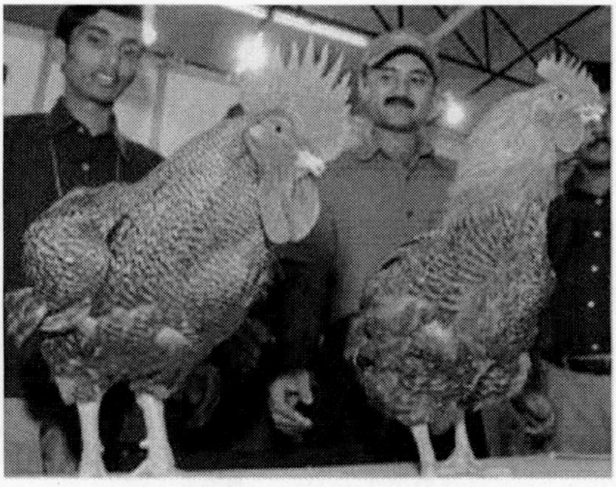

Fig. 5.34 Sawarandhara
(*Source:* http://vikaspedia.in)

5.7.3 Rajashree

Rajashree, a prolific egg laying chicken variety has been developed by Sri Venkateswara Veterinary University, Tirupati to boost the backyard poultry production. It was evolved by the university using three exotic breeds and desi birds. The bird is medium in size and is capable of producing 160 to 180 eggs per year. It weigh 25 per cent heavier than the desi bird. The birds weighs 550-600 g at 9 weeks of age with average mortality of 3.12 %. The body weight at 20th week are 1000-1200 g under backyard farming with 10-15 % of supplementary feeding. These birds can lay about 100-140 eggs in a year with an average egg weight of 52 g (Fig. 5.35).

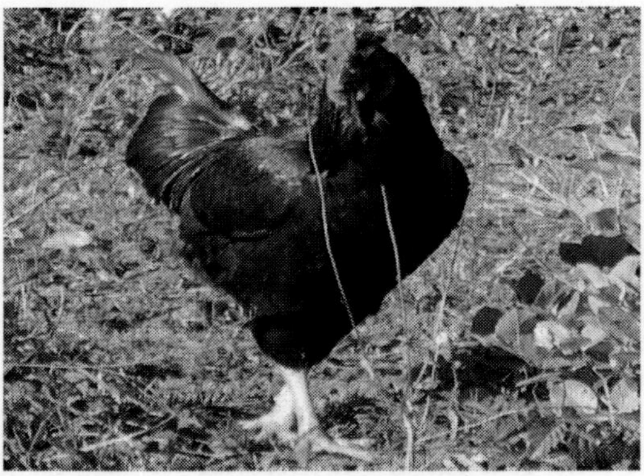

Fig. 5.35 Rajashree
(*Source:* roysfarm.com)

5.7.4 Gramalakshmi

A layer developed by Kerala Agricultural University has proved its versatility in the homestead farming situation. Homestead farming is a unique feature in Kerala egg production scenerio and therefore is an ideally suited bird for Kerala. Annual egg production is 180-200 eggs. Body weight at the end of lay is 1.7 kg. Colour of eggs is light brown. Mortality is less than 4%. These targets are achievable by feeding birds with household food waste and 40-50 g of compounded feed per bird per day and adopting timely immunization.

5.7.5 Athulya

A hybrid layer bird evolved at the All India Co-ordinated Research Project on Poultry Breeding, Mannuthy Centre. A product which has surpassed all other entries in performance testing programmes conducted by Government of India. Athulya has a potential to give 270-280 eggs under intensive management conditions. The feed conversion efficiency is excellent. Livability is also excellent. The average egg weight is 53g.

5.8 Germplasm Developed By Department of Animal Husbandry, Dairy and Fishery (DAHD&F), New Delhi

Chabro: It is a multi-colored meat type bird developed at Central Poultry Development Organisation (North Zone), Chandigarh. Chick has a body weight of 40 g at hatch, whereas at 7 week of age, 1400-1500 g with a FCR of 2.48 kg. The average dressing percentage is 74 %. It has a good livability of (97 %) upto 7 weeks of age. A dual type bird, known as **Chadual** is also been developed at this centre Fig. 5.37 and 5.37).

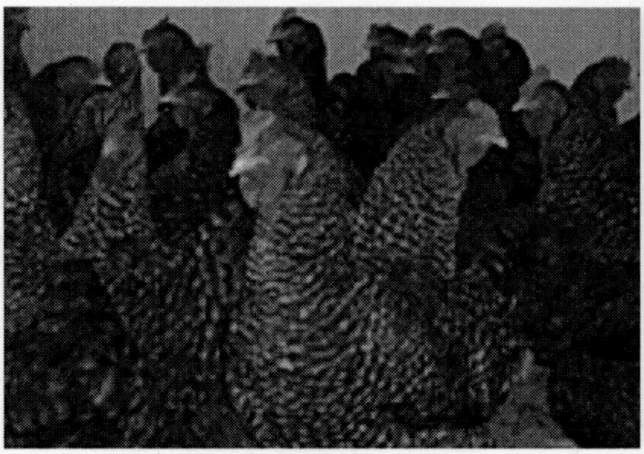

Fig. 5.36 Chabro birds (*Source:* cpdoti.org)

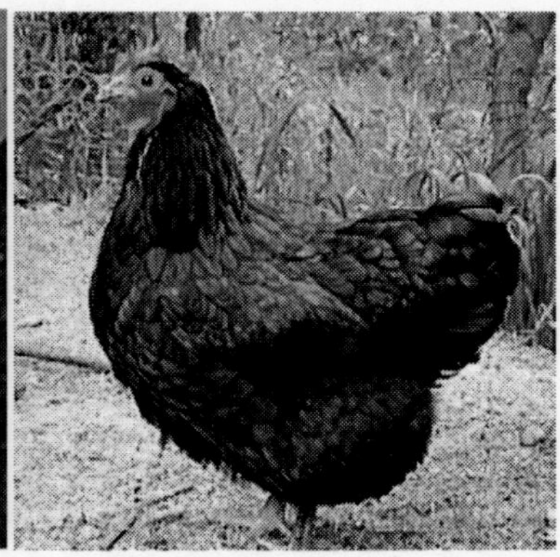

Fig. 5.37 Chadual (*Source:* backyardpoultrymag.com)

5.9 Germplasm Developed By Private Sector

Private sector has also developed germplasm for rural poultry production system such as Kalyani DK, Satpuda Desi and Kuroiler. Anant D. Samant of Mumbai developed new meat strain "Kalyani DK" to cater to the market in Maharashtra by utilizing desi birds. It is a synthetic hybrid prototype which resembles indigenous fowl in body conformation, and has multi coloured plumage, dull shanks, pink skin and single combs. It has generated new opportunities for poultry production in rural areas. Satpuda Desi chickens were introduced in

2002. They have multi coloured feathers, dull bluish shanks, pink skin and a single comb. It has an indigenous fowl body confirmation for meat and egg production. The Satpuda Male Desi attained 1.0 kg body weight in 8-9 weeks with 2.45 kg feed. Satpura - Desi chickens, have been able to capitalise on its acceptance as an indigenous breed in the local meat markets.

The Kuroiler was interoduced by Kegg Farms in 1990s and is a cross between coloured broiler male with Rhode Island Red female. It was developed as a dual-purpose germplasm both for meat and eggs and can live on a diet of kitchen and agricultural waste, and produce around 150 eggs per year, whereas; native Indian hens lay only 40 per year. The meat yield per bird of Kuroilers is also greater; males weigh approximately 3.5 kg and females about 2.5 kg whereas the native male bird weighs 1.0 kg and females 0.9 kg. Due to its unique genetic features, the Kuroiler is resistant to diseases. The kuroiler is resistant most avian diseases chick is a potential bio-converter of low cost agricultural/ household and natural waste abundant in villages into human protein food and substantial incomes for rural households.

5.10 Genetic Improvement Programmes in Layers and Broilers Involving Intra-Population Selection and Hybridization Leading to Evolution of Commercially Viable Layer and Broiler Stocks

5.10.1 Egg type germplasm for commercial farming

The AICRP on Poultry for egg and poultry for meat and subsequently an additional project on rural poultry production have been in operation over a long period. New high producing strains of layers and broilers have been evolved at different centers of AICRP using intra-population selection and involving predicting breeding value on the basis of individual, full sib and half sib information for egg production upto 64 weeks of age with superimposed independent culling level for egg weight at 28 weeks of age and layer house viability. This has led to evolution of high yielding strains which include IWD and IWF at SVVU, Hyderabad IWN and IWP strains at KVSU, Mannuthy and AAU, Anand, IWH and IWI strains at CARI, Izatnagar.

The poultry for meat component has evolved coloured synthetic broiler lines (CSML-sireline and CSFL-damline) and corresponding control at CARI, Izatnagar and OUAR, Bhubneshwar. A synthetic sire (PB1 and damline PB2 at GADVASU, Ludhiana and KVAFSU, Bangalore. As mentioned earlier, all the populations are being subjected to selection.

The rural poultry component involves ICAR Research Complex for NEH region, Agartala center, MPPVCVVU, Jabalpur, AAU, Guwahati, BAU, Ranchi MPUAT, Udaipur and CSKHVV, Palampur was added in March 2009 considering the importance being given for enhancing poultry production in rural areas.

Two pedigreed random bred control populations, separately for layer and broiler are being maintained and evaluated. Samples of hatching eggs are supplied to different centers of AICRP on poultry breeding. The commercially viable layer and broiler populations arising from different AICRP centers are being provided either as hatching eggs or day old chicks for commercial production. Each of the strains is maintained at two centers to reduce chances of accidental extinction and for making three and four way crosses.

5.11 Poultry For Egg

At KVASU Mannuthy, 26 generation of IWN and IWP strains have been studied the hen housed egg production up 72 weeks of age was 308.2 and 297 eggs in the two strains respectively and there was an annual increase by 3.5 and 4.8 in the two strains. The hen day production was 313.7 and 301.4. The average genetic gain for egg production up to 64 weeks was 3.70 and 2.35 eggs in the last 9 generations. The egg weight at 64 weeks however slightly decreased. Fertility and survivability were highly satisfactory.

The S10 generation of IWN and IWP strains were evaluated. The egg production upto 72 weeks was 288 and 277 in the two strains respectively. The egg weight at 64 weeks increased by 0.49 and 0.24 gram at 64 week of age in two strains. The hatchability and surviabiliyt were satisfactory.

The performance of IWD and IWF population at SVVU, Hyderabad showed a decline in fertility and hatchability. The egg production upto 40 weeks of age was 103 and 109 and egg weight 50.3 and 51.1g. The genetic response in egg production up to 48 weeks over 12 generation of selection was 0.57 and 0.45 in egg weight of 0.14g.

The S32 generation of IWH, IWI and control populations and IWH X IWI and IWJ x H1 and JGI crosses showed an increase in fertility and hatchability.

5.12 Poultry For Meat

The AICRP Center at Bangalore evaluated S13 and S18 generations of PB2 and S4 and S5 generation of PB1 along with PDP controlled population. The average live weight at 5 weeks was 1022 and 1041g in PB2 and PB1, respectively with an average genetic and phenotypic gain in PB2 of 7.32 and 6.07 g respectively over the last 7 generations. The age of sexual maturity decreased by 7 days in PB1 but increased by 4 days in PB2 over the last generation. The hatchability and mortality were satisfactory.

There was a decline in age of sexual maturity in PB1 but an increase in PB2. The survival and hatchability were satisfactory. The GADVASU, PB2 has completed 37 generation of selection and PB1 5 generation of selection. The body weight at 5 weeks was 1189,1178 and 975g in PB2, PB1 and control population respectively. Over the last 6 generations, the 5 week live weight improved by 25.68 and 25.80g per generation on phenotypic and gentic gains. There was improvement in FCE. Fertility, hatchability and survivability were satisfacorty. The age of sexual maturity decreased by 6 days in PB2 and increased by 10 dyas in PB1. The control population showed a decrease by 23 days. The egg production up to 40 week of age declined in both selected population but increased in control.

At CARI Izatnagar CSML, CSFL and control population were evaluated. The genetic response was 4.28g in CSML and 3.62g in CSFL for 5 week body weight per generation over the last 8 generations. The corresponding phenotypic responses were 16.45 and 15.79. The fertility and mortality were satisfactory.

❑❑❑

CHAPTER-6

Commercial Poultry Breeding

More than 90 percent of the commercial layers, broilers, turkeys, guinea fowls are crosses such as strain within breed crosses and inbred hybrids. Hybridization not only utilizes the additive genetic variance of the two lines but also the non-additive genetic variance. Where characters which are negatively related cannot be selected in the same population, it becomes necessary that separate populations are selected for different characters and crossed to incorporate the genetic superiority for a character. The crossbred progeny not only has the superiority in negatively related characters inherited from both the parents but also likely to express non-additive genetic effects. In case of layers it is a common practice to use four grandparent lines intensively for the major important traits some of which may have negative relationship or may be difficult to record at an early age. The crossing of grandparents leads to creation of male and female parent lines which are then supplied to the franchise breeding farms to be crossed to produce commercial layer and broiler chicks. This has led to large international poultry breeding concerns which maintain a large number of lines selected for different economic characters and test them in crosses in all possible reciprocal crosses. The inbreeding and hybridization has become an important approach in commercial poultry production necessitating very large poultry breeding establishments to maintain a large number of pure lines selected on the basis of their own performance and performance of their reciprocal crosses which helps in exploitation of superior genetic merit for specific economic characters in a particular line. Such lines are selected for a single character and thus the genetic gains are large and when such lines are combined, the additive genetic superiority for variable characters of economic importance are combined into a single breeding stock. In addition, non-additive variance also contribute to the superiority to the crossbred leading to improvement in all production traits even if they are negatively related.

Commercial crosses are tested at a number of locations and over a number of years to identify pure lines which will provide commercial stocks with higher efficiency of production.

In India, the Ministry of Agriculture and Farmers' Welfare, Department of Animal Husbandry, Dairying and Fisheries (DAHD&F) conducts random sample tests for layers and broilers where the commercial chicks marketed by various Government and private poultry breeding farms are tested under uniform conditions of feeding and management and results are published annually and provide guide to commercial poultry breeders in selecting lines for multiplication and use in production of commercial chicks through crosses. The centers are located at Bangaluru, Mumbai, Bhubaneshwar and Gurgaon.

The birds must be regularly culled on the basis of their performance to ensure better economic returns to a commercial poultry keepers. This requires that some records on performance must be maintained by the commercial farm and the birds which show poor growth; late age at first egg upto certain days of lay such as 100 day egg production, low egg production, poor egg size and shape should be culled as early as possible. Moulting refers to shedding of feathers which also provides some indication about laying capacity. Good layers not only molt later but also complete molting quickly and sometimes continue laying even during moulting. The beginning of moulting can be determined by counting stiff primary feathers in the wings. It takes about six weeks for the first new primary feathers and two weeks for each additional full grown feather. The birds can be in molting for 12 weeks and can restart laying.

The breeders do also cull some birds on the basis of external appearance and pigmentation. The latter has importance in heavy layers which tend to have bleached shanks indicating the bird having layed well for 3 to 4 months after start of laying.

There are a number of qualitative characters which follow Mendalian laws of inheritance and are governed by a few genes with a small numbers of alleles. The comb type is one such character. The quantitative characters are determined by a large number of genes with alleles located on each of the pair of chromosome following the Mendalian inheritance. There are a number of genes affecting a quantitative. These genes interact with which have small effect and interact with genes affecting the same trait and located on the same chromosome with which they are linked and tend to go together depending upon the distance of their location and result in linkage disequilibrium. If these alleles are located at the same locus they may have additive or dominance effects and if located on different chromosomes they have epistatic effects. Most quantitative characters have a large environmental variation resulting from feed and management and interfere with the determining the breeding value or additive genetic merit of an individual and thus in selection and genetic improvement. It is easier to make genetic progress through intra-population selection based on individual phenotype (performance), if a large part of genetic variation is additive in nature. In case of non-additive genetic effects, the selection based on individual performance (mass selection) is not very effective and would require information on relatives and follow more complicated selection and mating system such as reciprocal and recurrent reciprocal inbreeding and hybridization.

The genetic variation is measured on the basis of the differences among relatives, as close to the individual as possible, performing preferably contemporarily, and under similar feeding and management conditions. Generally performance on parents, collaterals (full and half sibs) and progeny separately or collectively is used in determining genetic merit of an individual specially in sex limited like in egg production where the selection of sire be based on the performance of its parents, collaterals, and sequently or in a combined manner. Most economic characters related to breeding chicken are egg production, and meat are egg production, egg weight, body weight and efficiency of feed conversion and carcass yield and quality, viability, fertility and hatchability.

The quantitative traits are generally expressed in terms of their means and variances. The former is expressed mostly as an arithmetic mean and the latter in terms of standard deviation/coefficient of variation. In addition the correlations and regressions among various characters affecting the economics of production are also considered while selecting for over all production efficieny. This requires that selection be based not on individual character but on a number of related character determining the economics of production or which are related to the character of interest and can help in improving predictability of genetic merit in that character. This would require that in genetic improvement of a population the phenotypic and genetic parameters in terms of means and variances, heritabilities, phenotypic and genetic correlations among the characters determining the over all genetic merit and the economics of production and the contribution of each character relative to others and overall genetic merit are available and are combined into an index weighed by their relative economic values in determining the independent weightage to be given to each economic character included in selection for improvement of overall genetic merit.

Basis of selection

For highly heritable characters such as body weight and egg weight, selection can be based on an individual's own performance and is called individual / mass selection. However for characters which are sex limited or have low heritability such as egg production or require slaughter of an animal such as carcass yield and quality, the selection is generally based on the relatives such as paternal/full/ half (paternal or maternal and progenies) and is called family selection. Larger the family size and closer the genetic relationship with the individual whose breeding value is being predicted, the breeding value would be determined more accurately. The selection in breeding males for egg production is generally based on the egg production of their female relatives viz parent, female collaterals and female progeny. With the availability of large national and multinational commercial breeding companies and large data storage and computation with computers, it is easier to handle vast data and determine the breeding value/ genetic merit of the sires more accurately and thus an increase in accuracy of selection and also intensity of selection by determining the breeding value of a large number of sires. Alternatively more elaborate selection schemes such as reciprocal/ reciprocal recurrent selection with or without a tester line maintained to make comparison where sires are selected on the basis of their pure line performance and performance of their crosses which will allow the utilization of both their additive and non-additive genetic variation, although this will increase the generation interval.

The selection can be based on individual's own performance for a character (mass selection) or based on independent culling levels where more than one character is of economic importance or using a selection index based on a number of characters of interest together, giving each a proper weightage in determining genetic merit or over all breeding value of an individual. The latter is most efficient in bringing genetic improvement in the aggregate breeding value/ genetic merit but requires information on a number of related characters and estimates on their phenotypic and genetic variances in and co-variances among and their relative economic value. Construction of a selection index combining different economic characters is generally recommended when a number of genetically negatively related characters are involved in determining overall genetic merit such as egg production and average egg weight, body weight gains and reproductive efficiency. The efficiency of index selection increases as the number of traits increases. Of the three systems of selection, tandem selection is the least efficient as it may eliminate genetically superior individuals for more important economic traits which are expressed later in life. Similarly selection based on individual culling levels can reduce the rate of improvement a more important traits which may be expressed later in life. However, index selection increases generation interval and this make lower per unit genetic gains. Further, since genetic and phenotypic parameters change over time due to selection and environmental and managemental effects, the selection index may have to be reconstructed at least every generation.

Selection of the individual within a population is called "mass selection" / "intra-population selection"/ "closed flock selection". Selection may be carried out for different economic traits individually in two different populations specially when they are negatively related which may subsequently crossed to combine the genetic merit of the two populations for two different economic characters and may allow not only utilization of additive genetic superiority in different traits for which the two populations have been selected but also the non-additive genetic variance arising from dominance and epistasis. The physical environment and management in terms of housing, feeding and health cover also determine variation in economic characters and such variation should be reduced by reasonably uniform feeding and management or statistically corrected the performance for environmental effects.

In case of egg production since there is a large non-additive genetic variation, more complicated selection schemes such as selection on the basis of deviation from a random bred contemporary control population and following reciprocal selection/ recurrent reciprocal selection or inbreeding and hybridization are followed.

After the parents selected for producing next generation, decision is required how they should be mated. The mating system involves breeding among phenotypically alike/ different- phenotypic assorted mating or mating on the basis of genetic relationship i.e. closely related birds-inbreeding or breeding among unrelated birds-outbreeding (cross breeding). The inbreeding leads to an increase in homozygosity at all loci related to a trait which may be desirable where the alleles have a positive effects or to a decrease where they have undesirable effects. A large number of lethal genes or genes with deleterious effects are generally recessive and continue in a population and have depressing effect on the mean performance as a result of higher incidence of diseases or abnormal phenotypes on the maturity rate. They can be purged out of a population only if they are allowed to express which is only possible in an homozygous state and can be created through inbreeding. The inbreeding thus leads to a decline in mean performance of the population more particularly for fitness traits related to reproduction and survival. However, it is necessary to eliminate undesirable alleles/genes and also create a certain degree of homozygosity as when such lines /populations are crossed the heterozygosity or hybrid vigor is expressed in the crossbred progeny, thus improving its survival rate, reproductive efficiency and overall production efficiency. Utilization of non-additive genetic variances through reciprocal / recurrent reciprocal selection started in breeding of corn in USA and subsequently adopted in poultry breeding for egg production and to a limited extent in broiler production.

Mating systems

Flock and pen matings are the two commonly used methods for mating selected males and females. Pedigree records cannot be maintained in a large flock mating but currently where the A.I. is used with freshly collected and preserved semen it is easier to identify the sire. Normally one male is used for mating with 8 to 10 females in broiler and 10-15 females in layers. In the cage housed birds generally breeding is done through A.I using freshly collected and diluted or undiluted semen and generally a single insemination maintains fertility for a week.

Egg production is the most important economic character in domestic fowl whether layer or broiler. A modern commercial layer starts laying around 20 weeks of age and continues to do so till it dies, however the rate of egg production (lay) declines below the economic level after the first laying cycle. Commercial layers therefore are not normally maintained after 72 weeks of age or 56 weeks of lay.

Commercial layers lay as high as 350 eggs in a first laying cycle but the average is around 320 eggs. Peak production in a flock is usually reached at about six to eight weeks after the first egg is laid and the egg production starts declining after nine months of lay. Egg production is measured either as number of eggs layed during a period or percent of lay. It can be expressed as hen housed, hen day and survivors. Hen housed egg production is calculated by dividing the total numbers of egg laid by the number of hens housed in a laying pen. Hen day egg production is calculated in a similar manner but after elimination the birds which die before the completion of the period of lay. Survivor egg production refers to the average numbers of eggs laid by each survivor and is a function of the eggs laid and the number of birds surviving the period of lay. Hen housed egg production is a better indicator of economics of egg production. Genetic factors such as age at first egg, persistency, intensity/rate of lay, broodiness and pauses and environment factors like year and season of lay, age of bird, nutritional conditions, disease incidence and duration and intensity of light affect egg production in chicken may be used in comparing merit a bird and its selection based on such merit.

□□□

CHAPTER-7

Poultry Production Management

Management of poultry production involves different management techniques that helps in improvement in production efficiency (productivity) and thus economic returns from poultry production. It involves brooder management, grower management, layer management and management of breeding males in case of commercial layer and broiler production.

7.1 Brooder Management

Brooder house (Fig. 7.1) should be draught proof, rain proof, and protected from insects and predators. Brooding pens should have windows with mesh for adequate ventilation. Excessive dusty environment which leads to respiratory ailments should be avoided. Besides, dust is one of the vehicles for transmission of infectious agents. Too much dusty atmosphere also results from fumigation with ammonia which irritates the respiratory tract and eyes and should be avoided. Good ventilation provides a comfortable environment without draught. Sanitation and hygiene are important for disease prevention and comfort of birds. All movable equipment like feeders, waterers and hovers should be removed from the house at regular intervals/ the birds have been removed and before the next hatchs has to be housed. The interior of the shed should be cleaned and disinfected. The litter should be scraped and removed. The interior as well as exterior of the poultry house should be cleaned with water containing a disinfectant under pressure. It should be further disinfected with any commercial disinfectant solution. Insecticides should be sprayed to preferably under pressure to eliminate ticks and mites. Malathion spray/ blow lamping or both can be used for prevention of ticks and mites. New litter should be spread after each cleaning of the shed. The insecticides should be mixed with the litter in recommended dosages. Most poultry diseases are highly contagious and all-in and all- out system or spraying disinfectant will help in the control and prevention of diseases. If this is not possible, the chicks should not be allowed to be brooded closer to older birds. The movement of workers and equipment from one building to other should be restricted to the extent possible. Attendants should change their cloths and wear clean overalls and disposable protective shoe covers. A footbath with recommended disinfectant such as phenol should be kept at the entrance of each building and people should walk through the disinfectant. Normally visitors should be restricted from entering inside the farm where layers and broilers are maintained. Suitable litter material like straw dust and paddy husk should be spread on the floor of poultry shed up to a depth of 5 cm depending upon the availability and cost. The litter should be stirred at regular intervals to prevent the development of mould and caking. Wet/caked litter should be removed immediately to prevent ammonia odor.

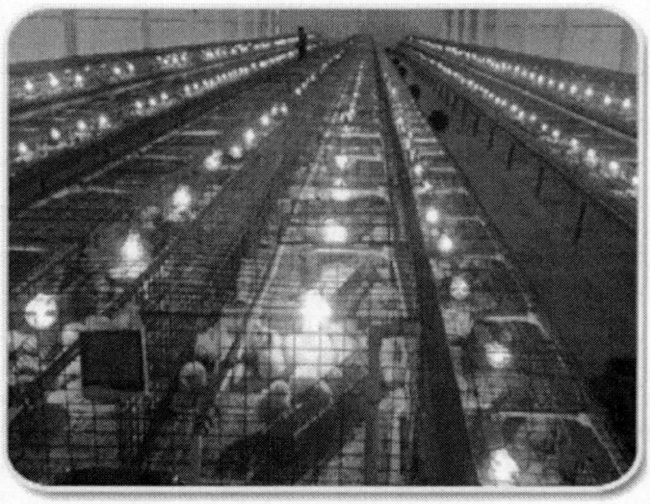

Fig. 7.1 A Brooder House
(*Source:* agridr.in)

Provision of right temperature in the brooder house is necessary. Too high or too low temperature slows down the growth of chicks and results in excessive mortality and morbidity. During the first week of placement of chicks, the temperature should be 95 °F (35 °C) which may be reduced by 5 °F every week till 70 °F (21.1 °C). The temperature in brooder house should be approximately 20 °F below the brooder temperature. It is necessary to have a maximum and minimum temperature thermometer in each shed to regularly record the temperature and adjust the heating/cooling arrangement accordingly. The behavior of chicks provides a better indication of whether they are getting desired amount of heat. When the temperature is less than required, the chicks tend to gather around brooder and when it is too high, they tend to move away from the source of heat and pant/ gasp. With a proper temperature the birds tend to properly spread and appear comfortable. In hot weather brooders are not necessary after the chicks are three weeks old. Several devices for providing artificial heat are available. Hover type electric brooders are most common being thermostatically controlled. The height and number of infrared lamps can be adjusted as per the temperature required in the brooder house. Brooder space of 7 sq. inch (45 sq. cm) is recommended per chicks. An 1.8 sq. meter hover can hold 500 chicks. The dimensions of the house must be taken into consideration as overcrowding results in starvation and thus require excessive culling due to poor growth and increased disease incidence. Chick guards should be provided to prevent the chicks straying away from the source of heat. These guards should be placed 60-75 cm from the edge of the hover. Guard should be removed after one week.

Floor space of 0.05 sq. meters should be provided per chick in the beginning and should be increased by 0.05 sq. meters per males after every four week until the pullets are about 20 week of age. For broiler at least 0.1 meter sq. of the floor space for females and 0.15 meter sq. for males should be provided till 8 weeks of age. Broiler pullets and cockerels are raised in separate pens. Provision of plenty of clean and fresh water is necessary. A 50 linear cm of water space per 100 chicks should be provided in the first two weeks and should be increased to 150-190 linear cm at six to eight weeks, while changing the chicks water trough should be disinfected and filled with fresh water and place it properly. However water trough should be continued for a few days when the chicks are getting accustomed to drinking from automatic water trough. Height of the waterers should be maintained at 2.5 cm above the height of the chicks to avoid spoilage. Antibiotics and other anti-stress medicines should be added to the water. All waterers should be cleaned daily.

The feeder space varies from 2.5 to 3 cm per bird from 0 to 8 weeks of age. Chick should be fed only for 3 to 4 hour after arrival in the brooder house. The feeders should not be more than 1/3rd to full to avoid feed wastage.

The brooding equipment should be spaced around the hover. Sound management practices and judicious use of disinfectants and medicines is essential to prevent occurrence of diseases. Nitrofurazone and coccidiostats should be given in the feed in recommended dosages as per the requirement. All night lights should assure uniform distribution of light up to a week of age. For broilers all night light is essential for the first two days for them to find their way to feeders and waterers. The lighting program can be varied according to the judgment of the poultry keeper.

Floor, feeder and water space recommended for a grower are 950-2350 cm^2, 7.5-12.5 cm and 2.0-2.5 cm respectively. Water consumption is influenced by temperature, humidity, air movement, age, dietary composition, and activity which is emitted in cage house birds. Water consumption increases with an increase in ambient temperature. Deworming is essential once in two months to reduce parasitic load specially if birds are kept in deep litre. It should be done preferable in the morning or late evening. 0.6 cm of litter should be scraped and removed to prevent re-infection. Increasing lighting schedule should be followed for growers upto eight weeks of age. Growing pullets should not be exposed to increasing lighting schedule. Debeaking is recommended between 12-16 weeks of age although it can be done earlier and even after hatching. For broiler breeder, feed restriction is essential during growing period to control body weight gain and age at maturity. Improper restriction can, however; result in an increase in feed cost, reduced egg production and hatchability.

7.2 Layer Management

For layer management, the flock should be transferred from grower to layer house (Fig.7.2) at 18-20 weeks of age. In a breeding flock, males should be placed 1 to 2 days prior to housing of females if they have grown separately. Floor space of 0.23 to 0.28 m^2, feeder space of 10 cm and watering space of 2.5 cm per bird is necessary and should be provided in floor house. In case of cage operations the space requirement is 46.5 cm^2 sq. per bird. One laying nest for every four pullets is necessary. A plateform in front of the nest entrance helps the birds to easily reach the nest.

Lighting of a layer house is very essential to optimize egg production. From 21 weeks onwards the lighting should be increased gradually till it reaches 16 to 17 hours per day and maintained at that level there after. It boosts egg production by 5 to 10 %. Irregular light causes depression of egg production. One 40 W bulb hanging 2.1 m above the floor for each 9.29 m sq of floor space should be provided along with the recommended intensity of light. The bulbs should be cleaned of dust regularly. The duration of light should be maintained uniformly throughout the laying period instead of using older type bulbs which produce more heat than light and have lower operative life. Florescent tubes or low heat producing electric bulbs should be preferred. These will save energy and provide similar amount of light as high voltage conventional bulbs/ tubes.

Breeder male management is similar to that of the layer management except that their diet should be fortified with extra calcium, magnesium, and vitamin E to ensure proper fertility.

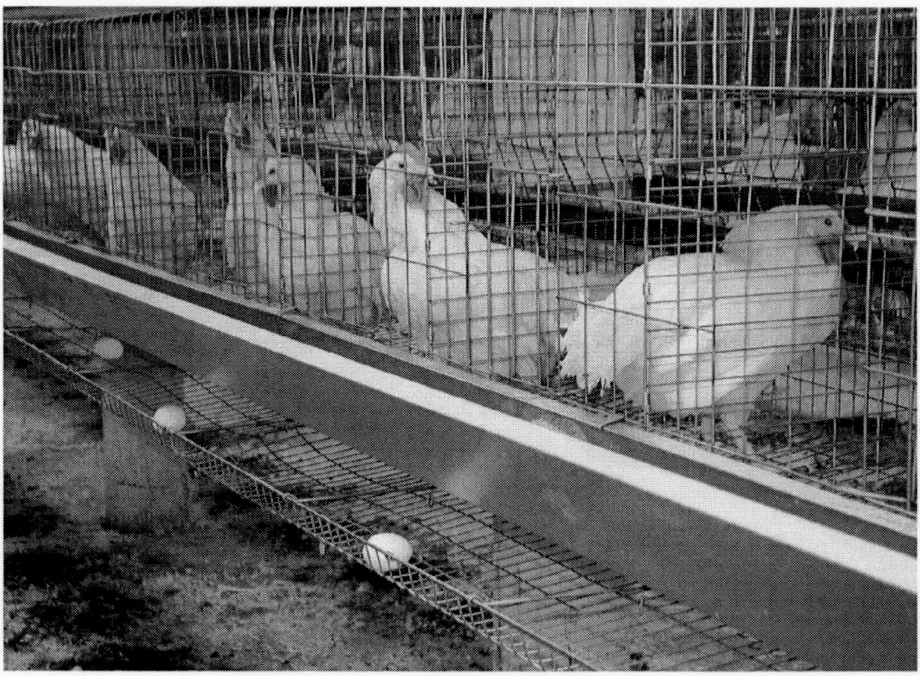

Fig. 7.2 A Layer House
(*Source:* http://agritech.tnau.ac.in)

□□□

CHAPTER-8

Poultry Shelter Management

Generally four systems of poultry shelter management are followed among the poultry keepers in India, depending upon the location of the poultry farm, the weather conditions and their seasonal variations and the type of birds and production system followed. They are: free range or extensive system, semi - intensive system, folding unit system and intensive system. Further there are two systems of management under intensive poultry production i.e. battery system and deep litter system.

8.1 Free-range / Extensive System

It is the oldest system of rearing chickens and other avian species and has been used for centuries by small poultry keepers in rural and peri-urban areas. This is primarily for managing a few indigenous chickens, where there is no shortage of land. This system allows a large room for each bird, where they can find a good amount of food and nutrition from natural resources in the form of herbage, seeds and insects (Fig.8.1). Birds may or may not be protected from predatory animals and infectious diseases including parasitic infestation. In general at night birds are protected from predators by covering them with a basket which allows free circulation of air. Presently due to advantages of intensive system of poultry production, the free range management system is becoming almost obsolete and is extremely limited even in rural areas. However, people concerned with animal ethics and welfare, require that the birds be maintained under extensive and free range system of management so that they can have total freedom of movement, natural feed resources etc.

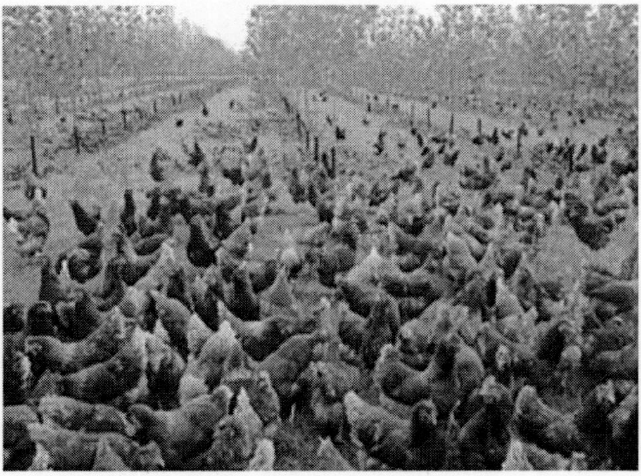

Fig. 8.1 Free-range or extensive system of poultry rearing (*Source:* wattagnet.com)

Even more productive layers and broilers are being raised under extensive system of management but are provided with adequate feed and health inputs.

8.2 Semi-intensive System

Where the amount of free space available is limited, semi intensive system is adopted, but it is necessary to allow the birds 20-30 square yards per bird of space run around freely. Wherever possible this space should be divided with a central partition giving a run on either side of 10-15 square yards per bird, thus enabling the birds to move onto a fresh ground to avoid infection arising from their own droppings. Such area can be provided with shady trees/shrubs and some leguminous fodder can be planted to provide leafy vegetation to the birds for meeting part of their nutritional requirement (Fig. 8.2).

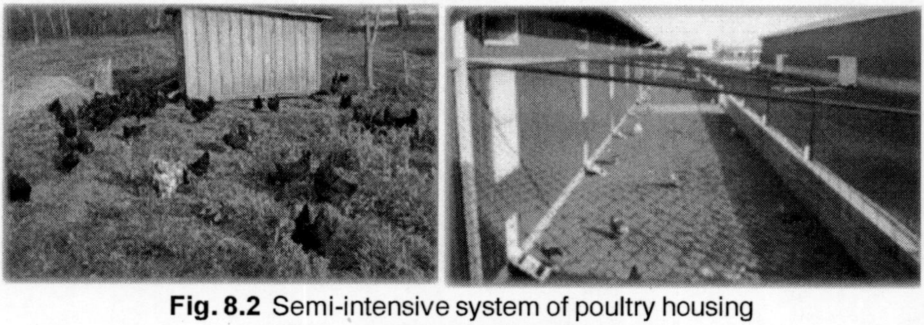

Fig. 8.2 Semi-intensive system of poultry housing (*Source:* http://www.slideshare.net)

8.3 Folding-unit System

This system of housing is an innovation developed during the recent years (Fig.8.3). In portable folding units, birds are confined to one small run, the position is changed each day, giving them fresh ground and the birds consume a considerable proportion of feed from the herbage and are healthier and hardy due to prevention of infection from their droppings. For the poultry keeper the beneficial effect of keeping the land open through scratching and fertilized through droppings gives an advantage for subsequent crop production.

The most convenient folding unit to handle is that which accommodates upto 25 birds. A floor space of 1 square foot should be allowed for each bird in the house, and 3 square feet in the run, so that a total floor space to the whole unit is 4 square feet per bird, as in the intensive poultry production system.

A suitable measurement for a folding house to accommodate 25 birds is 5 feet wide and 20 feet long, the covered the house being 5′ x 5′, one-third of the run. The part nearest the house is covered in and the remaining 10′ is kept open but is enclosed with a wire netting on all the sides and at the top to avoid predation.

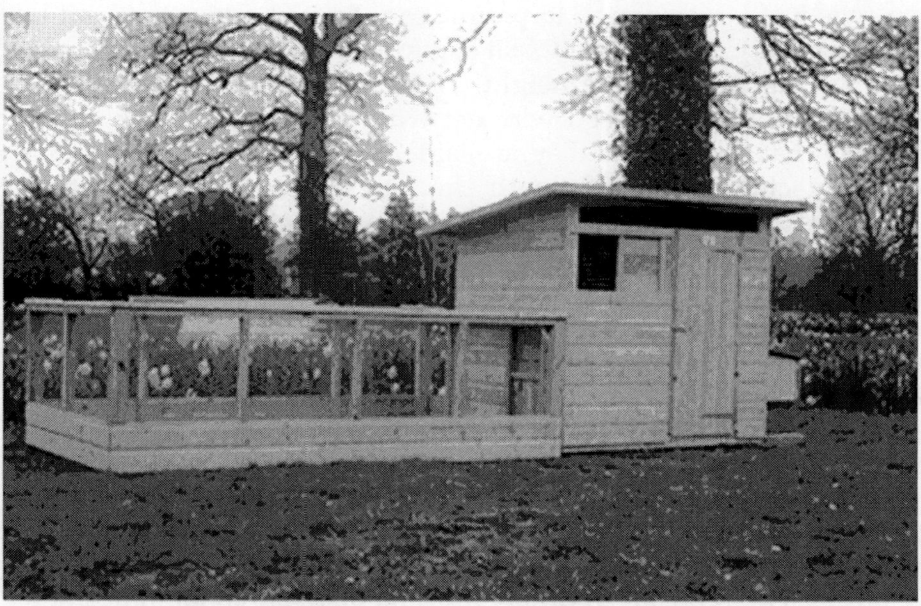

Fig. 8.3 Folding-unit system of poultry housing
(*Source:* www.poultryclub.org)

Disadvantages: The feeding and watering in this system must be carried out to the birds and eggs collected manually. This involves some extra labour in the regular moving of the folding units and some spoilage of feed.

8.4 Intensive System

This system is usually adopted where land is a limiting factor either due to high cost or non-availability as in urban areas. In this system the birds are confined to the house all the time, with no access to open area for exercising and social interaction with each other. There is a need to allow direct sun light to reach the floor of the house so that part of the windows should removable, which either can be folded or can slide down to permit the ultraviolet rays to reach the birds. Under intensive system, battery (cage system) and deep litter systems are most common.

8.4.1 Battery cage system of management

This is the most intensive type of poultry housing and is useful to those poultry producers with only a small piece of land floor space at their disposal (Fig. 8.4). In the battery cage system each hen is confined to a cage just large enough to permit very limited movement and to allow her space only to stand / sit comfortably. The usual floor space is 14 x 16 inches and the height, 17 inches. The floor is made of standard strong galvanised wire net with a slope from back to the front, so that the eggs as they are laid, can roll out of the cage to a receiving channel. Underneath the pen is a tray for collecting droppings. Both feed and water receptacles are held outside the cage. Many small cages can be assembled together; if necessary the cages may be placed in a multistoried manner. The whole structure should be made of corrugated metal and should be rust proof so that no parasites can be harbored. Further a thorough disinfection can be carried out as often as required. Batteries / cages should be set up in a place which is well ventilated, and lighted, is not too hot or cold and is vermin proof and that the feed meets all nutritional needs. This system provides the best comfort and production conditions to birds. It is now a practice to use a cage system to house a large number of birds in a cage, as much as possible. This, however is against animal welfare as it does not allow proper movement, freedom for interaction with other birds.

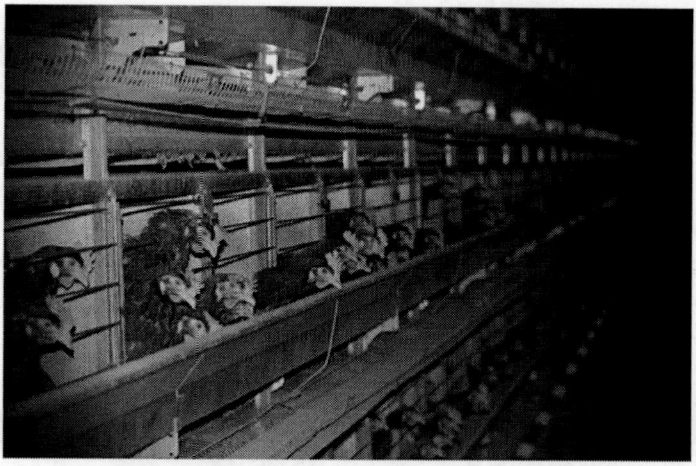

Fig. 8.4 Battery cage system of management
(*Source:* thepoultryguide.com)

The housing system has made remarkable success in poultry production for eggs and meat through battery cage system. It requires a minimum expenditure on energy of birds as they spend all time in the shade and being few in a cage with restricted movement will have no possibility of cometing with other birds for space, feed an water. It also lessens the load of excess body heat. The performance of such birds can be more easily recorded and the culling of the less productive birds can be carried out in time. The system is now being replaced by floor rearing which allows larger freedom of movement and social interaction.

8.4.2 Deep litter system

In this system, the birds are kept in large pens up to 250 birds or more in each pen, and on floor covered with litter like straw, saw dust or leaves up to depth of 8-12 inches (Fig. 8.5). Deep litter gets mixed with poultry droppings and constitutes an excellent manure where both the litter and the droppings can be used relative to the cage system where the droppings are collected once in a year or once in two years and such litter can be used as recycled ruminant feed or high grade organic manure. The litter is allowed to build up until it reaches a depth of 8 to 12 inches. The build-up litter has to be removed at a correct time to prevent transmission of any disease. Suitable dry organic matter like straw (which should be cut into two or three inch pieces), saw dust, leaves, dry grasses, groundnut shells, broken up maize stalks and cobs, bark of trees, in sufficient quantity to give a depth of at least six inches in the pen should be used. The droppings of the birds gradually mixed up with the bedding materials and is build up a high of organic fertilizer. In about two months, it usually becomes deep litter, and by six months it becomes built-up deep litter and after about 12 months it is moved. Wet litter should be removed from time to time and extra littre materials can be added to maintain sufficient depth and keep the bedding dry. After thorough disinfection and keeping the pen empty at least for a month, new litter is added before the new crop of pullets is housed and is continued for their entire laying period.

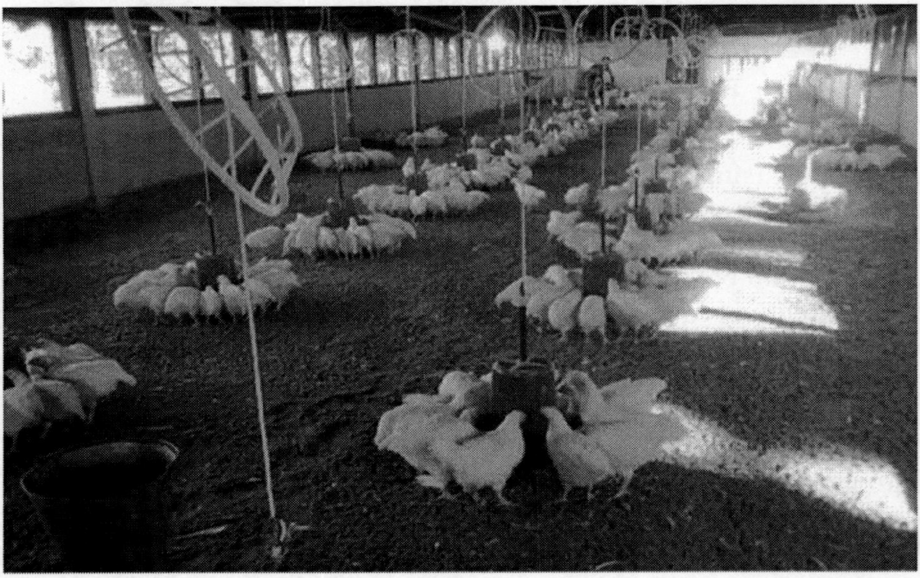

Fig. 8.5 Deep litter system of poultry housing (*Source:* asiafarming.com)

The advantages of this system are that the birds and eggs are safe as they are enclosed in deep litter pen, which has strong wire netting or expanded metal. Built-up deep litter also supplies some of the feed required by the birds. They obtain animal protein factor from deep litter. The level of coccidiosis and other parasitic load is much lower in birds kept on good deep litter which should be stirred regularly and the clumps or wet bedding is removed and replaced by fresh bedding material. Well managed deep litter kept in dry condition with no wet spots around waterer provide greater comfort and avoid spread of infection. With correct conditions observed with well managed deep litter, there is no need to clean a pen out for the whole year. The only attention requires is to regularly stir and remove the wet and clogged litter and often replace it with some fresh litter material as needed. Generally 35 laying birds can produce in one year about 1 metric ton of deep litter with droppings which can be used as organic fertilizer. The level of nitrogen in fresh manure is about 1%, but in well built-up deep litter it may be around 3%. It also contains about 2% phosphorus and 2% potash. Its value is about three times that of cattle manure.

The litter is also a valuable insulating agent, as it maintains its own constant temperature, so birds burrow into it when the air temperature is high and thereby cool themselves. Conversely, they can warm themselves in the same way when the weather is very cool.

The basic rules for deep litter system are that too many birds should not be housed in a single pen and each bird should be given 3 ½ to 4 and preferably 5 square feet of floor space which is comfortable for a bird. Sufficient ventilation should be provided to enable the litter dry and without clumps. Keeping the litter dry is probably more important in deep littre system. If the litter gets soaked by leaking from roofs or from watering troughs, it upsets the whole rearing process and the litter would have to be removed and replaced with fresh litter. All probable precautions should be taken to maintain the litters completely dry through stirring regularly. Turning the litter (just like digging in a garden) at least once weekly is very important in maintaining a correct built-up of deep litter.

8.5 Poultry House Equipments

The poultry house should be equipped with roosts, nests, feed hoppers, water containers and other items, which are essential for satisfactory poultry production and providing comfortable conditions for raising of birds for economic and ethical reasons.

8.5.1 Perches or roosts

Perches should be made (Fig. 8.6) from long wooden bars of two square inches rounded at the top and flat at the bottom, these perches may be fixed about 16 inches above the ground and near about the walls in such a way that they can be removed for cleaning and disinfection. At least a 12-inch space between two perches should be provided. Each bird will need about 8 inches of the perch to roost. Chickens start roosting when they are eight weeks old. Apart from catering to the natural instinct or desire of the chickens to get above the ground at night, perches help to keep the bird's feet and plumage clean. The rear perches should rest a little higher than those at the front, if they are arranged horizontally along the length of the house. This will encourage some of the birds that like to roost high will go to the back perches. Paint the perches occasionally with creosote to prevent insects.

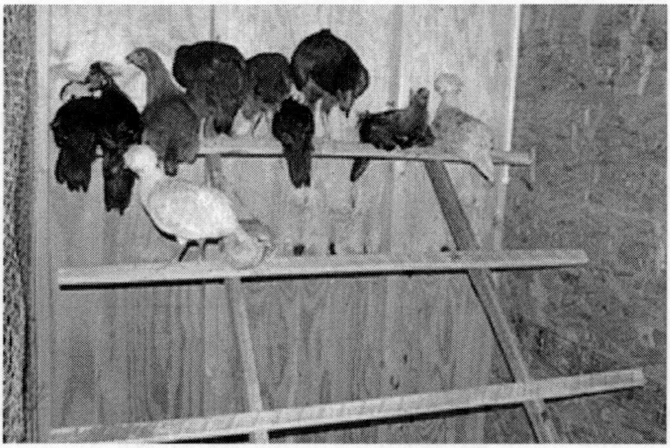

Fig. 8.6 Perches or roosts
(*Source:* raising-chicken,org)

8.5.2 Nest boxes

Each pen housing layer birds should be provided with nest boxes for laying eggs (Fig. 8.7). Nest boxes should be roomy, movable, cool and well ventilated, dark and conveniently located in the shed. Nests are usually 14 inches square, 6 inches deep and with about 15 inches head space. Metal nests are preferred to the wooden nests because of ease to clean and less chance of becoming infested with mites. Empty kerosene tins make excellent boxes. One nest should be provided for every 5 or 6 hens. Dark nest are desirable because they result in less scratching in the nest, less egg breakage and less egg eating. A wooden packing case 18 inches square or a wide mouthed earthen pot can be a suitable nest. Place some sand or soft hay or straw on the floor of the nest box. Nests sometimes are also placed inside a run but in that case care should be taken to prevent crows entering the sheds and consuming the eggs, etc. by covering the top of the run with wire netting.

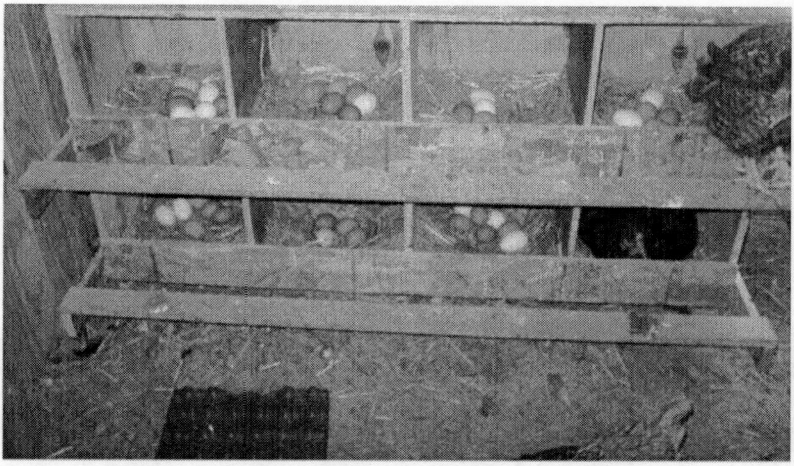

Fig. 8.7 Nest boxes
(*Source:* backyardchicken.com)

8.5.3 Trapnests

Each nest is provided with a trap door so that when the house keeper releases the hen from the nest he can identify her and mark her leg-band number on the egg (Fig. 8.8). There should be one nest for every 3 or 4 birds. Trapnests differ from regular nests in that they are provided with trap doors by which birds shut themselves in when they enter the cage for convenience of the labour, the nests should be placed 18 to 20 inches above the floor.

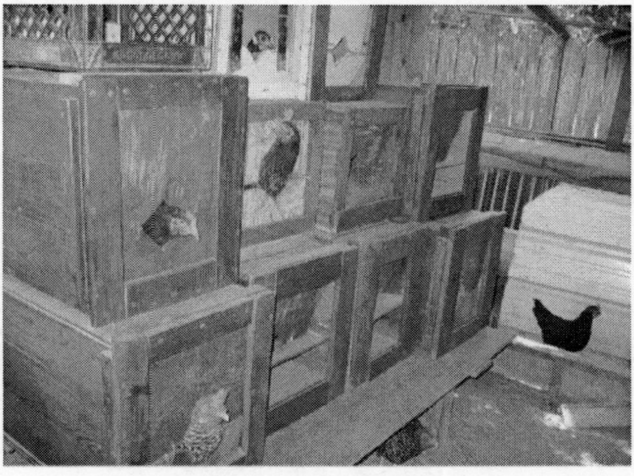

Fig. 8.8 Trapnests
(*Source:*backyardchickens.com)

8.5.4 Feed hoppers

The essential features of satisfactory feed hoppers are that they avoid wastage of feed, prevent the birds from getting their feet into the feed and from roosting on the hopper, further the hopper should be easy to clean and make it easy for the birds to eat even from the bottom of the hopper (Fig. 8.9). Troughs, pots and pans used for feeding should be of suitable size depending on the age, size and number of birds housed in a pen.

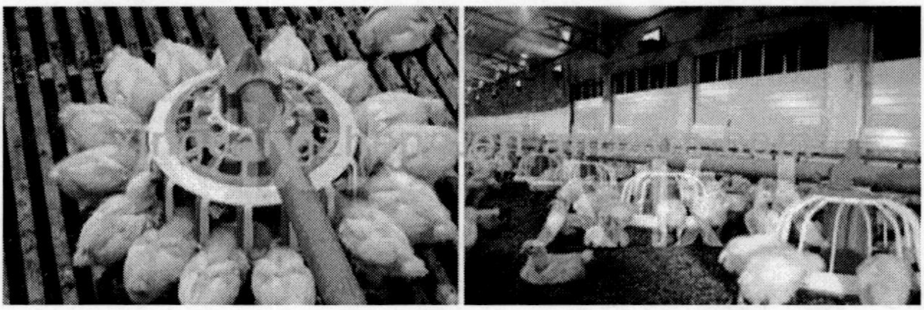

Fig. 8.9 Feed hoppers for poultry
(*Source:* xrpoultry.en.alibaba.com)

8.5.5 Watering devices

An ample supply of fresh water preferable cool during summer, should be made available at all times, otherwise egg production is liable to be affected adversely. The water containers should be cleaned often and filled with clean water, kept cool in summer, they should be easily cleaned because contaminated water tends to spread diseases among birds housed together (Fig. 8.10).

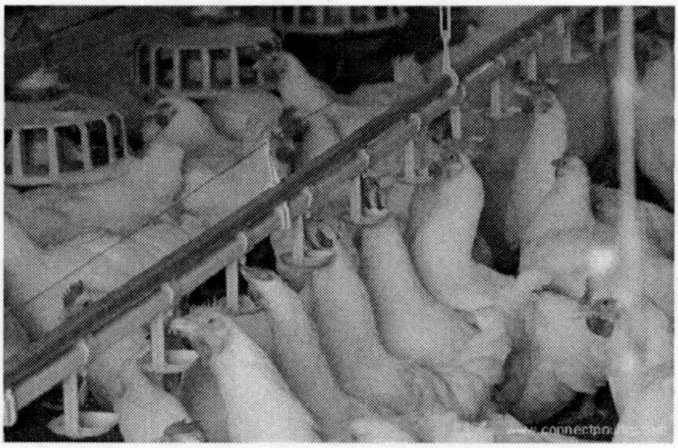

Fig. 8.10 Watering devices for poultry
(*Source:* connectpoultry.com)

8.5.6 Grit and shell container

Ordinary hoppers made either of wood or metal can be used for offering oyster shells or other form of grit (Fig. 8.11). It is advantageous as a source of calcium for egg shell formation and should be placed near the feed hopper.

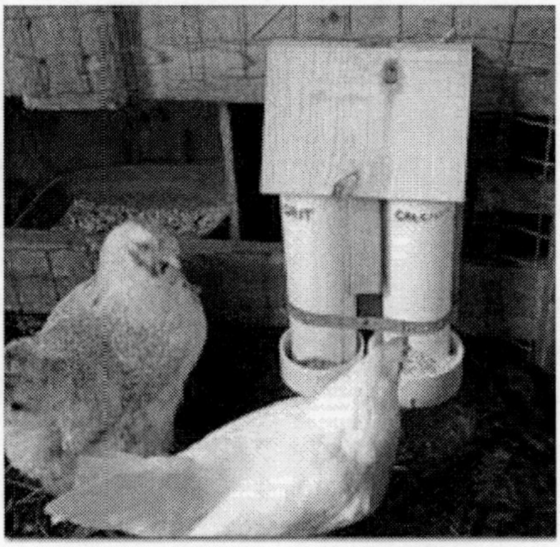

Fig. 8.11 Grit and shell container
(*Source:* pinterest.com)

8.5.7 Dust bath

An earthen pot or a hole in the ground, 2 ft in diameter, should be filled with dry, clean, sifted earth or ash and placed in the shed on the east side. The container should be continually refilled. Flavour of sulfur should be added to the ashes alongwith some dry coarse tobacco leaves. Coal ashes or cow dung cake ashes may be used alternatively (Fig. 8.12).

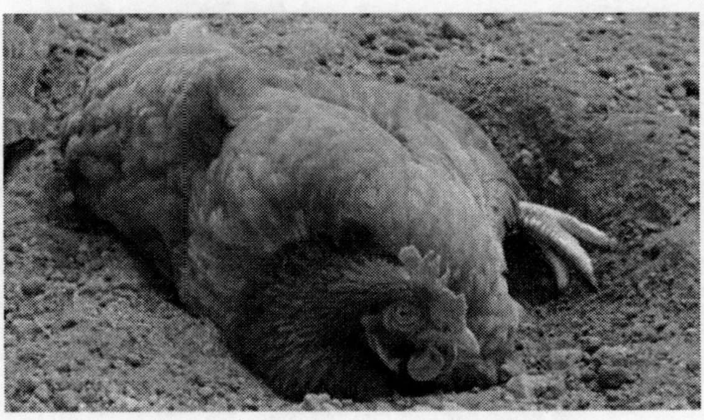

Fig. 8.12 Dust bath of poultry
(*Source:* accidentalsmallholder.net)

8.6 Poultry Housing Relevant to Tropical Countries

Poultry sheds should be designed in such a way that the space in between two sheds is sufficient (Fig 8.13). Plantation and shrubs in between can be helpful in keeping the shed protected from direct sun rays for maintaining low temperature (Fig. 8.14). Plants in the east side should be small in size so that the eastern side air can pass in the house. In the west side of the house, the plants should be comparatively taller than in the east side so that the hot air from west side should not enter the house. Provision of tunnel fans can further help in air flow in the poultry house, thus removing ammonia arising from the accumulation of poultry droppings and the heat accumulating from the metabolic activities of the birds. A simple poultry pen made with the support of bamboos or wooden rods and covered with a plastic sheet, preferably under shady trees to protect the birds from direct solar radiation can be highly cost effective and protect the birds from inclement weather.

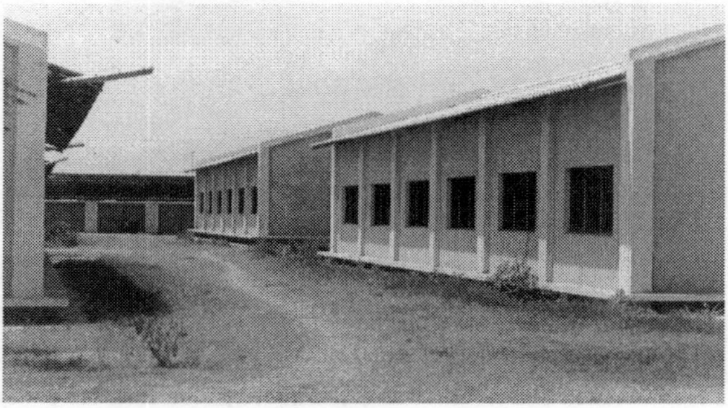

Fig.8.13. An ideal poultry shelter design

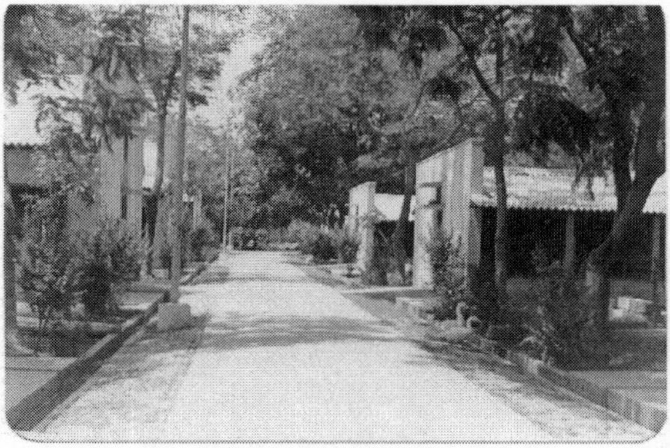

Fig. 8.14 Showing plantation along the poultry sheds

Plastic evaporative cooling pad is very useful for cooling (Fig. 8.15), flute angles should be (45° X 15° vs. 30° X 30°), edge coatings, and pad thickness (6" vs. 4"), but for the most part the traditional paper pad cools about the same as the plastic. The latter have a longer life and are easier to clean/sanitize, and more tolerant to poor water quality than paper pads. Therefore, the plastic evaporative cooling pad is traditionally used in comparison to paper evaporative cooling pads.

A six inch pad can be provided on the roof to keep the shed cool (Fig. 8.16). Fogging-pad system can be controlled by simply limiting the number of fogging nozzles operating; i.e., half the nozzles, half the cooling. But with six-inch pad system, controlling cooling is not that simple.

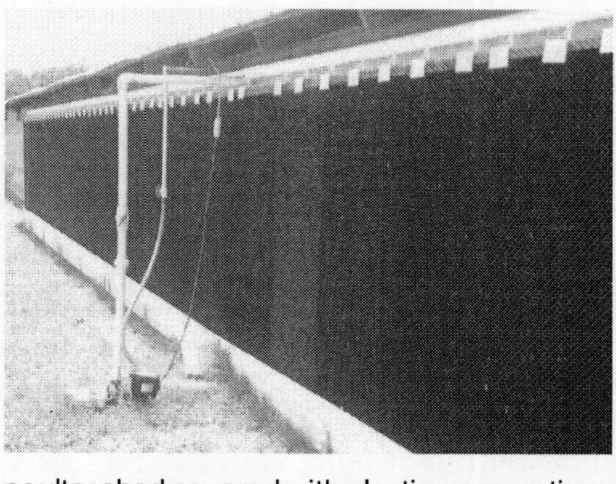

Fig. 8.15 A poultry shed covered with plastic evaporative cooling pads

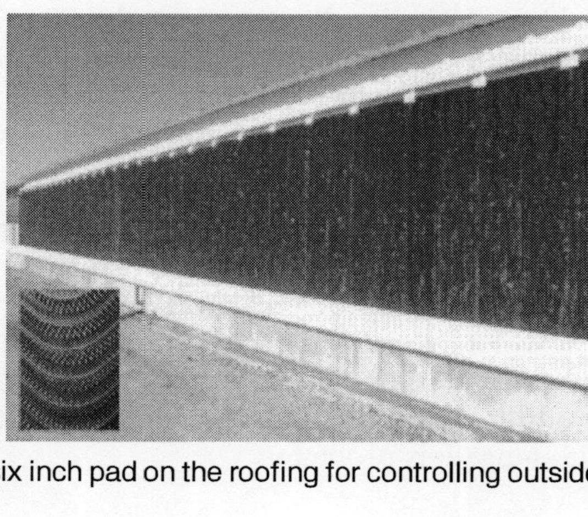

Fig. 8.16 A six inch pad on the roofing for controlling outside temperature

One problem is that a pad system's circulation pump can put a large amount of water on the pads in a very short period of time. For instance, the circulation pumps on the typical broiler house with six-inch pads can put approximately 100 gallons of water on the pads in less than one minute. 100 gallons of water is enough to drop the temperature of the incoming air by 10 °C or more on most days. Further complicating matters is that just because the circulation pumps shut off, does not mean that a pad stops cooling. In fact, cooling actually increases after circulation pumps turn off as the water which was previously placed on the pad slowly moves throughout the pads increasing the percentage of the pad which is wet thereby increasing the cooling produced. Being able to control the amount of cooling produced by a pad system is important for the following reasons.

Younger birds do not often need the full cooling potential of a pad system. A relatively lower house temperature (3-5 °C) on a hot day to produce the necessary level of cooling but not upto 20°F as most systems are capable of producing. Not only 20 °F cooling may be unnecessary, but often can cause other problems. For instance, excessive cooling can cause an environmental controller to take a house out of tunnel ventilation back to inlet ventilation and turn on the brooders/furnaces. Not only this is wasteful from an energy stand point, but can be stressful for the birds accommodated in the house.

Incandescent lighting, though effective in providing a wide level of control of poultry house light intensity, typically required for broiler production, is far from being energy efficient. Only 20% of the energy used by an incandescent light bulb, is utilized to produce light. The remainder is wasted in the form of heat. Though LED and fluorescent lighting are capable of reducing lighting costs by 70% or more they are not without problems. The amount of light produced by the typical LED bulb is not sufficient for the brooding phase of chickens while dimming a compact fluorescent light has proved to be very difficult, without sacrificing the life of bulb.

The galvanized ceiling inlets have proven to be effective in providing both air temperature and air quality during cold weather. However, they are not without problems. Air flow arising with minimal openings has a lower tendency to throw the air towards the floor during times of moderate ventilation, and makes a far tighter seal when closed. In addition the well insulated inlet would have longer life and fewer condensation problems.

As the urban population continues to grow especially at a higher rate in developing countries and land available for agricultural production is declining due to development of urban facilities like housing, roads, marketing facilities, education and medical facilities, recreation facilities etc., there is a need to intensify agriculture and DA production. Poultry production is a better alternative for urban production as it requires relatively less space and labour and have currently larger consumption of eggs and broiler meat, which are growing at a rate higher than other protein food resources. Further the problems of pollution due to poultry production are relatively less. Poultry droppings in case of caged birds can be built up for a whole laying period and can replace part of the ruminant feed after proper sterilization or can be used as high quality organic manure. Poultry production relative to other DAs impacts environment less through GHG emissions. The incidence of nuisance and complaints have however increased over the last few year. In particular, complaints about ammonia have become more prevalent, while odor is a byproduct of many agricultural and DA operations, ammonia is only one component of odor from DA manure management. Research and development is needed to determine what ammonia concentrations and at what distance from the typical poultry house is unavoidable. However, neighbors should consider the issues related to environmental pollution from the poultry farm with proper information to be used when such issues are raised. During cold weather, the concentrations of odor is generally lower than those observed in hot weather. Wind direction and wind velocity are factors that significantly influence downwind ammonia concentrations beyond 100 ft. At most times the ammonia levels exceed established ammonia odor threshold values.

The new sensor capable of accurately measuring ammonia levels for a longer period of time, say weeks, which has traditional been a major problem for most affordable ammonia sensors. Ammonia indictor strips, do an adequate job of accurately measuring long term ammonia concentrations, but may have a tendency to overestimate ammonia concentrations in a house where there are large variations in ammonia concentrations over the day.

8.7 Controlling Air Velocity in Poultry Shed

To produce optimal cooling of a large broiler shed during hot weather, the fans are designed to obtain a wind speed between 600 and 750 ft/min. It is important to realize that the air speed which is expected can be an average air speed. Air speed can vary significantly across the cross-section of a house. Air speed will tend to be higher in the center of the house than along the side walls and higher at the ceiling than near the floor. The reason for the variation is the fact that air will tend to take the path of least resistance, which is typically down the center of the house.

8.8 The Inverted-V Migration Fence

The corrugated black pipe (Fig. 8.17) is normally used for making a fence as it is easy to install. Birds can easily jump over it in case of crowding or when the handler is working or the producer is walking through the house on inspection, but can deflect the air movement off the floor when tunneling, and can be difficult to install around feeders and drinkers specially when the birds are smaller in size. The wire shelving material fence allows air to freely flow through it and virtually eliminates the movement of birds towards the tunnel inlet of a house, but is not free from problems, requiring efforts to be made, so that the birds do not pile against the fence when a handler is not extremely careful while walking in the house.

Air circulation fans (Fig. 8.18) have proved to be very effective in reducing fuel usage, promoting drier litter, and minimizing hot and cold spots in broiler houses during cold weather. The key to obtain maximum benefit from air circulation fans is making sure that they are installed in a circulatory system. Air circulation should be arranged in a way that it works as a unit together but gently and mix with the air in the house not only from ceiling to floor but from one end to the other end, on a continuous basis, without producing excessive air movement/draught at the floor level. All air circulation systems do not function well in all type of housing systems, for instance, though six 18" 1/15 hp circulation fans may do well in mixing the air in a 40' x 500' dropped-ceiling house, the same fans in a 40' X 500' open-ceiling house with exposed trusses will not tend to produce the same results. There are a number of reasons for this phenomenon. First, an open-ceiling house has a greater volume of air than a dropped-ceiling house, requiring heavy duty fan power to produce the same level of circulation. Secondly, stratification tends to be greater in a house with a higher ceiling which increases the difficulty in moving all the hot air down to floor level. Last but not the least, the exposed trusses in an open ceiling house reduce the distance a circulation fan will throw the air, which means a stronger fan is required to push the air to the same distance as that achieved in a smooth, dropped-ceiling house.

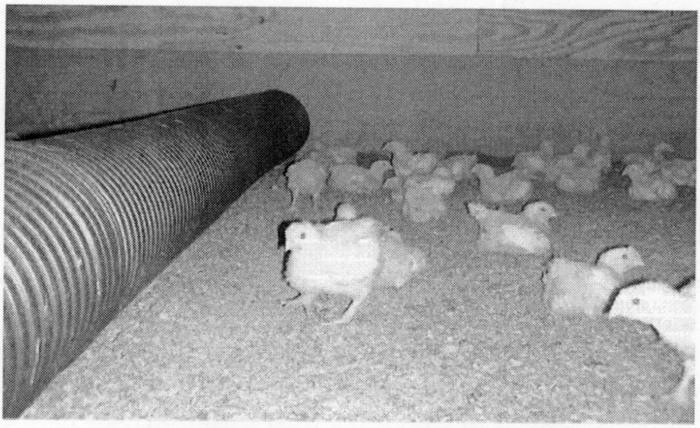

Fig. 8.17 Corrugated black pipe fence

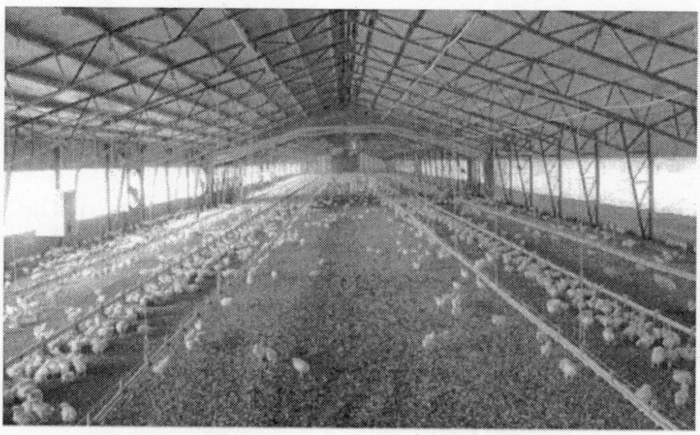

Fig. 8.18 Circulation fans for open ceiling houses

One of the key issue is to implement a successful lighting system is that the house is dark during the day so that the activity of the birds is kept to a minimum. Most broiler producers find that a light intensity between 0.2 and 0.01 ft-candles reduces bird activity to an acceptable level. To put this in perspective of the light intensity at floor level in a typical house with 40 watt light bulbs operating at full intensity is approximately 0.5 ft-candles. The primary challenge producers face when trying to keep a house dark is either direct or defused sunlight entering through side walls air inlets, even if the sun is high enough in the sky, so that there is no direct sunlight entering a house, light intensity at floor level can still easily exceed one ft-candle light (roughly equivalent to what one would expect to find in a house with 75-watt light bulb) when the side wall inlets are fully opened. If direct sunlight is to hit the upper side wall of a house early in the morning or late in the evening when the sun is closer to the horizon, light intensity in portions of the house can exceed 50 ft-candles. The net result is whether the sun is low on the horizon or high in the sky, if the side wall inlets are opened, light intensity and therefore bird activity, will be higher than what most producers would ideally like to have.

Care must be taken when installing light hoods because there are a number of hoods put on poultry houses these days that effectively reduce interior light levels if they are poorly designed. They also reduce the air capacity of the side wall inlets by 20% or more. As a result, even though a house may have been originally designed so that the producer would be able to pull half their tunnel fan capacity (four or five 48" fans) through the inlets, they may find that after hoods are installed, that operating just a two or three 48" fans causes the static pressure to exceed 0.12". If the producer tries to turn on additional fans the static pressure goes even higher resulting in dramatically reduced fan performance, excessive electric consumption as well as placing excessive strain on dropped ceilings

Though the opening of a hood may be roughly of the same size as the side wall inlet, because the hood is attached at the top of the inlet and extends downward at a 45°, house may have with poor lighting which is an impediment to production. Since the cross-sectional area of the light hood is 30% smaller than the side wall inlet, this reduces the amount of air that could enter through the inlet by roughly 30%.

The light hood is an improvement because the top of the hood extends down at a lesser angle, and it can still restrict air flow into a house, if not placed properly. If the hood has roughly the same cross sectional area as the inlet, the air velocity in the hood/inlet will tend to over 700 ft/min.

Setting up a modern broiler house is a more difficult task specially in a cold weather (Fig. 8.19). It requires a correct static pressure or minimum ventilation which is a critical consideration. Of course, there are other considerations related to the environmental control such as timer fans / cooling fans to minimize fuel usage but at the same time maintain the optimum brooding conditions. Decision on the sensors to be used to control house temperature would require that the sensors should be turned on relation to the target temperature. The proper time setting needs to be determined.

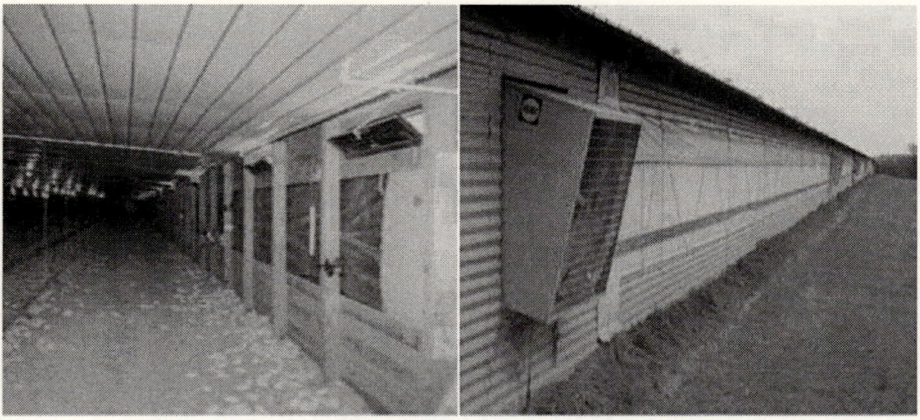

Fig. 8.19 A modern broiler house during cold weather

Air inlets are crucial for maintenance of an appropriate pressure in a broiler house which is crucial for environmental control. Air inlets allow air drawn in by exhaust fans to be directed along the ceiling to mix with the hot air produced by the birds and brooders/furnaces. It is important that 50% or more of the heat produced by brooders and furnaces ends up at the ceiling, which results in the temperature of the air at the ceiling being 20 °F or warmer than at floor level. As the air entering through air inlets moves along the ceiling it not only gets heated but also becomes "drier." This is because for every 20 °F the heat in the incoming air and the moisture-holding ability of the air doubles. So if it is 40 °F and raining outside (100% RH) and the incoming air has temperature of 80 °F while moving it along the ceiling, the moisture holding ability of the air quadruples resulting in the RH of air decreasing to 25%. When the incoming air moves down to the level of the bird, not only it will be warm, but also dry.

In order to ensure maximum heating and drying of all incoming air, it is necessary that all the air brought in by exhaust fans travels along the ceiling until it makes it to at least the center of the house.

❑❑❑

CHAPTER-9

Nutritive Requirements and Feeding Systems for Different Avian Species

There has been a large genetic group in different production traits related to egg and meat production and their quality of different production types, breeds within different production types and sire progeny groups which may require different feeding standards according to their level of production. Further differences in quality of different feed ingredients not only in terms of nutrients but also anti-nutritional factors, a common feeding standards may be difficult to be implemented. Feed is, however; the fundamental and a major production management input in any DA production systems, and accounts for 60-70 % of the cost of managing a flock. It is further a major determining factor in production cost and determines the efficiency of DA production system. Voluntary feed intake/appetite depends on the genetic constituents, age and live weight and in the manner feed is offered. There is a large genetic variation in voluntary feed intake which has been exploited in improving efficiency of feed conversion in to live weight gain/egg production. Thus requiring the birds to have a large body weight gain/egg production in a specified period. The nutrient requirements of the birds depend on a number of factors as mentioned earlier through selection for live weight gains and egg production not only there has been higher production but also higher efficiency of utilizing feed resources. The current day broiler reach the same live weight at six weeks which they earlier reached at eight to nine weeks. This has resulted in improvement in efficiency of feed conversion. The efficiency of feed conversion is ratio of live weight gain/voluntary feed intake or its reverse. Voluntary feed intake or appetite has a large genetic variation with a heritability around 0.4. Thus selection for body weight gain has resulted in improved efficiency of feed conversion and the birds reach a target production at an early age and thus have a lower maintenance requirement. In fact voluntary feed intake and live weight gain have been exploited in improving efficiency of broiler and layer production. This element has usually been ignored in determining nutrient requirements and feeding systems for commercial layers and broilers.

Commercial layers and broilers are more sensitive than ruminants DAs to composition of feed and quality of ingredients both in terms of nutrient content and their digestibility and to any incriminating factor such as mycotoxins, chemical and microbial pollutants that may be contained in the feed ingredient specially oil meals/ cakes. More than 40 macro-and micro-nutrients are required in poultry feed for economically efficient egg and broiler production. These can, however, be arranged into major classes according to their chemical nature, functions they perform, and ease with which they are chemically evaluated and are available in most commonly used feed resources. These are proteins, carbohydrates, fats, minerals, vitamins and water. Although water has no nutritional value like other feed ingredients but is extremely important for various body functions including feed intake and its digestibility, transport of nutrients, maintaining body temperature, etc.

Carbohydrates and fats are the principal sources of energy of which fats are more energetic and yield 2.0-2.5 time more calories than carbohydrates on unit weight basis. Fat also provide essential fatty acid that is linoleic, linolenic, and arachidonic. The requirement for the protein is essentially in terms of amino acids. The essential amino acids for poultry are arginine, glycine, histidine, leucine, isoleucine, lysine, methionine, cystine, phenylalanine, threonine, tryptophan, and valine. Out of these arginine, lysine, methionine, cystine and tryptophan are critical amino acids in poultry nutrition. They play an important role in several essential metabolic functions in the body. The minerals and vitamins that are critical in poultry diet are calcium, phosphorus, sodium, copper, iodine, iron, manganese, and zinc among minerals and Vitamin A, Vitamin B3, Vitamin E, pyridoxine, riboflavin, pantothenic acid, niacin, folic acid, B12 and choline. A balanced ration containing all required nutrients both macro and micro and in right proportion according to the requirement for maintenance and various productive functions at different ages and different sexes is essential for efficient egg / broiler production. Further the feed ingredients should be free from any incriminating factor and have the nutrient contents which will meet the requirements of the bird at various stages of its life and level of production.

9.1 Feed Ingredients

The ingredients used in compounding poultry rations under intensive layer and broiler production compete with human and other industrial uses as they include cereals like yellow maize, rice, wheat, oats, barley and cereal processing by products such as brans, polishes, and animal and vegetable protein like fish meal, meat meal, soyabean oil meal, groundnut cake etc. according to their availability and their nutrient value. The ration is fortified with minerals and vitamins in requisite quantities. As mentioned earlier, the feed is the costliest component in DA production as it reqire more dense nutrient containg feed ingredients and further with an increasing demand of DA products and services for internal consumption and export, especially in the expanding urban population with higher education, employment opportunities and incomes and nuclear families, there is a greater demand for food of animal origin because of their nutritive value especially essential amino acids, vitamins and minerals, and taste and satiety factor. The increasing availability of DA products and services would require for expanding livestock population and their higher and more efficient production through genetic and health improvement. Unfortunately there is a large diversion of limited feed resources especially coarse grains, oil cakes and brans/polishes through export to earn foreign exchange and to create bio-fuels. Molasses is also used for industrial purposes such as alcohol and is not readily available as an energy source for DA. This is further impacting DA production. Even the crop residues are being diverted to industrial uses such as paper, card board and as a fuel resource. Large number of technologies for improving the nutritive value, intake and digestibility of low quality forages and other agro-industrial byproducts has been developed in the last 50 years. Some of these technologies are being used by compounded feed industry and in some public sector organizations. Since a large percentage of DAs are maintained in rural areas in an unorganized manner most of these technologies have remained unused.

9.2 Conventional Poultry Feeds

Maize as a grain is highly digestible and contains little fibre. It is a major source of energy in poultry feed but is low in protein, especially in essential amino acids such as lysine and sulphur containing amino acids. The yellow variety is a good source of vitamin A and

Xanthophyll. The latter is responsible for yellow colouration in the skin of certain breeds of fowl as well as deep yellow colour of egg yolk.

Barley is not highly palatable because of higher fibre content and is not normally included more than 15% in poultry feed.

Oats is also not highly palatable because of high fibre content and should not constitute more than 20% in the poultry feed. Because of high manganese content it prevents hock disorders, feather pulling and cannibalism.

Wheat is a good source of energy but is low in protein especially most essential amino acids and can be used to replace maize.

Pearl Millet is a good feed stuff and as nutritive as wheat.

Broken rice can be used for replacing maize.

Rice polish is a good source of energy and can be used upto 50 percent. Because of high oil content it is likely to become rancid during storage under warm climatic conditions.

Deoiled rice polish has relatively low energy content because of removal of oil but is rich in protein and minerals.

Sorghum has similar nutritive value as maize and has higher protein content, is quite palatable and can replace maize in poultry feed. Sorghum meal is a good source of amino acids but is costlier than oil cakes.

Groundnut cake is a major source of protein in DA feed, is quite palatable and because of 40 % protein content is used in poultry feed.

Fish meal is best source of animal protein with essential amino acids and with 45-55 % protein content. The presence of fish scales and bones can decrease its nutritional value.

Lime stone is the major source of calcium but should not contain more than 5% magnesium.

Oyster Shell contains more than 38% calcium and is good substitute for lime stone and is more palatable.

A large number of non-conventional feeds have been identified, studied for their nutrient content, anti-nutritional factors and their intake and digestibility and have been incorporated in compounded livestock feeds. Extensive work has been carried out under the AICRP on agro-industrial and other non-conventional feed resources and also their incriminating factors and methods for their removal by treatment and dilution. As mentioned earlier, avian species are more sensitive to any incriminating factor in feeds compared to other non-ruminant species such as pigs and rabbits.

a) Common energy resources

1. **Deoiled Sal seed meal** is a byproduct from the processing of Sal fruits for oil and has similar composition as cereals but because of higher tannin content has not been used in poultry feed.
2. **Tapioca meal** is a byproduct of processed tapioca tubers and is good source of energy. Certain varieties of tapioca contain cyanogenic substances which can be removed through processing by sun drying or heating.
3. **Uncontaminated poultry droppings** such as from birds maintained in cages are dried through heating at high temperature or through sun drying. It can replace 10% of protein in the diet as it contains 10-12% true protein.
4. **Mollases c**an replace cereals as a source of energy up to 4-5% in poultry ration. High percentage results in loose excreta because of higher mineral content.
5. **Small millet** such as Kodon and Sawan can be used in place of maize up to 20% in poultry ration.
6. **Ragi, Kambu and Cholam** are available in Southern India and can replace maize in poultry ration up to 50%.

b) Common protein resources

b.i. Vegetable origin

1. **Mustard cake** is superior to groundnut cake in protein quality and lysine content. It is however used in limited quantity in poultry feed because of the presence of glycosides and goiterogens which can be reduced to some extent through treatment but limit the use in poultry feed up to 5% in chicks and 10% in laying hens.
2. **Soyabean meal** contains 35-40% protein and 18-21% fat. The oil is generally removed and the meal is used as DA feed. The oil can be removed through expeller or heat treatment, the latter reduces the

oil content but improves the protein quality of the meal. It is rich in lysine, arginine, glycine, tryptophan and cystine the limiting amino acid is methionine.

3. **Sesame meal** is a good source of supplemental protein and contains arginine, methionine and tryptophan but is a poor source of lysine, cystine and glycine.

4. **Cluster bean cake**- The byproduct of making gum from the seeds of the plants is rich in protein but is used in a limited quantity because of the presence of trypsin inhibitor.

5. **Sunflower seed meal** is superior to groundnut cake in its nutritional value but because of high fibre content has restricted use in poultry feed. It is richer in methionine and arginine but poor in lysine compared to groundnut meal. It is an excellent source of pantothenic acid and niacin.

6. **Sunflower meal** is good substitute for groundnut cake and can replace it in poultry ration up to 25%. Lysine deficiency is the major limitation in the utilization of the meal in poultry ration.

7. **Ramtil-cake** can replace groundnut cake satisfactorily up to 50 % and 100 % in chicks and layer ration respectively.

8. **Cotton seed cake** is high in protein content but is deficient in lysine and can be used upto 15 % as a substitute for groundnut cake. Continuous use causes yolk mottling on stored eggs due to the presence of gossypol in the cake.

9. **Maize gluten meal**: a byproduct of maize starch industry which is rich in protein and Xanthophyll but is deficient in lysine, tryptophan and arginine.

10. **Linseed meal** is a good source of tryptophan but contains cyanogenic glycoside and antipyridoxil factor. If not processed it is not used more than 5 %. The meal can be rendered nontoxic by boiling.

11. **Penicillin mycelium waste** is byproduct from the manufacture of penicillin. It is a good protein source and contains some residual antibiotic activity. It can be used at 5 % in poultry ration.

b.ii. Animal origin feed resources

1. **Blood meal**: it contains 80 % protein and is rich in lysine, arginine, methionine, cystine and leucine, but deficient in isoleucine. The

maximum dietary inclusion is not greater than 2 to 3 % due to unpalatability and low biological value protein.

2. **Liver meal residue**: it is a good source of lysine, methionine, cystine and tryptophan are excellent source of riboflavin, choline and vitamin B12. It can be satisfactorily used to replace all fish-meal.
3. **Silkworm pupae meal:** deoiled silkworm pupae-meal is a good protein supplement. Because of high fibre content and poor digestibility its use in poultry ration is restricted.
4. **Hatchery products meal**: this consists of infertile eggs, dead embryos, killed chicks and egg shells collected as waste during hatchery operations and have been cooked, dried and grounded with or without removal of part of its fat. It contains approximately 25-34% crude protein depending upon the material that goes into its making.
5. **Feather meal**: it contains 80-85 % crude protein and may be used 5 % in poultry rations.
6. **Poultry byproduct meal**: it is a product from poultry processing plants and includes heads, feet and entrails. It contains more than 16 % ash and no more than traces of feathers. The meal may contain 55 to 60 % protein and 12 % fat when not extracted.
7. **Meat and meat-cum -bone meal**: besides being a good source of high quality protein, it is a good source of calcium and phosphorus. The quality of the meal is variable depending upon the processing methods and the portion of gelatin it contains. The variable quality and phosphorus content limits the use of these meals not more than 5 to 10 % of the diet.

9.3 Low Cost Feed Formulation

Keeping the feed cost low and at the same time providing a balanced diet to poultry to meet the nutrient requirement for various body functions both maintenance and production, has been the main concern of both the poultry producers and the feed manufacturers especially Compounded Livestock Feed Manufacturers Association (CLFMA). Economization of feed cost without impairing poultry production can be achieved by formulating low-cost diets by appropriate selection of feed ingredients, by imposing feed restriction at the desired level, by minimizing feed wastage making nutritional adjustments during extreme weather conditions and by reducing stress and incidence of diseases.

9.4 Nutrient Requirements of Layer and Broiler Chicken at Different Ages/ for Different Production Functions

Nutritional requirements for various classes of poultry have been described in detail in ISI bulletins and also in several text books on poultry production and animal nutrion. There are no single feed formulae which can be claimed to be most satisfactory in all cases. The primary consideration in a compounded feed weather it fulfills the nutritional requirements given in the Table 1 and 2 as guidelines in formulating efficient poultry rations or not. However, numerous substitutions are possible depending upon the availability of ingredients and their comparative cost. Interrelationship among different ingredients and energy: protein ratio should be kept in mind while formulating rations.

Table 1. Suggested rations for various age groups of layers

Ingredient	Starter		Grower		Layer	
	1	2	1	2	1	2
Maize	32.00	4.10	27.10	-	35.00	20.80
Sorghum	11.00	-	-	41.00	-	-
Pearl Millet (white variety)	-	-	-	-	-	20.00
Rice Polish	16.80	18.00	40.00	40.00	30.00	30.00
Wheat bran	-	6.80	15.00	-	3.30	-
Salseed-meal (deoiled)	5.00	-	-	-	-	-
Groundnut-cake	11.00	-	-	11.00	10.00	7.00
Maize gluten-meal	-	6.00	-	-	10.00	12.00
Sunflower-cake	11.00	6.00	5.00	-	-	-
Mustard cake (solvent extracted)	-	6.00	5.00	-	-	-
Fish-meal	12.00	12.00	6.00	6.00	4.00	-
Meat-meal	-	-	-	-	-	2.00
Bone-meal	0.70	0.50	0.60	1.00	1.60	1.00
Lime stone	-	-	0.80	0.50	5.50	5.60
Salt	0.40	0.50	0.40	0.40	0.50	0.50
Mineral* and Vitamin mixture **	0.10	0.10	0.10	0.10	0.10	0.10
Total	**100.00**	**100.00**	**100.00**	**100.00**	**100.00**	**100.00**

* mineral mixture/ 100 kg: Ferrous sulphate 20 g; manganese sulphate 25 g; zinc sulphate 1.5 g and potassium iodide 100 mg.

** Vitamin mixture/ 100 kg: Vitamin A 800,000 IU; vitamin D3 100,000 IU; riboflavin 400 mg and folic acid 100 mg.

Table 2. Suggested rations for broiler

Ingredients	Starter		Finisher	
	1	2	1	2
Maize	43.75	57.10	65.10	44.10
Rice Polish	10.00	-	-	20.00
Groundnut-cake	14.00	-	-	11.00
Sunflower-cake	14.00	15.00	12.00	11.00
Mustard cake (solvent extracted)	-	10.00	10.00	-
Fish-meal (43 % protein)	10.00	6.00	5.00	5.50
Meat-meal (56 % protein)	-	7.00	5.00	5.50
Silk worm pupae-meal	-	3.00	1..20	-
Blood meal (73 % protein)	3.50	-	-	-
Animal fat	3.00	1.00	-	1.25
Bone- meal	1.15	-	0.60	0.60
Lime stone	-	0.50	0.60	0.70
Salt	0.50	0.30	0.40	0.25
Mineral* and Vitamin mixture **	0.10	0.10	0.10	0.10
Total	100.00	100.00	100.00	100.00

*, ** Same as in table 1

To meet the nutrient requirement for a production function, there is not only quantitative requirement of energy, protein, minerals, vitamins and water but there is qualitative requirement also. In DA, because of large requirement of grains (cereals and oil seeds), the animals primarily depend on agro-industrial by-products and to a limited extent cereals. In case of chicken, since the fibre digestibility is low and the feed intake is limiting depending upon the nutrient content and incriminating factors. The nutrient content of feed resources vary temporarily and spatially and inspite of the knowledge of nutrient requirement of body functions, it is difficult to prepare a compounded feed to meet the nutrient requirement of a bird for specific function. It is not only the nutrient content although it is highly correlated with nutrient content but these are not always in a desired balance limiting the intake and utilization. In case of chicken to overcome imbalances/ deficiencies of certain vital feed ingredients specially aminoacids, synthetic aminoacids which have better uptake and utilization are incorporated in the feed. There are additives which can improve the nutrient content and their utilization and thus improve production efficiency and health.

Probiotics

Probiotics are used for different functions for feed ingredients. Originally probiotic was usd to describe substances produced by one protozoan species when stimulated by another. It was however later used to describe animal feed supplements which had a beneficial effect on the GI tract of host animal. Probiotics are a source of live naturally occurring micro-organisms which include bacteria, fungi and yeast. FAO/ WHO defines probiotics as live micro-organisms which when administered in adequate amounts confirm a health benefit on the host. Therefore more precisely probiotics are mostly naturally occurring live micro-organisms, non-pathogenenic and non-toxic in nature, which when administered in sufficiently large number through the digestive route promote health in the receipient. It is known that there is a unsteady balance of beneficial and non-beneficail bacteria in the GI tract of normal healthy and non-stressed animal. However when a balance exists, the bird performs to the maximum of its efficiency determined by its genetic makeup and production environment. As already mentioned there is a large genetic variation in voluntary feed intake (appetite) and nutrient utilization and thus in addition to balancing the ration, efforts to improve a feed component utilization more efficiently through selection or manipulating genes responsible for synthesis of animal usable nutrients and their efficient utilization and when stress is imposed, the beneficial organism specially Lactobacilli has a tendency determined by its genotype to decline in numbers, increasing the growth of pathogeneic bacteria and predisposes the bird to diseases of GI tract such as diarrhea which negatively impacts growth, feed efficiency and overall production. In free range managed chicken, the chicks obtain complete GI flora from its mother's fecal matter. However in commercial reared, chicken has an incubators which are totally free from any organisms commonly found in GI tract of chicken. There is an effect of shell microbial contamination which may influence microflora in GI tract. Therefore, the use of probiotics in chicks at hatching is more important.

There is a change in brooding and hatching of chicks where the chicks after hatching stay for some time and with transparent doors given an insight of the process of hatching. The chicks therefore hatch in full light and have immediate access to feed and water, whereas; in conventional hatching it may take 48-72 hours before a chick gets access to feed and water as it takes this much time to travel from hatchery / breeding farm to the production farm. Further, the hatch window allows to take in account the initiation of hatching 30 hours before the chicks are removed and handled for transportation. However, reducing the size of hatch window increases the temperature and CO_2 levels in the hatcher which has an adverse effect on the chick growth and survival. Chicks get more space, a better air flow around the eggs with maximum 55% RH and 1500ppm CO_2 which are far more favourable than a normal hatchers. The chicks hatched in light are able to start consuming starter feed placed in specially designed crates and to consume water placed at the site of the hatcher. This not only reduces stress, the chicks are more uniform in body mass and weigh heavier and the residual yolk uptake is better. Yolk sac enables the chick to survive from the time it is taken out from the hatch to commercial farm. The early offering of feed and water saves the utilization of yolk which helps in improving immunity.

Generally live non-pathogenic bacterial strains belonging to genus *Lactobacillus, Streptococcus, Bacillus* or *Enteococcus* and the yeast Saccharomyces are used as probiotics. Strains of lactic acid producing bacteria (Lab) are specific in adhering to the intestinal epithelium aspergillus and confers beneficial impact on the performance of *Lactobacillus* and *Bifido* bacterium species which have been extensively used in human for improving innate immunity. These microbial probiotics are growth promoters. There are a large number of microbial species which are used as probiotics viz. *Lactobacillus, Streptococcus, Bacillus, Bifido* bacterium, *Saccharomyces, Enterococcum, Facium, Pediococcus, Escherichia, Lactococcus, Torulopsis* species, *Aspergillus oryzaa* and *Hawaiian spirulina* (blue green algae). However most commonly used organisms have probiotic are *Lactobacillus.*

There are many desirable traits for selection of functional probiotic. It should contain sufficient number of viable microorganisms which can withstand the hostile GI tract environment. They must be normal inhabitants of GI tract, capable of adhereing to the intestinal epithelium to overcome potential hurdles such as low pH. The presence of bile acids and the competition with other GI tract microorganisms, they should be non-pathogenic, non-toxic, preferably host specific beneficial microbes. In addition to the beneficial effect, these microorganisms should have the ability to produce antimicrobial compounds and exert their benefial effects that is enhancing nutrition and modulating immune responses to improve the body to stand against pathogenic microorganisms. They should be free of diffusible antibiotic resistant genes, be sufficiently stable during growth, processing and storage, do not under go recombination with pathogeneic strains and should not have any side effects. They must be viable under normal storage conditions and must be viable under normal industrial processing such as lyophilization i.e. overcome pelleting temperature and be compatible with most feed additives and not create any negative sensory feelings.

Their use in chicken helps in maintaining a balance of useful micro-organisms in the GI tract, improving efficiency of feed utilization, growth and overall productivity through stimulation of immune mechanisms to combat pathogens. Effective probiotics help in accelerating the development of normal microflora. Even spray application of probiotics has been found to be effective against Salmonella infection in chicks. A probiotic as a feed additive show a visible impact on the performance of broilers through increasing live weight gains and egg production. This happens through improved feed consumption and its conversion into products like eggs/ meat and improving immune system. They also reduce serum and egg yolk cholesterol level and further redue immunosuppressive diseases such as Infectious Bursal Disease, Infectious Anaema, Reoviral infection, Merck's disease, and Mycotoxic diseases. Their metabolites act as immunomodulatory agents by activating specific and nonspecific immune responses. Their consumption in sufficient quantity helps in preventing infections of bacteria , fungi, protozoa and viruses. To be effective, the probiotic should be administered regularly in feed. The GI tract is the largest immune organ as more lymphocytes are present than in any other tissues. The intestinal epithelium enterocytes provide a barrier to prevent passive loss of nutrient through pathogens and enable immune system to detect potential pathogens. The use of probiotics increases the amount of IgA found in the rumen through inceasing the number of IgA, IgM and Ig G producing cell and the number of T cells in the caecal lymph nodes. An increase antigen specific and body response following administration of probiotics and vaccination against new Castle Disease has been observed.

The salient features of probiotics are:

i) They should be used timely and regularly in feed more particularly in newly hatched chicks under stressful conditions such as during antibiotic therapy and even as an alternative to antibiotic growth promoters.

ii) Prevent diseases resulting in early chick mortality specially gastrointestinal disturbances resulting in diarrhea , loss of appetite, improper digestion and poor absorption of nutrients, pathogenic/ infectious conditions by fighting against the enteric pathogens.

iii) Improve intestinal microbial balance, nutrient absorption, increase digestibility, improve feed efficiency and growth, lower chick mortality, improve egg production and quality, fertility and hatchability, egg albumin quality and reduced yolk cholesterol concentration.

iv) Through quick detoxification of mycotoxins, nullifies the effect of enterotoxin, reduces ammonia in faecal contents, stimulate immunity and disease resistance.

v) It reduces stress after vaccination, antibiotic therapy, change in housing, transportation, change in feed and can augment the response to drugs and vaccines.

vi) Helps in synthesizing B vitamins, strengthening skeletal system, reducing carcass contamination, augmenting the effects of drugs and vaccines through maintaining healthy GI tract after antibiotic therapy.

vii) The use of pre-biotics can help in eliminating or reducing the use of antibiotics as feed additives/against infections.

In conjunction with antibiotics, probiotics can help in maintaining a desirable balance of intestinal micro-flora and reduce incidence of diarrhea. Probiotics should be administered immediately after hatching and subsequently on regular basis for optimum benefits. This is more important in intensive production where birds are always under stress and high pressure of infective agents. Commercially available probiotics may be single strains of yeast or/and a single strains of bacteria or their combination. Probiotics are available as powder or liquid feed supplements. The number of organisms in an ideal multiple strain probiotic should be in an order of 107 to 109 million or even higher and usual dose for chicks/layers/broilers is 0.5 to 1.0 kg/MT of feed. Probiotics can be given in feed or in water through mixing in drinking water or as top dressing in case of pelleted feed.

□□□

CHAPTER-10

Processing, Preservation and Marketing of Poultry Products

Poultry farms are increasing steadily in number and size although they are concentrated in a few locations in the country depending upon the availability of feed ingredients adequately and at competitive price and closeness of the market for eggs and particulry broilers. Many government agencies are encouraging poultry farming and even short term training is being imparted regularly. Such farms have generated considerable employment opportunities in peri- urban and rural areas. Marketing of poultry birds is expensive and death of birds during transit is an important bottleneck. This compels most of the poultry farms to concentrate in locations near the markets even if it means higher prices for production inputs but it allows a wider market and maintenance of live birds for slaughter. If these birds are processed after dressing and packed in tins, then transportation would become easier, shelf life of the product increases and the product is more hygienic. Mostly birds are purchased live essentially on the basis of size rather than live weight and are slaughtered in the presence of buyer and the meat is cooked and consumed before the carcass is set (rigor mortis is completed).

Number of non-vegetarian population is steadily increasing and because of changing social structure and other factors related to consumption of non-vegetarian food because of its taste and satity and nutritional factors, various food and snack preparations made from chicken egg and meat are very popular. Likewise, number of star hotels and eatries such as exclusive restaurants are also increasing in their number. Further, clubs, canteens, caterers and flight serve chicken and are resulting in growing market for broilers. Longer shelf life and hygienically packed poultry products would be preferred by most people especially in urban and peri-urban areas. Proper marketing network supported by publicity is very important but is still lacking in quantum across the whole country.

Poultry (chicken) meat is derived from the skeletal muscles of birds of various domesticated avian species and is a good source of protein, fat, vitamins and minerals for human consumtion. The fat content of poultry differs in several ways from that found in red meat. Poultry has a higher proportion of unsaturated fatty acids compared with saturated fatty acids. Both turkey and chicken contain about 30 percent saturated, 43 percent monounsaturated, and 22 percent polyunsaturated fatty acids. The high levels of unsaturated fatty acids make poultry meat more susceptible to rancidity through the oxidation of the double bonds in the unsaturated fatty acids. Saturated fatty acids, on the other hand, do not contain double bonds in their hydrocarbon chains and are resistant to oxidation. However, this fatty acid ratio has led to the suggestion that poultry may be a more healthful alternative to red meat. In avian species, fat is primarily deposited under the skin or in the abdominal cavity. Therefore, a significant amount of the fat can be removed from birds by removing the skin before eating.

Poultry provides an excellent medium for the growth of microorganisms. The principal spoilage bacteria found on poultry include *Pseudomonas, Staphylococcus, Micrococcus, Acinetobacter*, and *Moraxella.* In addition, poultry often supports the growth of certain pathogenic bacteria, such as *Salmonella.*

Potential causes of contamination of poultry during the slaughtering and processing procedures include contact of the carcass with body parts that contain a high microbial load (*e.g.*, feathers, feet, intestinal contents), use of contaminated equipment, and physical manipulation of the meat (*e.g.*,deboning, grinding). Prevention of microbial contamination involves careful regulation and monitoring of the slaughtering and processing plants, proper handling and storage, and adequate cooking of raw and processed poultry products.

10.1 Slaughtering Procedures

10.1.1 Pre-slaughter handling

When the birds have reached "harvest" time, they are generally taken off of feed and water. This allows their digestive tracts to empty and reduces the potential for contamination during processing. At night, the birds are caught by specially trained crews and placed into plastic or wooden transport cages. The birds are then transported to the slaughterhouse, where the trucks are often kept between sets of fans to ventilate the cages.

In the next step the birds are removed from the cages and transferred to continuously moving shackles where they are suspended by both legs. The transfer is often done in a dark room illuminated by a red light; the birds are not sensitive to the red light and this helps to keep them calm. The handling and transfer of birds both on the farm and at the slaughterhouse can be stressful. Stress can have negative effects on the quality of the final meat product.

10.1.2 Slaughtering

10.1.2.1 Stunning and killing

After the birds have been transferred to the moving shackles, they are usually stunned by running their heads through a water bath that conducts an electric current. Stunning produces unconsciousness, but it does not kill the birds. The birds are killed either by hand or by a mechanical rotary knife that cuts the jugular veins and the carotid arteries in the neck. Any birds not killed by the machine are quickly killed by a person with a knife assigned to the bleeding area. The birds are permitted to bleed for a fixed amount of time, depending on size and species such as (*e.g.*, 1.5 minutes for broilers).

10.1.2.2 Scalding

Following bleeding, the birds go through scalding tanks. These tanks contain hot water that softens the skin so that the feathers can be easily removed. The temperature of the water is carefully controlled. If retention of the yellow skin colour is desired, a soft-scald is used (about 50 °C or 122 °F). If a white bird is desired, a higher scald temperature is used, resulting in the removal of the yellow pellicle. Turkeys and spent hens (egg-laying birds that have finished their laying cycles) are generally run at higher temperatures -59° to 60° C (138° to 140° F).

10.1.2.3 Defeathering

The carcass then go through the feather-picking machines, which are equipped with rubber "fingers" specifically designed to beat off the feathers. The carcasses are moved through a sequence of machines, each optimized for removing different sets of feathers. At this point the carcasses are usually singed by passing through a flame that burns off any remaining feathers. An extra process, called wax dipping, is often used for waterfowl, since their feathers are more difficult to remove. Following the mechanical feather picking, the carcasses are dipped in a melted, dark-coloured wax. The wax is allowed to harden and then is peeled away, pulling out the feathers at the same time. The wax is reheated and the feathers are filtered out so that the wax can be reused. This process is usually performed twice. The blood and feathers accumulated during these early steps are generally collected and rendered to make blood meal and feather meal.

10.1.2.4 Removal of heads and legs

The heads of the birds go into a channel where they are pulled off mechanically; the legs of the birds are removed with a rotary knife (much like a meat slicer) either at the hock or slightly below it, depending on local custom. The carcasses drop off the shackle and are rehung by their hock onto the eviscerating shackle line.

10.1.2.5 Evisceration and inspection

The vent is opened so that the viscera (internal organs) can be removed. Evisceration can be done either by hand (with knives) or by using complex, fully automated mechanical devices. Automated evisceration lines can operate at a rate of about 70 birds per minute. The equipment is cleaned (with relatively high levels of chlorine) after each bird. The carcasses are generally inspected during the evisceration process. The inspection is generally performed by government inspectors / veterinarians, or plant personnel, the plant provides each inspector with an assistant who carries out any adjustments required by the inspector (*e.g.*, removing the entire bird or removing some part of the bird). The rejected parts are placed in a container marked "inedibles," and the contents are generally dyed (often a blue-purple), under supervision of the inspector, in order to prevent possible mixing with edible parts. Following inspection, the carcasses are further cleaned. The viscera are separated from the carcasses, and the edible offal is removed from the inedible offal. The heart, stomach, and liver are all considered edible offal and are independently processed. Stomachs are generally cut open and the inside yellow lining of the stomach along with its contents are removed. The lungs and kidneys are removed separately from the other visceral organs using a vacuum pipe. A final inspection is often carried out at this point, and the carcasses are then washed thoroughly.

10.1.2.6 Chilling

After the carcasses have been washed, they are chilled to a temperature below 4° C (40° F). The two main methods for chilling poultry are water chilling and air chilling.

10.1.2.6.1 Water chilling

Water chilling involves a pre-chilling step in which a countercurrent flow of cold water is used to lower the temperature of the carcasses. The carcasses are then moved into a chiller-a large tank specifically designed to move the carcasses through in a specific amount of time. Two tanks are used to minimize cross-contamination. Although this renders the chilling process very water-intensive, it helps to minimize bacterial cross-contamination by diluting the microorganisms washed off the carcasses, thereby preventing re-contamination. Water chilling leads to an increase in poultry weight, and the amount of water gained is carefully regulated.

10.1.2.6.2 Air chilling

In air chilling, the carcasses are hung by shackles and moved through coolers with rapidly moving air. The process is less energy-efficient than water chilling, and the birds lose weight because of dehydration. Air chilling prevents cross-contamination between birds. However, if a single bird contains a high number of pathogenic bacteria, this pathogen will continue spoiling the carcass remain on the bird. Thus, water chilling may actually result in a lower overall bacterial load, because many of the pathogens are discarded in the water.

The final temperature of the carcasses before shipment is usually about -2° to -1° C (28° to 30° F), just above the freezing point for poultry. In some cases a slight crusting on the surface occurs during the final chilling. For water-chilled carcasses this final chilling takes place after packaging, when the carcasses are placed in an air chiller.

10.2 Raw Poultry Products

Whole or individual parts of birds may be packaged raw for direct sale. Poultry package must include instructions about safe handling, including the need to wash all equipment that has come in contact with raw poultry and the need to wash one's hands before preparing other foods. Most raw turkey is sold frozen, while most chicken is sold fresh.

10.3 Frozen Poultry

Most frozen poultry is vacuum-packed in plastic bags and then frozen in high-velocity freezers. The birds are kept in cold storage until needed to be sold. Before freezing, poultry may be injected with various salts, flavorings, and oils in order to increase the juiciness of the meat. Injections are usually done with a multi-needle automatic injector, and information about the added ingredients is indicated on the package label. Frozen storage time (including poultry bought fresh and frozen in a home freezer) depends on the temperature of the freezer, the quality of the packaging, and the cycling of the freezer. For best results poultry should be used within three months. Frozen poultry products can be used directly in the frozen state or thawed first. Thawing should be done in the refrigerator or under running cold water to minimize the potential for microbial contamination.

10.4 Processed Poultry Products

Poultry may be further processed into other products. Chicken frankfurter and chicken bologna are finely comminuted products, which can be considered as raw-cooked products. Lean chicken meat provides the proteins and chicken skin replaces the fat to be finely dispersed in the sausage batter. Filled in small casings (18-22 mm), this typical raw-cooked sausage mix is the basis for chicken frankfurters. When filled in larger casings (40-60 mm), for chicken bologna, the mix also serves as the basis for products where coarse chicken meat (either diced or ground) is blended with batter and filled in casings of 60-80 mm or cans. These products may be named chicken or turkey ham sausage, chicken or turkey rolls etc. Chicken meat balls, a product in high demand in the Asian region, are also of the same category. They are manufactured based on the method used for traditional meat balls from red meat. Another chicken meat product, which resembles the cooked hams made from pork in both manufacture and appearance is called chicken ham (raw meat material may come from all parts of the chicken carcass) or chicken breast (in this case only chicken breast parts should be used). The meat material is tumbled together with brine containing curing salt, phosphates and spices, and either pasteurized when filled in casings or moulds or sterilized when filled in cans.

10.5 Other Chicken Meat Products

10.5.1 Coated / breaded products

In addition to chicken sausages, the chicken meat industry also developed new products, which have contributed significantly for meeting the global increase in demand for poultry meat. These can be compared to a few examples from the red meat and fish sectors, e.g. breaded and fried meat slices of pork or mutton known as "Escalope" or "Wiener Schnitzel" and in the fish sector as "fish fingers". The characteristic of such products is the coating of meat surfaces with flour, fat and flour mixes and/or breadcrumbs etc. In the poultry sector, similar products include chicken nuggets (ground meat mix), chicken sticks or fingers (muscle strips) or chicken schnitzel (breast muscle slices).

After the meat or meat mix is portioned, each portion is pre-dusted by applying a thin layer of dry flour on the meat surface. This serves to firmly absorb the batter and the breading in the following steps of the processing. Battering consist of dipping the meat pieces in a semi-liquid mixture of oil, eggs, water and spices. Breading is the coating with flour, fat/flour mixes and/or breadcrumbs. The final step in this process is heat treatment to stabilize the coatings on the meat surface. This short heat treatment in hot fat / oil (approx. +175°C) as part of the processing must be seen as a pre-treatment only and does not cook the product. The final heat treatment is carried out by the consumer right before eating.

In large chicken industries, the above processes have been automated by using continuous processing lines. This industrial level processing mainly focuses on comminuted and reconstituted meat parts, in some cases mechanically deboned meat (MDM) is used for cost reduction.

Even though the large poultry firms dominate the markets, there is still scope for small manufacturers to produce and successfully market similar products of high quality standards using manual processing methods. Examples of technologies and products suitable for the small-scale sector are:

10.5.2 Chicken burgers, chicken longganisa

These two products are easily made from spiced ground chicken/ poultry meat mixes. The mixture for the burgers is portioned into the desired weight and shaped using a hand-held moulding device. The longganisas are also portioned and rolled into plastic wrapping.

10.5.3 Chicken nuggets

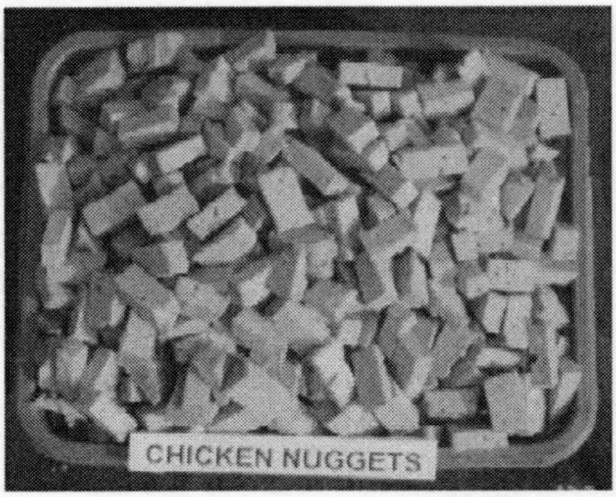

Chicken nuggets can be manufactured at the small-scale level. The meat selected for the chicken nuggets is mixed with spices, salt and herbs and ground to the desired particle size (1-5 mm). The ground mixture is spread in a tray to the desired thickness covered with plastic foil and frozen. After freezing the nuggets are cut out and breaded.

10.6 Battering and Breading

Some poultry products are battered (*e.g.*, with beer batter) or battered and breaded (*e.g.*, with cracker meal, bread crumbs, or cornmeal) for frying. The meat may be either cooked or raw prior to coating. For battered and breaded poultry, the pieces are passed through a flour-based batter containing leavening and then through the breading ingredients. Many types of baked breadings have been developed to meet different tastes. To hold the breading to the poultry, the product is deep-fried for a short time. If the poultry is fully cooked in this process, the consumer will only have to heat the product before eating it. Chicken nuggets are a battered and breaded product that is marinated before coating.

10.7 Tumbling and Massaging

In the manufacturing of many poultry products, the meat is mixed with a variety of nonmeat ingredients, including flavourings, spices, and salt. Tumbling and massaging are gentle methods that produce a uniform meat mixture. A tumbler is a slowly rotating drum that works the meat into a smooth mixture. A massager is a large mixing chamber that contains a number of internal paddles. Cured turkey products (*i.e.*, treated with sodium nitrite), such as turkey ham and turkey pastrami, are often tumbled or massaged during processing.

10.8 Smoking

Poultry meat may be smoked. Prior to smoking, the dresses birds must be brined (soaked in a salt solution containing certain flavorings) and then allowed to dry. Smoking can be done using real wood shavings or a smoke flavoring.

Further processed poultry products leave the backs, necks, and bones available for their own processing. These materials are run through a machine called a mechanical deboner or a meat-bone separator. In general, the crushed meat and bones are continuously pressed against a screen and the edible, soft materials pushed through the screen. The resulting minced product is similar in texture to ground beef and has been used for many poultry products such as frankfurters (hot dogs) and bologna. Poultry frankfurters and bologna are made using a process similar to that for beef and pork. The meat is combined with water or ice, salt, and seasonings and chopped to emulsify the materials. The mixture is stuffed into plastic casings and cooked in a smokehouse. The meat is then quickly chilled, peeled, and vacuum-packaged. Bologna is stuffed into a larger casing and is not necessarily peeled.

□□□

CHAPTER-11

Avian Diseases, Their Causation, Diagnosis, Control and Eradication

Poultry production has a high potential for employment and income generation and producing high quality food. In the last 50 years, tremendous progress in research and development has been made in poultry production and health but physical environment, availability of adequate quantity and quality of feed and diseases are impeding the efficiency of egg and broiler production. Ameliorative measures have been taken through better housing and management especially providing temperature and humidity control measures and feeding better balanced and compounded feed and undertaking disease prophylaxis. The poultry suffers from a large number of bacterial, viral and parasitic diseases which impact health and production and causes large mortality and morbidity. It is essential to undertake disease surveillance and monitoring and develop strategic control and eradication measures. The continuous introduction of exotic stocks inspite of their being subjected to quarantine is one of the causes of large incidence of poultry diseases in the country. The Government of India (GOI) has established four quarantine stations at the four major airports and also a large Central Institute for Disease Control and four regional surveillance and monitoring laboratories. It has also supported the strengthening of state disease investigation facilities. The ICAR had erlier established Centre for Animal Disease Research and Diagnosis (CADRAD) at IVRI by merging the Division of Avian Diseases with similar facilities with other Divisions for undertaking continuous surveillance and monitoring of livestock diseases for developing strategic control measures and advising the central and state disease diagnostic, control and eradication authorities about steps to be taken for control and eradication of infectious diseases in livestock including poultry. There also exists a National Institute of Veterinary Epidemiology and Disease Informatics (NIVEDI), a dedicated institute for veterinary epidemiology and disease informatics. The institute has played a vital role in eradication and control of various livestock diseases in India. With changing national and international scenario, the animal health is a priority for nation's economy and human health.

Diseases are often characterized according to their biology such as virus, bacteria, parasites, fungi and nutritional disorders. The importance of a disease is judjed by mortality rates and effect on production and will vary greatly from area to area and from season to season. Some less important diseases may interact with other diseases to create a more severe effect on the birds. This is the case for *E. coli* infections, nutritional deficiencies and internal parasites. Such diseases rarely kill the individual bird but have a remarkable effect on the immune system of the birds, thus creating the basis for easy infection by other diseases.

The important diseases affecting poultry are:

11.1 Aspergillosis

Epidemiology

- Aspergillosis is a fungal disease of chicken and turkeys
- The disease is of zoonotic importance especially in man associated with pigeon raising for support
- The disease is common in younger birds and results into high morbidity and mortality (90%)
- Transmission is through infected birds

Symptoms

- Clinical symptoms depend on the type of toxin and organs infected
- In acute form of the disease, it is commonly referred to as brooder's pneumonia typically seen in young birds
- Common signs are dullness, depression, anorexia followed by emaciation, increased thirst, accelerated breathing, gasping and prostration
- In chronic form, there is anaemia, anorexia, gasping, coughing and rapid loss of weight
- In turkeys, eyes may get affected resulting in inflammation and accumulation of cheesy materials under eyelids

- Brain is rarely affected resulting in nervous symptoms like lateral recumbency, in-coordination and muscle tremors

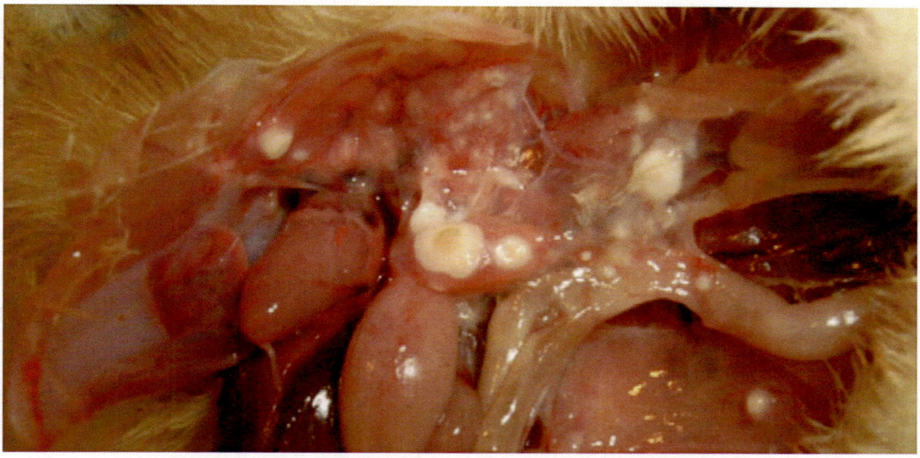

Fig. 11.1 Aspergillosis in the air sacs of a chick (*Source:* sandhillvet.co.uk)

Treatment

- Tetracycline sorbate and copper sulphate are advocated
- Treatment with Hamycin@20mg/ml in drinking water for 7 days, Ketocononazole @ 50 mg/kg body weight and Itraconazole @ 5-10 mg/kg body weight given orally are also advocated
- Cotrimoxazole therapy is also helpful

Control

- For prevention of aspergillosis, feed with low moisture content, provision of dry litter and avoiding moldy or spore bearing litter/ feed is essential
- Daily cleaning and other disinfection of feed and water utensils will help eliminating infection
- Affected birds should be removed and destroyed
- Strict hygiene in brooder house and hatchery is required management
- Litter can be treated with copper sulphate
- Increasing the frequency of egg collection to four times daily can reduce prevalence of the disease

- Decontamination of eggs by fumigation or application of QAT or phenolic disinfectants can help in reducing incidences of the disease
- Decontamination of setters, hatches and air ducts is reqired
- The efficacy of cleaning procedures may be monitored using an appropriate microbiological detection procedure such as an air samples on exposed pertiplates
- Infected litter and feed should be disposed off or preferably burnt and disinfection of brooder may be done with caustic soda (NaOH) solution
- Furthermore, an aqueous solution containing 1:2000 dilution of copper sulphate may be used in all drinking water to prevent the spread of the disease.

11.2 Avian influenza (Bird flu)

Epidemiology

- Contagious disease of domestic and wild bird characterized by respiratory illness and Central Nervous System (CNS) involvement and has zoonotic significance
- Caused by Influenzas A virus
- In highly pathogenic avian influenza (HPAI), mortality is very high (100%)
- Notifiable diseases as per OIE
- Transmissible to human being, particularly H5N1 strain
- Transmitted by air borne virus particle from respiratory tract, fecal materials, contaminated water, clothing and shoes and contaminated equipments

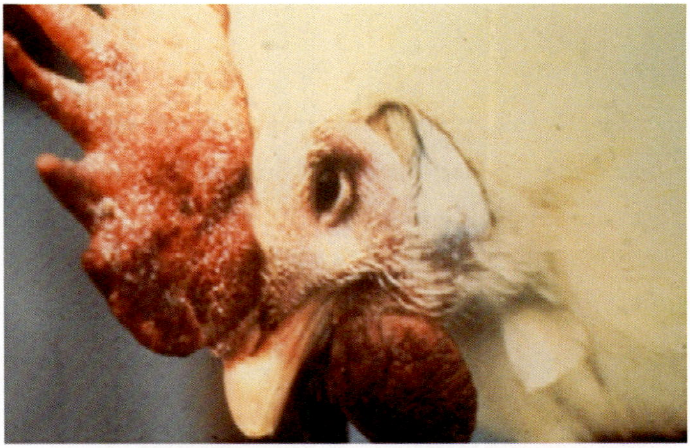

Fig. 11.2 A bird suffering from Avian influenza (Bird flu) with swelling of skin, wattles and combs (*Source:* www.poultryhub.org)

Symptoms

- Birds found dead (>75%)
- Drop in egg production
- Depression, huddling, anorexia, ruffled feathers
- Respiratory signs such as nasal discharges, coughing, snicking and dyspnoea
- Cyanosis and swelling of skin, wattles and combs.
- Conjunctivitis, swelling of the sinuses, head and reduced vocalisation
- Nervous signs and diarrhoea
- Wide spread hemorrhages in shanks, breast muscles, visceral organs and brain
- Severe hemorrhagic enteritis with greenish-white contents

Treatment

- Contact immediately for identification of disease
- There is no specific treatment
- Use of antibiotics can help in control of secondary infection

Control

- Strict biosecurity
- In case of outbreak, intensive control program with rapid diagnosis
- Slaughter and disposal of affected flock, quarantine of the affected area
- Restriction on movement of flock and products from infective area
- Immunization although no satisfacotrity vaccine is availanble in India

11.3 Infectious Bronchitis (IB)

Epidemiology

- Infectious bronchitis (IB) is an acute highly contagious disease of chicken characterized by respiratory signs and tracheal rales
- Economic important disease, as affected birds generally show poor weight gain and layers have significantly reduction egg production
- Caused by RNA virus (Genus *Corona*)
- Transmitted through aerosol and transovarian routes

Symptoms

- Incubation period varies between 18-36 hours
- Chicks up to 6 weeks of age are highly susceptible
- Respiratory signs like gasping, sneezing and coughing followed by tracheal rales and nasal discharge are common in chicks
- Tracheal rales, sneezing and hoarse cough are prominently audible
- Decrease in feed consumption and weight gain
- The growers over 6 weeks of age reveal less severe respiratory signs and slight depression, ruffled feathers and general weakness
- Broiler chickens infected with nephropathic viruses may recover from respiratory phase but show wet droppings, increased water intake and ruffled feathers
- In adult birds, drop in egg production with inferior quality of eggs in addition to respiratory signs are seen
- Hatchability of eggs is generally low

Treatment

- There is no treatment for the disease
- Complication due to secondary bacterial infection may be prevented by treating the infected birds with antibiotics
- Increasing temperature of the broiler house and under the hover by 5-10 °F may lower mortality in growing chicks

Control

- Proper ventilation and provision of air filters in the poultry houses along with adequate cleaning and disinfection of houses are important in preventing the infection
- The birds of different age group should be maintained separately and overcrowding must be avoided
- Strict bio-security measures must be practiced
- Under intensive poultry production, it is necessary to immunize the birds with freeze dried live vaccine. The primary vaccination is done at the age of 21 days through instilling a drop in eye/nostril followed by booster at 6th and 14th weeks in drinking water
- Immunity in laying flocks may be boosted further by administering live attenuated IB vaccine in drinking water or as a course spray during their production period
- Broiler chicks in the endemic areas are vaccinated by aerosol spray at 1-4 days post hatching and subsequently by course spray or in drinking water between 15-20 days depending on their maternal antibody transfer pattern of IBV challenge

11.4 Fowl Coryza

Epidemiology

- The disease is caused by *Haemophilus paragallinarum*, a gram negative, polar staining, and non-motile bacteria.
- Infection occur by contact. Chronic or healthy carrier birds are the source of infection.

Symptoms

- Affected birds show depression, nasal discharge, conjunctivitis, facial oedema, swollen wattle, coughing and gurgling.

- It causes drop in egg production.
- Air sacculitis and pneumonia may also occur, though the morbidity rate is high, the mortality is low and the birds can recover in 2-3 weeks.

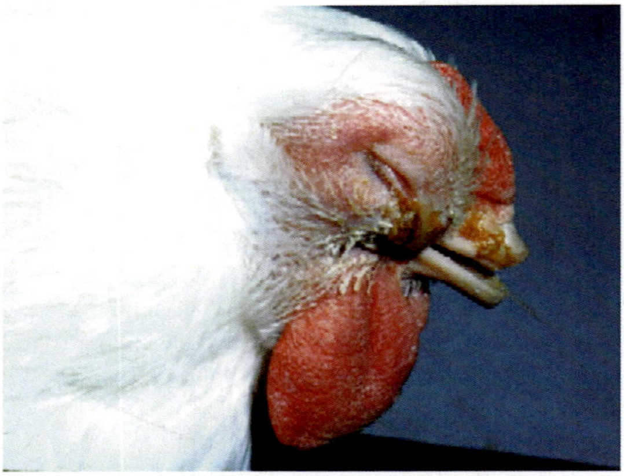

Fig. 11.3 A bird suffering from Fowl Coryza showing depression, nasal discharge, conjunctivitis, facial oedema and swollen wattle (*Source:* www.poultrydisease.ir)

Treatment

- Treatment with sulphathiozole, streptomycin and tetracycline for 7 days is effective, but the bird continues to be a carrier.

Control

- A monovalent and polyvalent vaccine can be tried. It can be administered along with Ranikhet Disease and Infectious Bronchitis vaccination.

11.5 Infectious Laryngotracheitis (ILT)

Epidemiology

- ILT is a disease of respiratory system resulting in respiratory distress, gasping and expectoration of exudates with blood and occurs in acute or sub-acute form
- Infectious Laryngotracheitis is caused by a herpes virus
- Infection occurs by ingestion or inhalation.

- The infection is mainly from acutely infected birds than from clinically recovered birds. The incubation period is from 2-8 days.
- In acute outbreaks, the morbidity is up to 100% with over 20% mortality

Symptoms

- The incubation period is of 6-12 days in natural infections
- In acute cases, sneezing, coughing and rattling sounds, swelling of eyes, nasal discharge, gasping with head extended forward and upward at each inhalation
- Cough results in explusion of mucous or blood
- Cyanosis of comb and wattle
- Drop in egg production is recorded in laying birds
- The death occurs due to asphyxia caused by occlusion of trachea by bloody mucous
- In sub acute form, there are moist rales, slight coughing, nasal discharge, shaking of head, conjunctivitis, unthriftness and drop in egg production

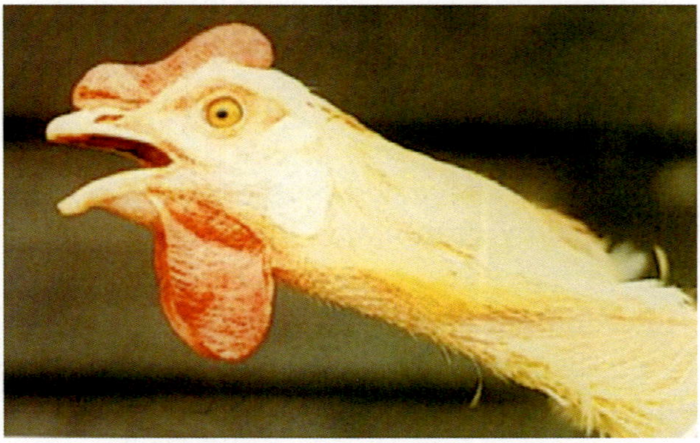

Fig. 11.4 A bird suffering from Infectious Laryngotracheitis showing gasping with head extended forward and upward (*Source:*eshop.bellsouth.com.au)

- In mild outbreaks there is lowered growth rate and feed conversion efficiency and little or no mortality in broiler
- Birds usually return to normal egg production within 3 weeks after exhibiting initial signs of illness in mild cases of ILT

- Recovered birds may become carriers and may shed virus up to one year
- Clinical symptoms, demonstration of type-A intra-nuclear inclusion bodies in epithelial cells of tracheal or conjunctival smears, postmortem examination for gross lesions, virus isolation from tracheal exudates/lung suspensions in chicken embryos demonstrate the virus antigens by fluorescent antibody technique.

Treatment

- There is no treatment for the disease
- Complication due to secondary bacterial infection may be prevented by treating the infected birds with antibiotics

Control

- Proper management to prevent introduction of infected birds in the farm is key point in prevention
- Quick diagnosis and isolation of infected birds are important in reducing the incidence of ILT
- Strict biosecurity measures have to be followed
- Rearing of different age groups of birds in the same premises is not desirable
- The recovered and vaccinated birds must not be mixed with susceptible birds
- The disease can be prevented by the use of modified live virus vaccine prepared by propagating the virus in chicken embryos or cell culture
- In an eradication program flocks may be vaccinated at 3-4 month interval until such time as eradication has been accomplished
- To stop further spread of infection, immediate vaccination is advisable even when an outbreak of ILT has been detected

11.6 Mycoplasma Gallisepticum "CRD"

Epidemiology

- Mycoplasmas are the smallest of all known free-living bacteria and can cause great concern to the poultry industry due to economic loss and disease

- Mycoplasma gallisepticum (MG) is the most important and can infect chickens, turkeys and game birds
- Mycoplasma gallisepticum (MG) infection is commonly known as chronic respiratory disease (CRD) in chickens and infectious sinusitis in turkeys
- MG infection causes significant economic losses to the poultry industry throughout the world. It causes a reduction in egg production of 10-20%, an increase in embryo mortality and chick mortality of 5-10% and a reduction in weight gain and feed conversion efficiency by 10-20%
- MG predisposes birds to other infections such as *Escherichia coli* and *Haemophilus paragallinarum* through the inhibition of immune functions causing aggravation of disease leading to further economic losses
- In the complicated infections, the severity of the disease is greatly affected by the degree of secondary infection with viruses such as newcastle disease and infectious bronchitis, and/or bacteria such as *Escherichia coli*

Symptoms

- In chickens MG may not cause obvious signs of disease unless the birds are stressed for example by respiratory viruses such as infectious bronchitis or newcastle disease
- The interaction between MG and pathogenic strains of *E. coli* is also well known
- Other stresses include overcrowding or excess ammonia in the poultry house. M. gallisepticum infections vary from asymptomatic to severe, depending on the infecting strain and other factors
- More severe infections are seen when the birds are infected concurrently with Newcastle disease virus, infectious bronchitis virus, *Escherichia coli* or other pathogens
- Infected chickens usually develop respiratory symptoms that may include rales, coughing, sneezing, nasal discharges and dyspnea
- Turkeys typically experience more severe disease, often accompanied by swelling of the paranasal (infraorbital) sinuses
- Conjunctivitis with a frothy ocular exudate is common in turkeys and occurs occasionally in chickens

- Production is lower in infected flocks, with decreased weight gain, feed efficiency and egg production
- The symptoms of Avian mycoplasmosis are typically slow to develop, and the course of the disease can be prolonged. However, acute respiratory disease sometimes occurs in young birds, particularly turkeys
- Often appears close to the onset of lay. In older birds, the onset of a positive serological picture may precede the onset of clinical signs

Treatment

- For the prevention of clinical diseases in broiler breeders, tiamulin can be used in water as 15 mg/kg for 1 week
- For the prevention of clinical diseases in laying hens - till the 17th week, tiamulin can be used in water as 15 mg/kg for 1 week
- For the treatment of clinical disease in broiler breeders, tiamulin can be used in the water as 30 mg/kg for 3-5 days
- For the treatment of clinical disease in laying hens - till the 17th week, tiamulin can be used in the water as 30 mg/kg for 3-5 days

Control

- *M. gallisepticum* can be introduced into a flock by live birds or hatching eggs, as well as the movement of people and fomites. Subclinically, infected small backyard flocks can be a source of infection for commercial poultry. The lateral transmission, for example; is one of the most common means of introduction, as the disease has been eradicated from most primary and multiplier breeding flocks
- *M. gallisepticum* - negative breeding stock can be identified and maintained by serologic testing. Heat treatment or Tiamulin can eliminate egg transmission from valuable breeding animals
- Biosecurity measures are important in preventing transmission on fomites
- Wild or pet birds can also carry *M. gallisepticum,* and should be excluded from poultry operations
- Infections can be eliminated from a farm by depopulation of the flock, followed by thorough cleaning and disinfection of the premises. Most commonly used disinfectants are thought to be effective for M. gallisepticum

- Recommended disinfectants for buildings and equipment include phenolic or cresylic acid disinfectants, hypochlorite, and 0.1% glutaraldehyde
- Mycoplasmas are typically fragile and survive in the environment only for a few days; birds can be reintroduced after two weeks. The fragile nature of the mycoplasma means that infected premises can be successfully cleaned and disinfected between flocks
- The importance of good biosecurity in maintaining mycoplasma-free flocks cannot be overstated. Primary and commercial breeding flocks are monitored regularly for M. gallisepticum by blood testing for antibodies
- Vaccines are generally used to prevent egg-production losses and reduce the impact of respiratory disease in commercial layers, but they can also aid eradication, or reduce egg transmission in breeding stocks

11.7 Mycoplasma Synovie

Epidemiology

- *M. synoviae* was first recognized as an acute to chronic infection of chickens and turkeys that produced an exudative tendinitis and synovitis (infectious synovitis); it now occurs most commonly as a subclinical infection of the upper respiratory tract, especially in multi-age layer flocks
- *M. synoviae* infection is also a complication of airsacculitis in association with Newcastle Disease or Infectious Bronchitis
- It is seen primarily in chickens and turkeys, but ducks, geese, guinea fowl, parrots, pheasants, and quail may also be susceptible
- *M. synoviae* isolates vary widely in virulence, and suspected virulence factors include adhesins, sialidase, nitric oxide, cell invasion, and antigenic variation and immune evasion
- *M. synoviae* is egg transmitted (transovarian), but the infection rate in breeder hens is low, and some hatches of progeny may be free of infection
- Horizontal transmission is similar to that of *M. gallisepticum*, primarily via the respiratory tract, with direct and indirect routes
- *M. synoviae* infections of multiple-age layer flocks are common and may contribute to decreased egg production

Symptoms

- Although slight rales may be present in birds with *M. synoviae* respiratory infection, usually no signs are noticed. Birds under stress or with concurrent infections are more likely to be clinically affected
- The first signs of infectious synovitis include pale-bluish head parts and lameness in many birds with a tendency to sit
- The more severely affected birds are depressed and found resting around feeders and waterers
- Hocks and footpads are swollen, and sternal bursitis (breast blisters) may be seen.
- Morbidity is usually low to moderate with mortality of 1%–10%
- Effects on egg production are usually not apparent, but instances of transient egg production drops have occurred in layer flocks
- Respiratory lesions may be absent, or consist of mild mucoid tracheitis or sinusitis with airsacculitis when birds are stressed from poor air quality or challenged with Newcastle disease or infectious bronchitis
- Early in Infectious Synovitis, a creamy to viscous yellow-gray exudate is present in most synovial structures but most commonly seen in swollen hock and wing joints
- In chronic cases, this exudate may become inspissated; livers are enlarged and sometimes green, spleens are enlarged, kidneys are enlarged and pale, and birds may be weak and thin with breast blisters from sternal recombency

Treatment

- When *M. synoviae* involvement in airsacculitis is an anticipated problem, preventive antibiotic therapy during the time of respiratory reaction to Newcastle disease and infectious bronchitis vaccines may be helpful.

Control

- Chicks and poults should be obtained from *M. synoviae*-free breeders and raised with biosecurity to prevent introduction.

11.8 Ranikhet Disease or Newcastle Disease

Epidemiology

- Ranikhet disease, also known in the West as Newcastle disease is a contagious and highly fatal and ranks as one of the most serious virus diseases of poultry
- The disease is very common during dry season and is often seen in young chicks but also in adults
- The disease is also suspected to cause conjunctivitis among laboratory workers and persons handling infected birds.
- Acute infectious viral diseases of domestic and wild bird, clinically characterized by respiratory and nervous symptoms
- Transmitted through respiratory discharges of infected birds and contaminated materials
- Morbidity and mortality rate are high, up to 60-80 %

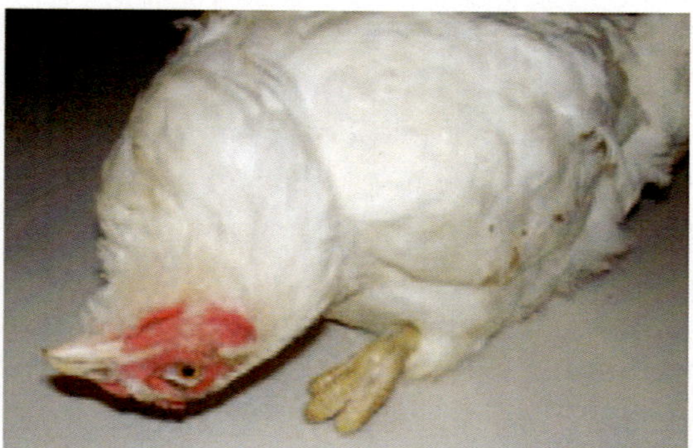

Fig. 11.5 A bird suffering from Ranikhet disease or Newcastle disease with drooping of wings, incoordination due to paralysis of legs (*Source:* thepoultrysite.com)

Symptoms

- Occur in various clinical forms
- In generalized form, bird become dull, febrile, ruffled feather, loss of appetite, restlessness and cyanosis of combs and wattles.
- Greenish diarrhea is characteristic signs of disease
- In Neurotropic form, drooping of wings, incoordination due to paralysis of legs

- Tremors, convulsions, twitching of neck and head, lack of swallowing reflex
- Torticollis is common
- In Pneumotropic form, respiratory distress is the main sign
- Dysponea, rales, gurgling and death are seen
- In laying hens, drop in egg production, small or shell less eggs occur
- Poor quality eggs are produced

Treatment

- No effective treatment
- Supportive treatment with saline and vitamins
- Antibiotic to prevent secondary infections

Prevention

- Proper hygienic management and maintenance of strict biosecurity measures
- Immunization of vulnerable flock. Lentogenic F strain in day old chick and mesogenic M at 6-8 week age are being used
- The vaccine consists of freeze - dried virus grown in chick embryos. Vaccination of birds 6 weeks old and above confers immunity for 1 to 3 years. Care should be taken to vaccinate bird's not carrying heavy coccidian infection. Birds with heavy worm infection or coccidiosis are not protected even with a good vaccine. There are sometimes complications side reactions following vaccination with 'Mukteswar' strain of Ranikhet disease vaccine. These consist of incoordination of limbs and sometimes paralysis in 1 to 3 per cent to the vaccinated birds. The reactions may become more acute if the birds are affected with roundworms, coccidiosis or are weak on account of malnutrition.

11.9 Marek's Disease

Epidemiology

- Marek's disease (MD) is the most common lymphoproliferative disease of poultry caused by herpes virus

- Chickens are the primary host but it also infect turkeys, quails etc
- Characterized by a mononuclear of peripheral nerves, gonad, iris, various viscera, muscle and skin
- This is a progressive disease with variable intensity of signs depending upon infection with MD pathotypes
- Acute form occurs in chickens of 2-5 months with high mortality (upto 50%) caused by highly pathogenic strains
- Disease is transmitted by infected environment

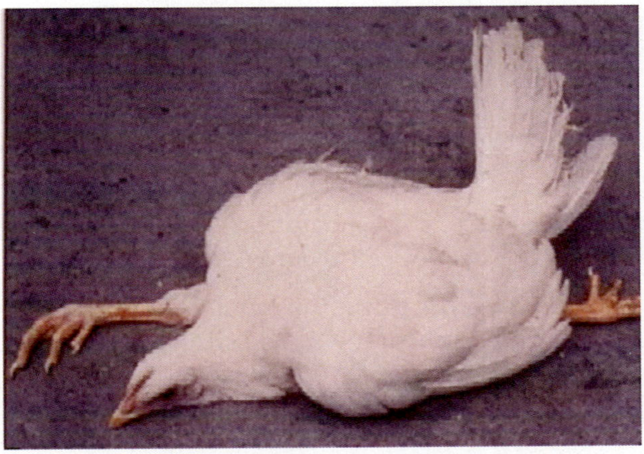

Fig. 11.6 A Marek's Diseased bird with paralysis showing a characteristic sportsman posture with one leg stretched forward and the other held behind (*Source:* www.poultryclubsa.co.za)

Symptoms

- Neural or classical MD involves peripheral nerves especially brachial and sciatic resulting in paresis of legs or wings
- Progressive paralysis showing a characteristic sportsman posture with one leg stretched forward and the other held behind
- Wing dropping and lowering of head and neck
- Cervical nerves are occasionally involved, results typical torticollis
- In ocular lymphomatosis leads to graying of iris of eyes giving the appearance of fish eye or pearly eyes due to lymphoblastoid infiltration resulting in partial or total blindness
- In cutaenous MD is usually recognized after plucking when round nodular lesions up to 1 cm are evident at feather follicles

- In the visceral form, there are neoplasms in various tissues and organs and as size of the tumour increases, clinical signs are observed
- Affected birds rarely recover
- Weight loss, depression and greenish diarrhoea are other signs
- Paralyzed chickens are unable to reach food and water, usually die from starvation or dehydration

Treatment

- There is no effective treatment for MD of either flocks or an individual chicken

Control

- Management and hygiene should be strictly followed, proper disposal of dead birds should be ensured
- Isolation of infected birds, operation of farms as single age units with all in all out cycles, selection of resistant breed of chickens
- Vaccination of embryos using the *in-vivo* technique at the 18th days of incubation or by subcutaneous administration of vaccine to day old chicks is an effective mean of control
- Three types of the vaccines are available
- Type-I attenuated chicken strain (Respen's), Type-II apathogenic chicken strain (SBI), Type-III apathogenic turkey strain (HVT)
- Type II allows vaccinated flocks to develop a solid immunity. It is essential to place day old chicks for not less than one week in the houses which have been thoroughly decontaminated
- Viral infections such as infectious bursal disease, chicken anaemia, reticuloendotheliosis or reovirus infections are known to interfere with the incubation of vaccinal immunity due to their immunosuppressive effect
- The vaccine HVT is widely effective

11.10 Egg Drop Syndrome

Epidemiology

- Egg drop syndrome (EDS) is an infectious disease of avian species that is mainly characterized by drops in egg production with poor shell quality

- Only laying hens are affected
- Transmission is through eggs

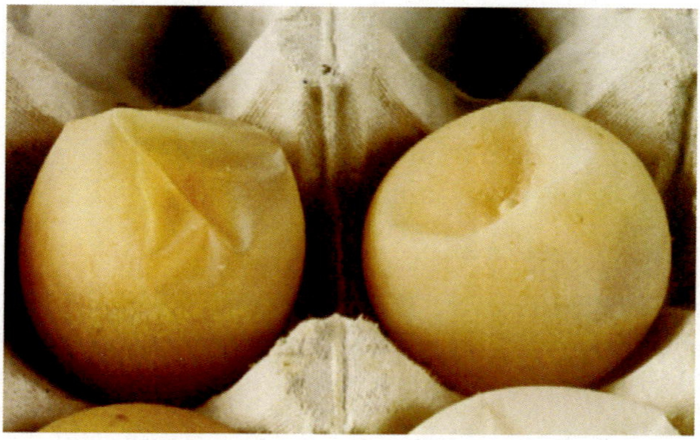

Fig. 11.7 Egg Drop Syndrome with soft, broken and thin shelled eggs (*Source:* www.worldpoultry.net)

Symptoms

- Incubation period varies from 7-9 days
- The affected birds reveal diarrhoea at the start of laying period
- A loss of shell pigment and production of shell less, soft shelled, broken and thin shelled eggs
- Eggs have a chalky appearance
- Internal egg quality, fertility and hatchability of these eggs remain unaffected
- The chickens infected at 19 weeks of age show delayed onset of laying
- Poor interest in food intake
- Reduction of egg production up to 5-50%
- In older chickens, infected at 26 and 47 weeks of age, the production may remain unaltered
- Total serum protein, globulin and calcium values in the serum of infected birds are increased
- Chemical analysis of eggshells reveals significantly higher levels of calcium, magnesium, iron, copper and zinc

Treatment

- There is no effective treatment
- Vitamins, calcium and protein supplementation helps in restoring production performance

Control

- Purchase of birds from uninfected flocks
- Hygienic management
- Vaccination :Immature breeding and laying flocks should be vaccinated with an oil adjuvant inactivated EDS virus vaccine at 14-16 weeks of age
- Vaccinal antibodies can be detected up to one year

11.11 Fowl Pox

Epidemiology

- Fowl pox is an acute viral disease
- It commonly occur in domestic fowl, turkeys, pigeon, ducks and wild birds
- Characteristic nodular proliferative skin lesions on the featherless parts of the body
- Fibrino necrotic and proliferative lesions in the mucous membrane of the upper respiratory tract, mouth and oesophagus are common
- Transmission is by direct contact with diseased /carriers birds or through feed and water. Blood sucking arthropods may also transmit infection
- In general mortality is 20-50%
- The infection causes life long immunity

Symptoms

- Three clinical forms of the disease, cutaneous or skin form, contagious epithelioma, diptheritic or wet pox and ocular form
- Incubation period of the disease is 4-10 days and outbreaks persist for 2-3 weeks

- In general there is a lack of appetite, drop in egg production and growth rate
- In skin form typical pox lesions on the unfeathered parts of the head and legs, particularly on the comb, wattles, eyelids, corners of the beak, feet and skin under the wings
- Small white macule followed by vesicles and ultimately formation of grayish brown wart like scab in skin form are seen
- Dried Scabs after a few days removed leave a raw of bleeding surface
- Affected birds are more likely to recover if complications due to other infection do not arise
- In diphtheritic type, small caseous white patches inside the trachea, pharynx, mouth, at the sides of the tongues, on the roof of the palate and around the epiglottis
- The lesions coalesce to form large cheesy necrotic nodules occur which may prevent the birds from eating
- Death may result form suffocation by occulusion of the larynx
- Mortality may reach up to 50%
- In ocular form, lacrimation and conjunctivitis, cheesy exudates accumulates under the eyelids

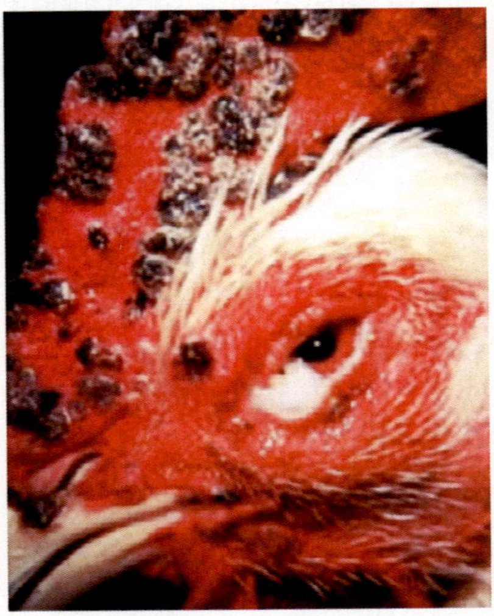

Fig. 11.8 Symptoms of Fowl Pox with pox lesions on the comb, wattles, eyelids, corners of the beak (*Source:* www.poultryhub.org)

Treatment

- There is no treatment
- Antibiotics may be used in drinking water to prevent secondary bacterial infection
- Treatment of local skin lesions with disinfectant and/or removal of diphtheritic membranes from the larynx to avoid suffocation is helpful in early healing
- Local dressing with gention violet, concentrated sodium chloride solution or lime juice of the lesions of the combs and wattles after removing the scab aids speedy healing of the wounds
- Plain white petrolium jelly smeared on the eyelids may aid in keeping the lids open and make birds able to see feed and water

Control

- Proper hygienic management
- Vaccination : Egg adapted freeze dried fowl pox vaccine may be used at 4-6 weeks of age followed by second dose at 12-14 weeks of age
- The attenuated fowl pox virus vaccines of cell culture origin can also be effectively used in day old chicks along with Marek's disease vaccine
- Vaccinated birds must be protected as far as possible from exposure to concurrent pox virus and other infection at least for 2 weeks to develop immunity
- Regular observation of the flock for removal of fresh cases is advisable
- In areas where flocks are affected with vertically transmitted mycoplasmosis, adverse vaccine reaction can be avoided by administration of a pigeon pox vaccine

11.12 Infectious Bursal Disease (IBD)

Epidemiology

- IBD is an acute highly contagious immunosuppressive disease of chicken and is characterized by destruction of lymphoid cell in the Bursa Fabricus and other lymphoid organs

- IBDV, a double stranded RNA virus of the genus *Birnavirus* under the family *Birnaviridae* is responsible for the disease
- Chicken of 3-6 week age are mostly affected
- Transmission of the disease usually occurs through contaminated feed, water and litter

Symptoms

- Incubation period ranges from 2-3 days
- Birds may suffer from either clinical or sub-clinical infection
- There is acute onset of depression and the birds sit quietly with closed eyes and ruffled feathers
- Affected birds peck at their vents and pericloacal feathers are stained with urates
- There is whitish or watery diarrhoea and feed intake is reduced
- Birds may show sternal or lateral recumbency with coarse tremor or shivering at terminal stage and finally death occur
- High morbidity and mortality rate in acute infection
- The birds may recover in a week but the reduction of antibody levels make the birds more prone to other infections
- In sub-clinical infection, the symptoms are less pronounced and the birds of less than 3 weeks of age remain dull and depressed

Treatment

- No effective treatment
- Supportive treatment with normal saline solution to prevent dehydration
- Vitamins, specially Vitamin-K is advocated to prevent haemorrhages
- Antibiotics are advocated to prevent secondary infections

Control

- In endemic zones, vaccination is recommended
- First vaccination within one week of age by mild vaccine followed by vaccinations at 12-14 days, 19-21 days, 28-32 days and 42-48 days using intermediate virus strain
- Maintain hygienic condition to prevent infection

11.13 Hydropericardium-Hepatitis Syndrome (Leechi diseases)

Epidemiology

- Hydropericardium hepatitis syndrome (HHS) is an acute, infectious viral disease of chickens
- Mostly occurs in 3-5 week old broiler with morbidity ranging from 10-70% and mortality from 5-80%
- Adult birds may also be affected
- Clinically the disease is characterized by high rate of morbidity and mortality. There is excess pericardial fluid, and multifocal hepatic necrosis
- Transmission of the infection is through contact and infected environment (faecal-oral route)
- Incubation period is 24-72 hours
- Flocks with HHS show no specific clinical signs

Symptoms

- Abrupt onset of mortality, lethargy, huddling with ruffled feathers, and yellow, mucoid droppings are characteristic symptoms
- The affected birds have decreased haemoglobin, packed cell volume, erythrocytes, and total leukocytic count

Treatment

- There is no specific treatment for the disease
- Use of an iodophor in the drinking water reduces mortality and severity of the disease
- Liver tonic supplementation helps in recovery

Control

- Strict hygienic measures like proper disposal of litter, avoiding over crowding, are important
- Appropriate vaccination program should be followed
- Inactivated live homogenate from natural and experimentally infected broiler chicks has been used as an effective vaccine

- A killed oil emulsified vaccine has been developed in India using IBH-HHS virus serotype 4 propagated in chicken embryo liver cell culture

11.14 Fowl Cholera

Epidemiology

- Fowl cholera is an acute contagious and septicemic bacterial disease of domestic birds including chicken, turkeys, guinea fowl, pigeons, pheasants and wild birds. Adult broilers are more susceptible.
- *Pasteurella multocida*, a gram negative non- motile, non- spore forming, capsulated, bipolar rod shaped organism is responsible for causing the disease

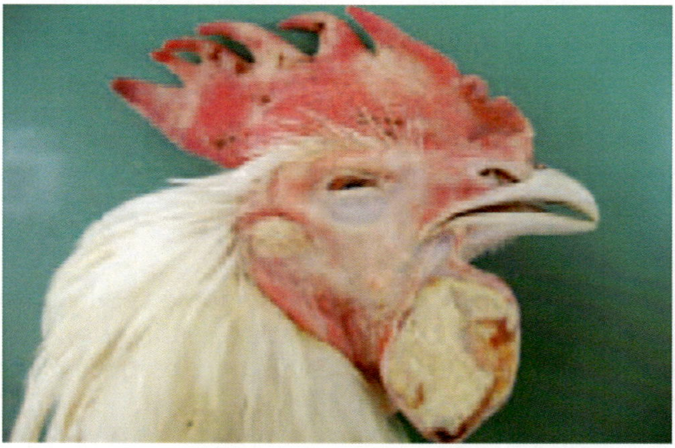

Fig. 11.9 A bird suffering from Fowl Cholera with oedema of wattles, combs (*Source:* thepoultrysite.com)

- The serotypes isolated from domestic animals can not produce disease in birds
- Common route of infection are oral, nasal, conjuctival though contact with infected bird

Symptoms

- The affected birds may show per acute or chronic symptoms
- In per acute form, death may be the first indication of the disease and large number of birds may die within 6 hours

- In acute form, some birds may show a rotational movement for few minutes keeping the legs in position, suddenly jump up, fall aside and die
- In other cases, there may rise in body temperature, anorexia, ruffled feather, mucous discharge from mouth, diarrhoea, which is first watery and whitish but later become greenish and contain mucous
- The respiratory rate increases initially followed by retardation before death
- Cyanosis often occurs immediately prior to death
- In chronic form, seen in terminal stages of an outbreak or in sporadic cases and is associated with localized lesions
- Most common symptoms are oedema of wattles, combs and sometimes otitis, conjunctivitis, arthritis or pharyngitis, etc

Treatment

- Sulfonamides and antibiotics like, penicillin, streptomycin or a combination of the two are generally recommended

Control

- General hygienic measures should be adopted at the farm and dead or affected birds must be isolated from healthy flocks as quickly as possible. The litter of the shed housing the affected birds should preferably be burnt
- The birds of different age groups must be reared separately and new birds should be introduced after removal of old stock
- Effective ticks and rodent control should be constituted
- Vaccination with killed live attenuated vaccines may be used
- Inactivated (killed) fowl cholera vaccine is commercially available in the country, which is given initially at the age of 8 weeks and repeated after 6 weeks. A combined inactivated fowl cholera infectious coryza vaccine is also available in the country

11.15 Necroenteritis

Epidemiology

- Necroticenteritis is an acute enterotoxemia.

- The clinical illness is usually very short, and often the only signs are a severe depression followed quickly by a sudden increase in flock mortality.
- The disease primarily affects broiler chickens (2–5 wk old) and turkeys (7–12 wk old) raised on litter but can also affect commercial layer pullets raised in cages.
- Early mortality is often related to coccidiosis vaccination programs, with *Eimeria* cycling in these flocks.

Symptoms

- Most often the only sign of necrotic enteritis in a flock is a sudden increase in mortality. However, birds with depression, ruffled feathers, and diarrhea may also be seen.
- The gross lesions are primarily found in the small intestine (jejunum/ileum), which may be ballooned, friable, and contain a foul-smelling, brown fluid.
- This pseudomembrane may extend throughout the small intestine or be localized.
- The disease usually persists in a flock for 5–10 days, and mortality is 2%–50%.

Treatment

- Treatment for necrotic enteritis is most commonly administered in the drinking water, with bacitracin (200–400 mg/gal. for 5–7 days), penicillin (1,500,000 u/gal. for 5 days), and lincomycin (64 mg/gal. for 7 days) most often used

Control

- Avoiding drastic changes in feed and minimizing the level of fishmeal, wheat, barley, or rye in the diet can also help prevent necrotic enteritis. When higher amounts of wheat, barley, or rye are necessary, use of enzymes for nonstarch polysaccharides in the feed has reduced the level of necrotic enteritis in flocks fed these cereals
- Administration of selected probiotics or competitive exclusion cultures has been used successfully to both prevent and treat clinical necrotic enteritis

11.16 Pullorum Diseases

Epidemiology

- Pullorum disease is a septicaemic disease of chickens and turkeys
- Quail, pheasants, ducks, sparrows, peacocks, guinea fowls, etc may also be affected with the disease
- The disease is caused by bacteria, *Salmonella pullorum*
- In acute form of the disease, the affected chicken seen with heavy mortality, while chronic cases in adult birds show a low mortality
- Infected bird, eggs are common source of infection in birds

Symptoms

- In chicks there is continuous mortality which may vary from 20 to 80% and seen in chicks of 14 to 21 days of life
- Mainly respiratory distress, ruffled feathers, drooping of wings, drowsiness, weakness, anorexia, chalky white coloured diarrhoea, increased thirst, lameness are common symptoms
- Characteristic chirping sound and typical shrill cry while voiding droppings is also seen
- The adult birds do not show any typical signs of the disease but there is reduction in egg production and fertility and hatchability of eggs. Further, inappetance, dullness and paleness of comb, dropping of wings and head, ruffled feathers and greenish brown diarrhoea are observed in affected birds

Treatment

- Furazolidozone, sulphonamides and chlortetracycline are quite effective against the disease
- Co-trimoxazole, ampicillin and ciprofloxacin are now generally recommended to avoid the cases of drug resistance
- Use of vitamin and mineral supplementation helps in early recovery and reduces risk of medication stress

Control

- Strict hygienic measures and sanitation procedures can help in controlling the disease, the flocks should be routinely tested with rapid plate agglutination test and reactor birds should be isolated and should not be used for breeding purposes

- After removal of reactors, the premises should be properly cleaned with disinfectants and new birds should be introduced after testing only
- The infected eggs should not be allowed in incubators and incubators should be properly fumigated before incubating the eggs, the waste from incubators should be burnt properly
- A sound bio-security program should always be maintained

11.17 Fowl Typhoid

Epidemiology

- Fowl typhoid is an important infectious disease of domestic birds and is characterized by acute septicaemia and high mortality rates resulting in heavy economic losses to poultry farmers
- The disease can also occur in chronic form
- The disease is caused by *Salmonella gallinarum*, gram negative bacteria and is highly infectious
- Transmission from infected birds to other bird is common

Symptoms

- The disease can occur both in acute and chronic forms
- The affected birds may die suddenly without showing any specific signs in the acute form of the disease
- There is severe diarrhoea and dropping are greenish yellow in colour
- There is dejection, anorexia, drooping of wings, ruffled feathers and pale comb and wattle are seen
- In adult birds, there is reduction in egg production, poor body weight gain and reduced feed intake

Treatment

- Co-trimoxazole, chloramphenicol and ampicillin are highly effective against these organisms and are used in drinking water

- The birds that do not show recovery through the administration of these drugs should be treated after performing drug sensitivity and gentamycin and ciprofloxacin have been found useful in such outbreaks
- Use of mineral and vitamin supplements along with medication is helpful in early recovery of the affected birds

Control

- General hygienic and strict sanitary measures are important in preventing the disease
- The carrier birds should be removed
- Factors responsible for stress should be avoided

11.18 Para-typhoid Infection

Epidemiology

- The disease is caused by Salmonella group of bacteria other than *S. pullorum* and *S. gallinarum*.
- The common organisms causing paratyphoid are *S. typhinurium, S menston, S Virchow, S hadar* and *S enteritidis*. Of these *S typhinurium* is most common in chicken, turkey, pheasants, ducks and geese.
- Transmission can occur through infected embryos, contaminated feed, equipment, litter, soil and utensils are responsible for disease transmission.

Symptoms

Treatment

- Treatment can be attempted through new generation antibiotics like Furazolidone/ Chloramphenicol.

Control

- Isolation and identification of the organism is the only method of diagnosis.
- Continuous screening and elimination of reactors with better flock management can help in controlling the disease.

11.19 Coliform Infection

Epidemiology

- *Escherichia coli,* a gram negative bacterium is responsible for disease which occurs in birds of age group of 5-10 weeks.
- Mortality and morbidity are variable but are 5 and 50 %.

Symptoms

- It causes loss of appetite, respiratory distress, diarrhea and weakness
- The gross lesions occur in air sac, peritoneum, liver and heart
- Pericarditis may be fibrous with thickened pericardial sac

Treatment

- Must be done after sensitivity test to choose the most suitable drugs to reduce the severity and mortality
- It is necessary to start treatment for 5 days
- *E. coli* may be sensitive to quinolones, streptomycin, ampicillin, neomycin, chloramphenicol, tetracyclines, nalidixic acid and sulfonamides

Control

- Sanitation and sound management
- Chicks must be from a source free from mycoplasma also have been vaccinated against IBD, IB, ND and any other disease that is a local threat
- Cleaning and disinfection of equipments
- Suitable temperature and humidity
- Good ventilation; avoid pockets of stagnant and build-up of ammonia fumes
- Cleaning and disinfection of houses between floks
- Avoid contamination of food and water with good feeding
- Eradication of rodents

- Good litter hygiene and management; it must be kept dry but not dusty
- Avoid stress factors especially MG infection
- Hatching egg saniation clean source, fecal contamination of the egg may result in the penetration of E. coil through the shell and it has been estimated that in some cases 0.5 -6 % of eggs may contain the organism, frequent collection, exclusion of dirty eggs, cleaning, disinfection and fumigation of eggs, boxes, incubators and hatcheries
- Successful trials with oil emulsified multivalent vaccines and other types of vaccine

11.20 Egg Peritonitis

Epidemiology

- It is a condition in chicken caused by *E coli* and shows peritonitis, salphingitis and some times impaction of oviduct
- Egg peritonitis is characterized by fibrin or albumen-like material with a cooked appearance among the abdominal viscera. It is a common cause of sporadic death in layers or breeder hens, but in some flocks may become the major cause of death before or after reaching peak production and give the appearance of a contagious disease
- The condition may be associated with vent picking and cannibalism

Symptoms

- Peritonitis follows reverse movement of albumen and *Escherichia coli* bacteria from the oviduct into the abdomen
- If the incidence is high, culture should be done to differentiate between *Pasteurella* (fowl cholera) or *Salmonella* infection
- When hens have too many large ovarian follicles, a problem described as erratic oviposition and defective egg syndrome (EODES) is seen in broiler breeders. This condition is accompanied by a high incidence of double-yolked eggs, prolapses of the oviduct, internal ovulation, and/or internal laying that often results in egg peritonitis and mortality
- EODES is prevented by avoiding light stimulation of underweight pullets too early and by following guidelines for body weight and uniformity, and lighting recommendations for each breeder strain

- Overweight hens may also have a higher incidence of erratic ovulations and mortality associated with egg peritonitis

Treatment

- Antibiotic treatment of peritonitis caused by *E coli* infections is usually ineffective

Control

- Management of body weight and uniformity, reproductive development (ovary follicle growth and maturation), and drinking water sanitation are the best preventive strategies

11.21 Omphalitis or Yolk sac infection

Epidemiology

- Omphalitis is a condition characterized by infected yolk sacs, often accompanied by unhealed navels in young fowl.
- It is infectious but noncontagious and is associated with poor regulation of incubation temperature or humidity and marked contamination of the hatching eggs or incubator.
- If young poultry are placed in contaminated transportation boxes before their navels are completely closed, bacteria can migrate up the patent yolk stalk and infect the yolk sac.
- The navel may be inflamed and fail to close, producing a wet spot on the abdomen; a scab may be present.
- Opportunistic bacteria (coliforms, staphylococci, *Pseudomonas* spp, and *Proteus* spp) are often involved, and mixed infections are common.
- Proteolytic bacteria are prevalent in outbreaks.
- Mortality often begins at hatching and continues to 10–14 days of age, with losses of as much as 15% in chickens and 50% in turkeys.
- Chilling or overheating during shipment may increase losses. Persistent, unabsorbed, infected yolks often produce chicks or poults with reduced weight gain.

Symptoms

- The yolk sac is not absorbed and often is highly congested or may contain solidified pieces of yolk material; peritonitis may be extensive. Edema of the sternal subcutis may be seen.
- Affected chicks or poults usually appear normal until a few hours before death. They have little interest in food and water and are often found severely dehydrated.
- Depression, drooping of the head, and huddling near the heat source usually are the only signs.

Treatment

- There is no specific treatment; antibiotic use is based on the prevalent bacterial type involved. Even then, treatment may not result in satisfactory outcomes, because severely affected chicks and poults often die, and unaffected birds are unlikely to be aided by antibiotic treatment.

Control

- The disease is prevented by careful control of temperature, humidity, and sanitation in the incubator. Only clean, uncracked eggs should be set. If it is necessary to set dirty eggs, they should be segregated from clean eggs.
- Sanitizing detergents must be used according to directions if eggs are washed. Time, temperature, and frequent changes of water are as critical as the concentration of sanitizer in both wash and rinse water.
- The rinse should be warmer than the wash water (which should be warmer than the internal temperature of the egg) but should not be >60°C.
- The incubator should be cleaned and disinfected thoroughly between hatches. If fumigation is to be done with formaldehyde, vents should be closed.
- Thirty ml of 40% formaldehyde/0.6 m^3, or paraformaldehyde (in the strength recommended by the manufacturer), should be allowed to evaporate in the closed incubator or hatcher.
- The machines are readily contaminated after fumigation unless the exterior of the machines and the rooms in which they are located are also cleaned and disinfected.

11.22 Duck Septicemia

Epidemiology

- It is caused by *Pasteurella anatipastifer*
- The disease affects ducklings during 1-8 weeks of age
- It can also be by faecal contamination of feed, water or the environment where survival of the infectious agent may be prolonged
- Adverse environmental conditions and pre-existing disease are predisposing factors

Symptoms

- The affected birds may die without showing any symptoms
- There can be ocular and nasal discharge, mild coughing, sneezing, greenish diarrhea and tramers of head and neck, mortality ranges from 1-70 %. Disease can be recognizing from clinical symptoms and postmortem
- The isolation and identification of organism provides final diagnosis

Treatment

- Sulphonamides and potentiated sulphonamides are the products most commonly recommended for drinking water application. Subcutaneous injections of penicillin + dihydrostreptomycin, or streptomycin + dihydrostreptomycin are also highly effective

Control

- Good husbandry and hygiene, rigid depopulation and disinfection, adequate protection, 'hardening off', correct house relative humidity, sulphonamides in feed
- Inactivated and attenuated vaccines available in some countries
- Autogenous bacterins sometimes used

11.23 Avian Tuberculosis

Epidemiology

- Caused by *Mycobacterium avium* and leads to unthriftiness, loss in egg production and death

Symptoms

- There is progressive loss of weight, gross emaciation, and anaemia has seen from comb, wattles and ear lobes
- It may also cause jaundice and persistent diarrhea and soiling in vent region
- Liver may also be enlarge and show fatty degeneration.

Treatment

- The disease can be treated with the administration of ethambutol and rifampicin

11.24 Erysipelas

Epidemiology

- An acute fulminating disease caused by *E. incidosa*, a gram negative bacteria which affects turkeys, ducks and quails and chickens are less susceptible

Symptoms

- It causes sudden death without any apparent symptom, however diarrhoea, cyanosis of the head and unsteady gait. Lameness is seen in recovered birds

Treatment

- Affected birds can be treated with short acting penicillin

Control

- Inactive vaccine can also be used in turkeys

11.25 Coccidiosis

Epidemiology

- It is a disease of intensive poultry production
- There are seven species of Coccidia showing different symptoms and pathological lesions
- *Eimeria tenella* causes caecal coccidiosis characterized by blotchy haemorrhagic lesions in the caecum causing dysentery

- *E. mexica* is responsible for focal haemorrhagic lesions in the mid intestines, the faeces is soft, mucoid and pink coloured
- *E. acervulina* produces white irregular necrotic lesions
- *E. necatrix* produces disease both in older and younger birds, dysentery is a common symptoms

Symptoms

- The lesions are mainly seen in the middle third of the intestine, which appears to be excessively dilated, marked congestion, haemorrhage and necrosis may be seen in the mucosa. Sudden increase in mortality and soft mucoid droppings sometimes with blood are indicative of the disease.

Treatment

- Treatment involves use of sulphadimidine, nitrofurazone, sulphaquinoxaline, sulmet 12.5%, cordinal and amprolium hydrochloride
- Sulphaquinoxaline, Amprolium hydrochloride, Clopidol, Monensin, Decoquinate, Dinitrotoluamide drugs can be used for prophylaxis

Control

- The prevention and control involves immunization with live unattenauted vaccines/ live attenuated vaccines

11.26 Chicken Anaemia

Epidemiology

- Caused by Chicken Anaemia Virus. Diagnosis is by clinical symptoms

Symptoms

- No clinical signs are seen in parents, however chiks born from infected birds may show mortality up to 60%. Anaemia, alaplasia of bone marrow and atrophy of thymus, bursa of Fabricius and spleen are observed

Treatment

Control

- A crude live vaccine is used in breeder flock to prevent egg transmission of the virus

11.27 Duck Plague / Duck viral enteritis

Epidemiology

- Duck plague (Duck viral enteritis) is caused by Herpes Virus
- The incubation period is 3-7 days
- A sudden high and persistant mortality in ducks of all ages is indicative of the disease
- Adult breeder ducks may show higher mortality. Otherwise the mortality rate can range from 5-100%

Symptoms

- The birds may die without showing any clinical symptoms
- Nervous symptoms such as paralysis of wings and legs, failure to swim in water and greenish diarrhea are other clinical manifestations
- There is a large drop in egg production in laying flocks. The diagnosis is from clinical symptoms and should be differentiated from influenza, pasteurellosis and aflatoxicosis
- The demonstration of intra-nuclear inclusion bodies in hepatic cells from the cut surface of the liver, isolation and identification of the virus, demonstration of viral antigens confirm the disease

Control

- Vaccination with a modified live virus vaccine adapted in chicken embryo is effective. It is administered subcutaneously to ducklings above 2 weeks of age

11.28 Avian Leukosis/Sarcoma

Epidemiology

- Highest incidence is observed at sexual maturity

Symptoms

- Clinical symptoms are paleness of comb, inappetance, emaciation and weakness
- Enlargement of liver, bursa and kidneys results in distention of abdomen are also major consequences of the disease
- The disease is to be differentiated from Marek's disease. It is based on history, clinical symptoms and histopathological lesions and Virus isolation

Control

Genetic selection and flock management can reduce the incidence

11.29 Thrush (Candidiasis)

Epidemiology

- Caused by *C. albicans* which is contained in contaminated feed

Symptoms

- The affected chickens become dull, look ruffled and are found at resting and sleeping stage most of the time
- Lesions are mostly located in the crop, but may also occur in upper respiratory tract
- The mucous membrane is covered with grayish white, thick and fibrinous coat
- The diagnosis is from gross symptoms and histopathological examination

Treatment

- Nystatin in feed or drinking water is found to be effective in preventing the disease

Control

- Maintenance of good hygiene and overcrowding can prevent the disease

11.30 Aflatoxicosis

Epidemiology

- Aflatoxicosis is defined as the intoxication that results from consumption of feed stuffs contaminated by one or more poisons of fungal origin the aflatoxins
- Secondary metabolite of fungus (*Aspergillus flavus and A parasiticus*), which grow in feed stuffs like groundnut cakes, maize, cottonseed oil cakes in presence of higher humidity
- Causal aflatoxins are B1,B2, G1, G2
- Contaminated stored feed with moisture and fungus is source of Mycotoxicosis

Symptoms

- The signs of aflatoxicosis in poultry are non specific, however they may show symptoms after 2 weeks following ingestion of toxins more than 02 ppm
- Impaired growth and poor feed conversion efficiency is also observed
- Loss of pigmentation and passage of undigested feed particles are also observed

Treatment

- Stop feeding of feeds suspected to have been infected by fungus especially when they have been stored in humid environment
- Supplement feeds with lipotrophic factors, liver tonics and biotin
- To increase the detoxifying potential of the birds, supplement the birds with sulphur containing amino acids like 400 gm lysine and 200 gm DL methionine and 400 gm 50% choline chloride mixture per 500 ton of feed
- The use of certain B vitamins, vitamin E, selenium, enzyme produced by yeast and bacteria, absorbents and antixidants also are capable to reduce and facilitate the decomposition and detoxification of mycotoxins within individual birds

Control

- Prevention of fungal growth on crops in the field, at harvest of crop, during storage of Food stuff and during processing of feed can help in reducing the incidence
- The raw materials should be dried thoroughly before storage to contain moisture levels well below the minimum threshold levels
- Feed should be stored allowing sufficient space for the air movement in the storehouses
- Stored compounded feed must be utilized within two weeks applying the concept of first in first out
- Heating at less than 300^0 C can not destroy aflatoxin but be degraded by exposure of feed to heavy sunlight in thin layers for 12-14 hours
- Ammonia gas can be used to destroy aflatoxin but it reduces the nutritive value of feed
- Adding mold inhibitors in the feed has been found effective in reducing the occurrence of this condition

11.31 Coli granulamatosis

- Coligranuloma (Hjarre's disease). It is characterized by multiple granulomas in the intestinal tract, the mesentery and the liver, but not in spleen. The lesions are similar to these observed in tuberculosis.

11.32 Avian Chlamydiosis

The affected birds appear sleepy, show fits, shivering, ruffled plumage, nasal discharge, watery greenish diarrhea and marked wasting of pectoral muscles. The mortality is high and occurs in a short period. The disease is diagnosed from postmortem lesions and identification of microorganisms on staining. Treatment with broad spectrum antibiotic is effective.

11.33 Listeriosis

The disease is transmitted through faeces. There are no specific clinical symptoms; however there may be depression, ataxia and torticollis. There is hepatic necrosis, spleenomegaly with miliary necrosis, nephritis, enteritis, mycorditis and conjunctivitis. There is no control except to avoid potential source of infection.

11.34 Ulcerative Enteritis

Can occur in chicken quails, pheasants and partridges. It is caused by *C. colinum*. It leads to depression, anorexia and huddling. Diagnosis is from postmortem and prevention is through avoiding predisposing factors.

11.35 Gangrenous Dermatitis

Primarily occurs in broilers at four weeks of age or in replacement pullets. It is caused by *Clostridium sapticum* and *Clostridium perferingens.* Sudden increase in mortality and rapid decomposition of carcass are important clinical symptoms. There is a reddening of skin under the wings, between the thighs, over the ribs and flank region. Avoidance of overcrowding and good management and hygiene can drastically reduce the incidence.

11.36 Spirochaetosis

Is a tick borne disease and is characterized by anorexia, depression and cyanosis of head and anaemia. Paralysis is seen before the bird die. The disease can be diagnosed through examination of blood and the affected bird can be treated with antibiotic.

□□□

CHAPTER-12

Other Avian Species (Evolution, Speciation, Domestication and Breed Formation, Their Performance and Systems for Improvement of Productivity)

12.1 Ducks

The duck belongs to family Anatidae and is distinguished from other avian species by relatively smaller size, shorter neck, flatter body, shorter legs and broader bill. The male ducks are known as drake and the female as duck. The immature young are known as ducklings, the term is used till the feathers are grown. Most breeds of domesticated ducks have originated from wild mallard. Ducks occupy second place to chicks in their economic importance and spread especially with respect to the contribution to table eggs. Ducks are mostly concentrated in coastal areas and in states in eastern and southern regions viz. Tripura, Assam, West Bengal and Odisha, Tamil Nadu, Andhra Pradesh and Kerala besides parts of Jammu & Kashmir. Although it is more economical to raise ducks for egg and meat purposes since they can be raised in a number of free range management systems such as along the coast line, along the large rivers, running water channels and lakes and can consume natural feed resources, are more resistant to common poultry diseases, and therefore can be more profitably raised for rural egg and meat production. They are more economical than chicken as they produce more eggs. Duck eggs are 15-20g heavier than chicken eggs. Duck require less management inputs (housing and health cover), meet their nutritional requirement through foraging and eating insects and snails, the latter helps in reducing incidence of liver fluke infestation for which snail is an intermediary host and related diseases in ruminant livestock, they can inhabit marshy and wet lands, have less aggressiveness and cannibalistic tendencies, lay most of the eggs during the night and early morning which can be more easily collected with least amount of expenditure on time and labour. They are intelligent and can be easily trained to reach the pond from their shelters and back. They go together like a sheep in a flock and follow the leader and therefore, are easier to manage. Duck cum fish culture is extremely popular as the droppings of the ducks provide organic matter for the growth of phyto-and zoo-planktons which provide the feed for fish. It is a common practice to have some poultry and duck sheds built on or along fish ponds.

Hatching

The optimum size of the hatching egg varies from 70-75g compared to 50-58g in chicken. Duck eggs are more porous and can be easily fumigated after collection. The incubation period is 28 days. However, Muscovy duck requires 32-35 days for eggs to hatch. Ducks require less temperature (99 to 99.5 °F) and less ventilation and more humidity (70-75%) compared to chicken during incubation period. High humidity is generally maintained by sprinkling the eggs with luke warm water twice during the 2nd week and every alternate day during 3rd and 4th week. Duck eggs are required to be turned at an angle of 180° against 90° in chicken eggs. Duck eggs require cooling during incubation. Cooling for a maximum period of 30 min per day starting from 5th day of incubation to a temperature of 90 ^{o}F. The duck eggs have usually lower hatchability than chicken eggs.

Breeds of ducks

Khaki Campbell and Indian Runner are the most common indigenous breeds for egg production and Buff Orpington is a dual purpose breed although is primarily utilized for egg production. In selection for egg production, attention must be given to physical appearance especially upright carriage and light weight. Laying ducks may be identified like layer chickens. The egg type ducks start laying by 20-22 weeks of age. One drake for 5-6 ducks is sufficient for assuring fertile eggs. In the beginning and the terminal part of breeding season the males are slightly less active and increase in their number can help in improving fertility. Stud mating is very popular although individual has distinct advantage over trap nesting for the purpose of pedigree hatching. Breeding ducks do perform relatively better under free range management with water bodies available for bathing and drinking, than under confined. These facilities are dispensable and ducks are now being managed more intensively almost like layer/ broiler chicken.

White Pekins, Aylesbury and Muscovy are important duck breeds for meat. White Pekin are creamy white in colour with yellow flesh and long, broad and deep body. It grows very fast and reaches 2.2–2.5 kg in 7 weeks of age. Under confinement and intensive feeding they produce a large number of eggs with reasonable fertility. Aylesbury breed has been regarded as a deluxe table bird because of light bones and large percent of creamy white flesh. Muscovy ducks when crossed with other breeds produce all sterile progeny known as mule ducks. They graze like goose and the males have no coloured feathers which is sex linked character. There are no feathers on the face and the drake has a knob on the head. The males are twice the size of females.

Green ducklings are produced from 2 to 3 way crosses. The commercial ducklings are generally produced through crossing medium sized females having high reproductive efficiency and males with high growth potential. Male lines are derived from Aylesbury or Pekins and female lines from Pekin or White Pennine. The preference of hybrid ducks is due to higher viability and also some superiority in production traits.

Economic and social aspects

Duck farming has an important role in poverty alleviation through providing employment and and incomes in areas which are more prone to floods. In such a situation duck farming can ensure supplementary income and provide a viable option to improve the economic and nutritional status of rural poor in areas affected by recurrent floods. The duck and geese love water and are called water fowls. India has 5700 km of coast line and a very large area with low lying and marshy land. Generally indigenous chicken are reared in most rural areas for egg and meat production but in states along the coast line ducks are raised for meat and eggs. Ducks have advantage for rearing in coastal marshy wetlands waterways and ponds, because they love water and consume vegetable and animal material available in it. They are suitable for mixed farming such as deep water paddy cum duck culture, deep water paddy-fish-duck farming. They require less care and management and can sustain on foraging insects, snails, weeds etc. They can be used as a biological control for liver fluke for which the intermediary host is snail. They have got excellent growth and egg production, lay larger number of eggs than indigenous chicken (160-180 vs. 50-100) with hard shell and thus have longer shelf life without preservation. The birds can continue laying during the second year of their life, most eggs are laid at night and in early morning and are thus easy to collect and being hardy and resistant to most avian diseases can be more easily managed extensively. Little shelter and supplementary feed is further required and being raised under free range require little attention. They improve soil fertility through removal of weeds and through their droppings. The droppings of 20 ducks can provide sufficient organic manure for an acre of land. The droppings contain 16% N, 23% P and 10% K. The day old body weight averages 60 gm, 4 weeks 1.2-1.4 kg, 6 weeks 2.0-2.2 kg with feed required upto six weeks of around 4.5 kg. The mortality is low upto six weeks (2-6%). Age at fist egg averages 120 days, 50% egg production is attained at 140 days of age, Average egg lay 300 eggs annually with an weight of 60-66 g. Body weight at 40 weeks is 1.8 kg, daily feed intake is 120-140 g, duckling mortality (0-8 weeks) is 2-3%.

The ducks are generally reared in backyard/free range/ scavenging system or integrated with agriculture (vegetables and food crops), and aquaculture. Pig-duck-cattle-vegetable-aquaculture is a common practice. Ducks consume aquatic plants and other animal species and provide fertilizer which promote the growth of phyto and zoo-planktons used by fish as feed. The help in reduction of weeds in paddy fields and increase paddy productivity both through removal of weeds and providing organic fertilizer. They can be raised under intensive management under confinement with proper housing, feed and health management. In India, intensive duck farming like intensive poultry production for eggs and meat is not still practiced. Incubation period in ducks is 28 days i.e. 7 days more than in chicken. 6-8 ducks are allotted to one drake in case of egg type and 4-6 ducks in broiler type. Hatching eggs are collected 15 days after introduction of drakes for hatching of eggs, temperature should be between 37-37.5°C and humidity between 70-75%. Humidity can be increased by splashing of lukewarm water on alternative days. Turning of eggs is at 180°C and not 90° as in chicken eggs. Ducks has generally a lower hatching percentage than in chicken. Ducklings can be bred on free range after 3 weeks of age, a brooder used for chick brooding can also be used for brooding ducklings.

Management

Normally little attention is required for feeding and watering of ducks raised under free range system but some supplementary feeds based on household food waste such as wheat bran, rice bran/polish, broken grains, kitchen waste, snails and fish can help in improving production. Under intensive rearing palleted feed offered early morning or late evening is preferred, for meat type ducks starter, grower and finisher feeds should be given in first two weeks, three to six weeks and seventh week to market, respectively. For layers, supplementary feed should be provided one month prior they come in egg laying. Feed restriction to layers is similar to that in chicken. The feed conversion ratio in meat type ducks is 3.0. Ducks suffers from aflatoxicosis. They suffer from virus apitycus and pasteurolosis. Ducks should be vaccinated against duck plague and duck cholera.

Constraints and their solution

The major constraints in duck production are lack of proper training facility to rural duck keepers, non-availability of genetically superior ducklings, non-availability of balanced compounded feed, total lack of bio-security, facilities for institutional finance, organized marketing and support from central and state governments.

12.2 Turkey

Turkey is mainly reared for meat which is one of the choicest white meat famous for its leanness and delicacy. Turkey meat is very much popular in North America and European countries compared to broiler meat because of its leanness and delicacy. Ninety percent of the World's Turkey Industry is located in North America and Europe, but the production locations are limited within these areas. The three states in USA (North Caroline, Minnesota and California) have 46% turkey, whereas France, UK and Italy constitute 85% of total turkey production of Europe. Domestication of turkey and its diffusion is relatively well known. The ancestor of the domestic turkey is the true wild turkey (*Meleagris gallopavo*). The wild turkey is indigenous to much of the eastern and southwestern states of USA, northern Mexico and southeastern Canada. Seven subspecies of the wild form have been distinguished by geographic range and plumage differences have been reported viz. Eastern (*Meleagris gallopavo silvestris*), Florida (*M. g. osceola*), Rio Grande (*M.g. intermedia*), Merriam's (*M.g. merriami*),

Gould's (*M.g. mexicana*), Southern Mexican (*M.g. gallopavo*) and Moore's (*M. g. oneusta*). The ocellated turkey (*Agriocharis ocellata* or *Meleagris ocellata*) is considerably different because of its size and coloration and is considered as a separate species entirely. It is native to the Yucatán peninsula of Mexico and is more difficult to domesticate. Out of these, only three have role in domestication. It is generally accepted that the first ancestor of the domestic turkey was the Mexican subspecies. The eastern wild turkey later hybridized with Mexican domestics to form the modern commercial turkey. Merriam's wild turkey was involved in a separate domestication in southwestern USA which has not persisted. Turkeys have been known domesticated in Mexico between 200 B.C. and 700 A.D.; neither date nor location are precisely established. The wild ancestor was the Mexican subspecies (*M. g. gallopavo*). Two breeds of turkeys, different from those of Mexico, were being raised in pre-Columbian southwestern USA. Mexican turkeys were taken to Europe immediately after the discovery, perhaps as early as 1500 AD. Diffusion through Europe was very rapid and by mid 16th century they were no longer a curiosity. Rate of diffusion is estimated at 40-50 km/yr. Colonists brought turkeys from Europe to Eastern North America early in the 17th century. The birds hybridized with the Eastern wild turkey (*M. g. silvestris*) resulting in the American Bronze breed, the foundation of modern commercial turkeys.

Genetic variance

Turkeys are not classified into breeds; however, there are 7 standard varieties such as White Holland, Bourban Red, Narrgansett, Black, Slate, Bronze and Beltsville Small White.Turkeys with white plumage have a better performance due to higher heat tolerance and carcass yield and quality. Vent system in hatching chicks can be used for sexing. Males are usually heavier than females. The mature males have conspicuous black beard attached to the skin of the upper region. Dubill or Snood, a fleshy protuberance near the base of the beak is relatively large, plump and elastic in males and relatively small, thin and non-elastic in females. The two sexes also differ in breast feathers. Male poults strut even at one day old stage and continue do so through out their life. Both strain/variety crosses are used in commercial turkey production. Mostly they are two to three way crosses although five way crosses are not uncommon. The higher crosses arise due to poor fecundity of pure stock under more intensive management use.

Reproduction

Since the breast meat is most preferred, being white and dry with extremely low fat, turkeys have been selected for breast meat leading to distortion in body conformation and consequently difficulties in natural mating and poor semen quality and fertility. Specialized male and female lines are more common in producing commercial stocks. Male lines are selected for growth and conformation and female lines for egg production and fertility. Conformation does seem to be related to lean meat yield or distribution of meat in the carcass. Conformation traits play an important role in selection of male lines because of demand for certain cut up parts.

Production and reproduction traits are the major characters in the female lines which are selected for these traits, although some emphasis is also laid for growth. There is a negative correlation between growth and conformation traits on one side and fertility on the other. Separate male and female line have been developed through selection for different economic characters. Most of the modern turkeys are selected for rapid growth and wide breast. While it has been possible for breeders to successfully achieve desired conformation, as mentioned earlier, it has led to serious problems of male fertility especially under natural mating although AI has been introduced to obtain desired fertility although the semen quality in males is still adversely affected by selection for broad breast.

The number of eggs per hen housed in a season depends on the genetic merit of the stock and management conditions related to feeding and housing and climatic conditions including light and temperature. The average age at first egg is around 30 weeks. Egg production is adversely affected when it commences too early. With artificial light turkeys can produce 100 eggs in 24 weeks after laying of first egg or reaching age at sexual maturity. Strain and variety crossing improve egg production.

Turkey eggs weigh approximately 85g with a noticeably pointed end and strong shell. Turkey eggs are as palatable as chicken eggs. The hatching period is 28 days which is lower by 12 to 24 hours in light bodied strains. With optimum fertility and hatchability, 60-70 poults can be obtained from each breeder compared to 100-120 chicks in case of broiler chicken. Because of reduced fertility the toms are rarely used after first year, whereas; hens can be used to the extent of 20-25% based on their first year annual egg production.

Turkey poults weighing around 4kg are in great demand. Given proper environment, feeding and health cover, the weight can be attained by 12-14 weeks of age. Further increase in body weight leads to reduction in efficiency of feed conversion for live weight gains. Turkey hens can also be sold as roasters approximately 20-24 weeks of age at a weight of 8-9kg. Feed efficiency is poor in small sized turkeys.

Management systems

Cage system of rearing of turkeys is not popular except in small flocks maintained for experimental purposes. Rearing in confinement on deep litter is preferred to provide better management but it increases labour cost. Deep litter system has higher efficiency but has better management efficiency and is more effective in disease control as it prevents exposure to predators and unfavourable environmental conditions.

The optimum floor space when the birds are housed at breeding time should be 1.02 m^2 per bird for larger breeds and 0.83 m^2 in smaller breeds. Floor space can be reduced to half in debeaked hens and where ample ventilation is provided. Under range management the space can be reduced to almost $1/3^{rd}$. Range management is possible when the weather condition is mild and rains are not heavy. Turkeys should be rotated from one range to the other and more or less the same age group should be managed in a range at a time. Turkey poults require double the hover space as compared to chickens. They are not self reliant and should be prevented by guards in the beginning. They need to be forced fed in the beginning. Feed should be placed under bright light. Coloured marbles may be placed in the feed and the water to attract the turkey poults. They are of nervous temperament and get easily panicky.

Diseases of Turkeys

Turkeys are relatively more resistant to common avian diseases such as Marek's Disease and IBR. New Castle Disease, Fowl Pox and Coccidiosis do occur in turkeys in milder forms. The most common diseases are Fowl Cholera, Fowl Typhoid, Mycoplasmosis, Blue Comb, Erysipelas, Hexamatiasis, Arizona infectionand ring worm infections. The breeding stock should be routinely tested for Arizona infection, Fowl Typhoid, Paratyphoid, Mycoplasma and Pullorum diseases and those free from these diseases should be used to reproduce the next generation. The birds need protection against Fowl Cholera and Erysipelas through vaccination. To avoid Mycoplasmosis, the hatching eggs should be routinely dipped in tylosin solution.

Although the feed ingredients are similar to those in chicken, the feeding requirement is different from that in the chicken. The turkeys require more protein, minerals and vitamins to allow faster growth. It is desirable to separate turkeys by sex at the time of hatching. The turkeys must be fed in troughs or hoppers and not on the ground.

Weight by weight basis turkey meat is costlier than broiler meat and is primarily due to low survival of poults. Flock size is important in determining the economics of turkey meat production.

CARI-VIRAT Turkey

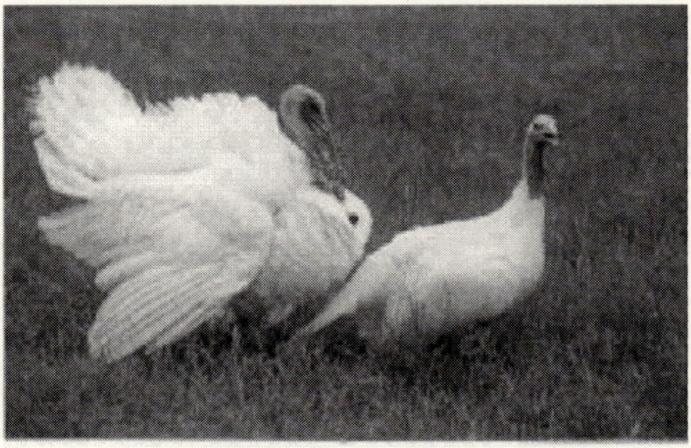

(*Source:* icar.org.in)

It is broad breasted white type turkey. Marketed as broiler at approximately 16 weeks of age when hens usually reach a live weight of about 8 kg and toms weigh approximately 12 kg. Smaller, fryer roasters can be produced by slaughtering at an earlier age as per the demand of the local market.

12.3 Guinea fowl

Guinea fowl is found in a reasonably large numbers in a wild state and has only been domesticated recently as a broiler. Guinea fowl meat is slightly darker in color and tender than the chicken meat.

It has the flavor of a game bird. It is a hardy species, gregarious in habit, moves in a flock and is adaptable both to tropical and temperate climate and thus can survive under extremely poor feed resources and can live on scavenging and eating low set natural forages. Because of little attention has been received towards its domestication, history of guinea fowl is very imperfectly known. Guinea fowl was perhaps domesticated for aesthetic appeal and for religious rites and as a sacrifical animal to the deities; it has been recorded that the guinea fowl was offered as sacrifical animal in the past in Athens. Historical records and writings strongly suggest that in the period of antiquity guinea fowl was a common barnyard poultry in Greece and Greek islands of the Roman Empire. With the fall of the Roman Empire guinea fowl almost disappeared from the European scene till the Middle Ages. It is generally agreed that two different guinea fowl species were independently domesticated but the African people initiating domestication is not known clearly. For all practical purposes, the return of Protuguese from the West African explorations in the later-half of fifteenth century mark; guinea fowl had its advent into Europe, West Indies, Central America, India and Malaysia. In a way, all presentday guinea fowl are the descendents of these reintroductions from Gambian regions. The present English name the 'guinea fowl' also suggests its African origin. Guinea (pronounced as 'GINHEE') referring to part on the western coasts of Africa has been possibly derived from a 'Berber' word meaning the 'Land of Blacks'. Though not clearly defined the 'Guinea' region include Ivory Cost, Gold Coast (Ghane) and Slave Coast (Benin and Nigeria). In these regions guinea fowl in wild state is still available in large number. In India, the induction of guinea fowl might be along with that of black African ethnic group slaves in 13th century A.D. Later, Portugues brought more negroid ethanic group slaves from Mozambique and Ivory coast.

Genetic Variants

Unlike chicken, not many varieties are known of guinea fowl. The existing varieties are classified according to plumage colour. The three principal well known varieties are the Pearl, White and Lavender. Pearl variety appears to have developed originally from the wild African type and has uniformly dark grey plumage, regularly sprinkled with dots which give it the characteristic pearled appearance. Lavender birds are light gray or lavender in colour and always uniformly dotted with white. White variety is characterized by presence of completely white plumage.

White breasted variety is characterized by pearl plumage with white breast feathers. This plumage pattern is produced by crossing the white and pearl or lavender varieties, hence these variety do not breed true. Other varieties are Buff, Coral-blue, Dundottes, Isabellia, Liliac, Royal -Purple and other plumage patterns.

Sexing and reproductive performance

Sexing on physical appearance is not possible before 12 weeks of age. The guinea fowl chicks are known as keets. It is a seasonal breeder and mostly breeds from March to September. The male to female ratio should be 1:4 - 5. Hatchability reduces if eggs are held for more than 7 days before incubation. Incubation period is 4 weeks. The birds start laying at 36 to 38 weeks and lay around 50-100 eggs during a year. Varieties through selection can produce 180-200 eggs and mature at 28 weeks of age. Eggs are smaller in size than of chicken and are yellow to brown in color with a thick shell. It is a nervous type bird and is shy of man and needs protection from predators. Young keets need coaxing for eating of feed and drinking of water. Under good management, the bird can attain 1.2 kg live weight at 13 weeks of age. Only recently R&D efforts have been initiated at the Central Avian Research Institute for studies on various aspects of guinea fowl production and their improvement.

Guinea fowl are highly free moving birds. These are best suited for marginal and small farmer. Three available varieties are KADMBARI, CHITAMBARI and SWETAMBARI

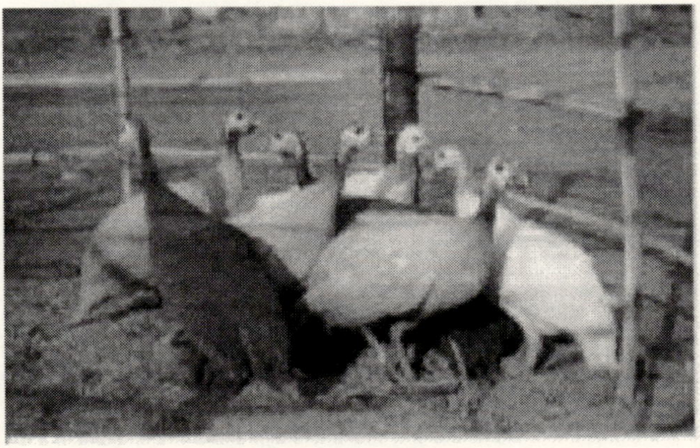

KADAMBARI
(Source: http://www.icar.org.in/cari/varieties_deve.php)

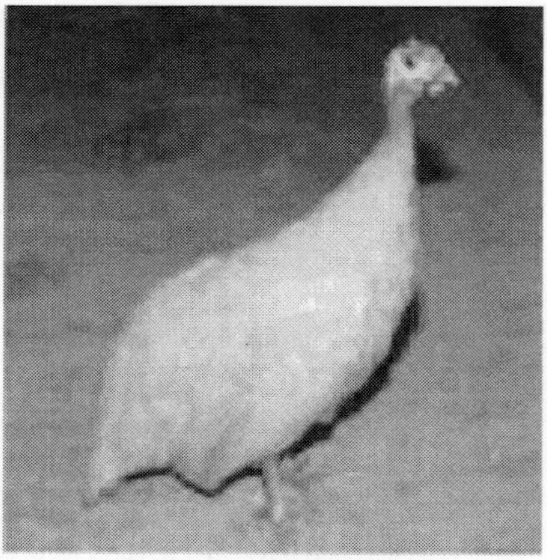

CHITAMBARI
(*Source:* http://www.icar.org.in/cari/varieties_deve.php)

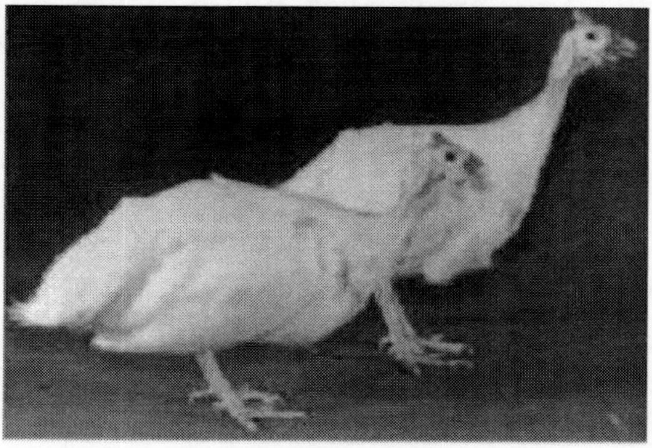

SWETAMBARI
(*Source:* http://www.icar.org.in/cari/varieties_deve.php)

Special features

- Hardy bird
- Suitable to all agro-climatic conditions
- Resistant to many common diseases of chicken
- No requirement of elaborate and expensive housing
- Excellent foraging capabilities
- Consumes all non-conventional feed not used for chicken feeding
- More tolerant to mycotoxin and aflatoxin

- Hard egg shell provides minimum breakage and long keeping quality
- Guinea fowl meat is rich in vitamins and low in cholesterol

Production characteristics

- Weight at 8 weeks: 500-550 g
- Weight at 12 weeks: 900-1000 g
- Age at first egg: 230-250 day
- Average egg weight 38-40 g
- Egg production (in one laying cycle from March to September): 100-120 eggs
- Fertility: 70-75%
- Hatchability on fertile eggs set basis: 70-80%

12.4 Japanese quails

The species belongs to the class Aves, family Phasanidae, and genus Qoturnix and the species is named as *Coturnix cortunix japonica*. The Bob white quails belong to a different family. The male is lighter than the female unlike in other avian species and is identified by the cinnamon color feathers on the upper throat and lower breast region. The female is similar to male in color except the feathers on the throat and the upper breast are longer, pointed and much lighter in color.

Egg production

They are prolific layers, start laying at 5 weeks of age depending upon the day length, the average age at first egg is around 40 days. The female attains peak egg production by about 50 days of age. The selection for egg production can reduce age at sexual maturity to 7 to 8 weeks and reach peak production by about 10 weeks. Under favorable feeding and management conditions, the birds can lay for a longer periods and can produce on an average 250 eggs per year. Domesticated quails are similar in sexual development and egg production like high yielding strains of chicken. Research done at University of California at Los Angels in USA shows that Japanese quails require 14-18 hours of day light for optimum production, 75 % of eggs are layed between 3 to 6 pm and 20 % during night. Eggs are multi colored ranging from dark brown, blue and white to buff, each is heavily mottled with black, brown and blue colour spots. Individual hens lay eggs of a characteristic size shape and color pattern. The weight of the egg averages 10 g with range from 7 to 14 g. This is about 7 % of the body weight of the female. Hatchability decreases at a fairly constant rate of 3 % per day. Age of the hen at lay has a pronounced effect on hatchability. Maximum hatchability occurs from 8 to 24 weeks of age.

Domesticated quails lay eggs throughout the year. Young females mate more frequently than older ones regardless of the age of the males. Special care is required in collection and handling of hatching eggs because of their thin shell which breaks easily. The bird should be 10-24 weeks old for obtaining optimum fertility. One male per 3 females should be used and egg should be collected four days after the introduction of males. The hatching eggs should be fumigated for 20 minutes before storage. The hatchability decreases with the age of female, however has no effect of the age of male. Medium sized eggs have better hatchability. It takes about 18 days for eggs to hatch. The incubator and hatchers for quail egg similar to those used for chicken with a small modifications considering the size of the eggs.

Adaptation to Climatic factors and Disease Incidence

Quails are extremely sensitive to abrupt changes in physical environment especially during first 2 weeks of life. They also need better care during breeding. The disease pattern is similar to that in chicken, but the quails are more resistant to the most common poultry diseases and are therefore not vaccinated or dewormed.

Nutrition and feeding

For optimum growth up to 3 weeks of age, 27% protein with 2800 k.cal ME/Kg of feed is recommended and 24 % protein with same energy level during 4 to 5 weeks of growth. During laying, the requirement is 22 % protein and 2900 K.cal ME/ kg live weight.

Production management

High ambient temperature and humidity in tropical ecologies depress performance of layer and broiler poultry as reflected by poor growth, feed efficiency, carcass yield and quality and egg production and egg size. Similar are the effects in quails. The environmental stress also results in higher mortality which requires ameliorative measures. Modern management requires environmentally controlled housing facilities but it is costly especially for poor rural poultry producers. There is a need to develop alternative management strategies which will ameliorate environmental stress and make the production in tropical conditions more efficient. This can be done through environmental control which is costly to create and maintain especially in countries with poor and irregular electric supply. Some of the genes express phenotypically and help in reducing the environmental stress. There is a major gene in poultry- Naked neck-Na which reduces the feathers by 30-40 % with a total loss in the neck region in homozygous genotype and has a favorable effect on growth rate under environmental stress conditions. The birds with naked neck have higher survival rate in fluctuating temperature and humidity conditions. The birds with naked neck gene also have better growth rate, feed efficiency and dressing percentage. The gene acts by reducing plumage around the neck and thinner and lighter skin. The meat of naked neck bird has slightly higher crude protein and appreciably lower ether extract. Biochemical parameters related to blood indicate higher total cholesterol content in na/na compared to Na/Na and Na/na. It is known that Na gene reduces cholesterol content in the blood especially triglyceride and VLDL compared to the normal feathered bird. There is also better immuno-competence. The less fat content especially in the abdomen has been recorded in Na due to utilization of higher proportion of lipid for thermoregulation. Pure broiler line with Na gene is more suitable for rearing in an open housed management system without any cooling arrangements.

Japanese quails have created a big impact in recent years and many quails farms have been established throughout the country both for egg and meat production. It is due to fact that increasing consumer awareness for quality meat.

The following are the factors which made quail farming as economically viable and technically feasible-

- Very short generation interval
- Quails are very robust and less susceptible to diseases
- No vaccination is required
- Low space requirement
- Easy to handle

- Early maturity
- Very high laying intensity- female starts laying at an age of 42 days

There are a number of varieties of quail evolved through selection to perform better egg/ meat production. These are

i) CARI Uttam (Broiler Quail)

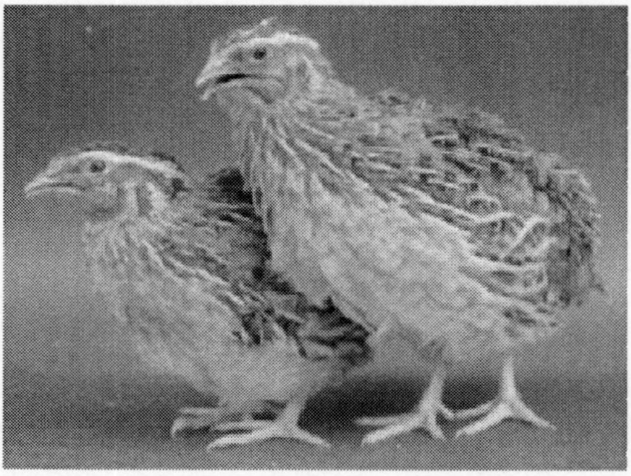

(Source : www.icar.org.in/cari/varieties_deve.php)

- Hatchability on total eggs set: 70-75%
- Weight at 4 weeks: 150 -155g
- Weight at 5 weeks: 240 g
- Feed efficiency at 4 weeks: 2.51
- Feed efficiency at 5 weeks: 2.60
- Daily feed consumption: 25-28g

ii) CARI Ujjawal (White breasted quail)

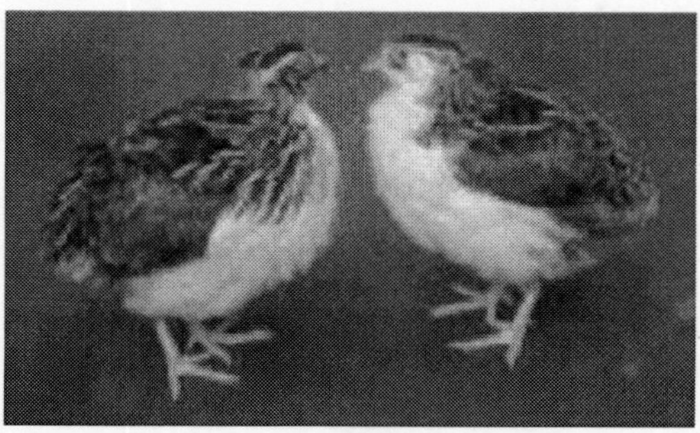

(*Source:* www.icar.org.in/cari/varieties_deve.php)

- Hatchability on total eggs set: 65%
- Body weight at 4 weeks: 140 g
- Body weight at 5 weeks: 175 g
- Feed efficiency at 5 weeks: 2.8
- Daily feed consumption: 25-28 g

iii) CARI SHWETA (White feathered quail)

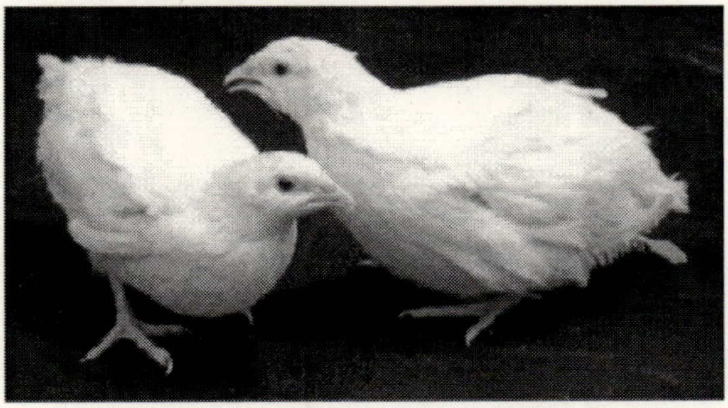

(*Source:* www.icar.org.in/cari/varieties_deve.php)

- Hatchability on total eggs set basis: 50-60%
- Body weight at 4 weeks: 135 g
- Body weight at 5 weeks: 155-165 g
- Feed efficiency up to 4 weeks: 2.6
- Feed efficiency up to 5 weeks: 2.7
- Daily feed consumption: 25 g

iv) CARI PEARL (White egger layer)

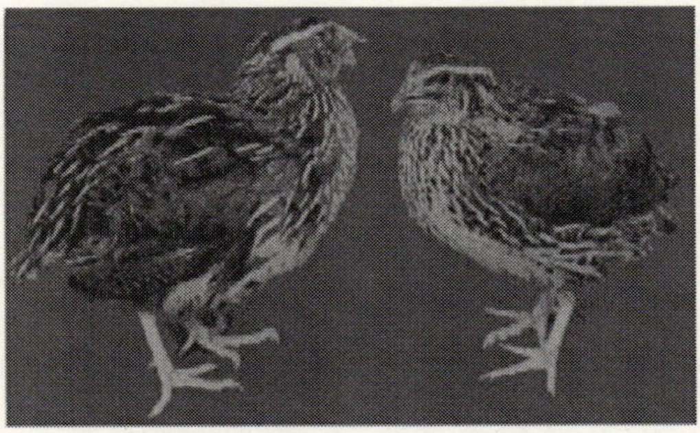

(Source : www.icar.org.in/cari/varieties_deve.php)

- Hatchability on total eggs set: 70-80%
- Weight at 5 weeks: 140 g
- Daily feed consumption: 20-25 g
- Age at 50% egg production: 8 weeks
- Age at 80% egg production: 10 weeks
- Hen day production: 285-295 eggs

❑❑❑

CHAPTER-13

Some Important Issues Related to Commercial Poultry Production

13.1 The Impact of Phytate as an Anti-nutrient Factor in Poultry Production

Phytate, also referred as phytin or phytic acid, is a major system for storage of phosphorus (P) in the seeds and is a part of a complex system in which potassium, magnesium and calcium are contained in plant tissues. It was originally recognized as a source of P during germination of seeds but is now known to play an important role in reducing oxidative stress during the germination and prevents plant embryo mortality.

Phytate is an anti-nutritional factor in animal feed and has posed a long term challenge. It was initially used as a potential source of P to be available through targeted use of phytase feed enzymes, the focus however has shifted to its anti-nutritional role and its demonstration in significant reductions in performance.

Even though the phytate has a higher affinity for cations such as copper and zinc, it is the molecule's affinity for calcium that is of greater concern in poultry nutrition. The dietry calcium requirement increases from 0.60% to 0.95% when the phytate-P level in the diet increases from 0 to 0.25%, equivalent to phytate concentration found in a standard corn-soybean diet. The impact on other minerals can be seen when assessing the impact of progressive phytate reduction through application of increasing doses of phytase feed enzyme. The selenium content rises when a diet containing no phytase is supplemented with a commercial phytase. The reduction in pepsin activates between pH 0.8 and 2.8 in the presence of phytate. Since the pH in the stomach contents is typically between 2.0 to 3.0, it can subsequently reduce the pepsin activity causing a less protein being initially broken down during the acid phase of the digestive process, leading to a lower overall protein digestibility. This is due to reduction in pepsin activation which may be overcome by higher production of its precursor, pepsinogen in the stomach. The presence of phytate also reduces protein solubility and subsequent digestibility. The presence of phytate can also reduce the activity of the sodium/ potassium pump, which is crucial to amino acid uptake across the gastro-intestinal wall.

The reduction in protein digestibility has further a negative effect on the production of the bird due to an increase in the level of undigested protein reaching the duodenum, increasing secretion of hormone gastrin and cholesystokinin, stimulating additional production of hydrochloric acid and pepsinogen in the stomach which reduces gastro-emptying. This results in a substantial increase in endogenous losses. A greater amount of sodium bi-carbonate has to be secreted to neutralize gastro-intestinal pH, whilst the additional irritant effect on gastrointestinal mucosa leads to excessive production of mucus to maintain protection level.

The elimination of phytate has a positive impact on performance through superdosing of phytate. This response is attributed to phytase breakdown and not phosphorus release. Not all phytates have similar activities at the pH normally found in the stomach or able to continue degrading phytase towards its elimination as concentration falls to a level to be effective for such super dosing. The anti-nutritional effect of phytate is causing very large economic losses in the monogastric animals like chicken through reducing performance and profitability so a high dose of phytase is required for the elimination of phytate.

13.2 Inclusion of Dried Distillers Grains with Solubles (DDGS) in poultry feeds

About 70% of the cost of poultry production is due to feed and there is a never ending effort for finding affordable feed ingredients. By-products from human food and also other non-ruminant domestic animals (DA) are used in feeding DA species. The majority of by-products of the dry grind ethonol industry are dried distiller grains with soluble DDGS. These can arise from different sources like maize, rice, wheat, sorghum and are highly useful as feed ingredients in DA including poultry. Among the corn, DDGS is an excellent feed ingredient for use in diet for layer, broiler, duck and turkey and contains approximately 85% of the energy value in corn, has moderate levels of proteins and essential amino acids and high in available phosphorus.

With growing demand for food and declining feed grain resources, the animals will have to depend essentially on cerial by-products not usable as human food. Corn by-products, DDGS from the ethanol industry are normally considered as waste but can be used as a feed ingredient because it is a cheap source of crude protein, crude fiber, available phosphorus, unsaturated fatty acids and essential amino acids, which can allow it to effectively replace soya and corn in the poultry feed and that too at a reduced feed cost. Further with an increased use of feed grains in ethanol production, utilization of by-products as animal feed will be economically and most feasible rather than their disposal as waste which also results in environmental pollution.

Ethanol production is continually increasing to replace the fossil fuels and therefore the availability of DDGS will be enormous throughout the season to be used in poultry diet with economic advantage. DDGS have a better feed intake, feed conversion ratio, live weight gains. DDGS also improve meat and egg quality by enriching it with Omega-3 fatty acids (linoleic acid) which helps in checking cardiac diseases in humans. The use of high quality corn DDGS in layer diets is an excellent partial replacement of corn, soyabean meal and inorganic phosphate and supports excellent layer performance and egg quality. These can be added in the feed of laying hen at a level of 10-20%, accounting for about 30% of the total dietary protein, without synthetic lycine supplementation and with no adverse effect on egg production and egg weight. Further, there is an improvement in internal egg quality (Haugh units). Due to high xanthophyll content, DDGS feeding improves egg yolk colour. The oleic acid content decreases and linoleic acid increases in the egg yolk, thus improving the food quality of eggs. Feeding of up to 15% DDGS does not adversely affect production.

In case of broilers, there is positive improvement in liveweight gains and carcass quality. The weight gain increases from 2.5% with DDGS up to 25%. However, quality DDGS is accepted in broiler diet upto 6% in the starters and 12-15% in growers and finisher.

Due to the use of sulphuric acid in ethanol production from food grains, the by-products have high sulphate content, increasing the risk of sulphur toxicity specially when fed in large quantities. A high concentration of H_2S inhibits the oxidation process in nerve tissues and results in central nervous system disorders. In addition, mycotoxins in feed are a risk factor. Maize, a major source of energy in poultry feed is susceptible to fungal infection producing mycotoxins. Due to an increased in concentration of the non-starch ingredients undergo during the distillery process, mycotoxin concentrations inceases three fold in corn distillers' grains compared to the original grains. There are also ways to alleviate mycotoxin problems such as removing damaged gains before they enter the process. Chemical treatments with NaOH, NH_4OH, H_2O_2, NaCl and CH_2OH need to be performed to detoxify mycotoxins.

Certain traditional liquor distilleries use copper rather than stainless steel for stills and pipes and thus their by-products have high level of copper, which is toxic. While copper content and biological copper availability are highly variable in liquor by-products, it is essential to determine the copper content in distillers' grain by-product. Copper is however is not an issue in industrial ethanol production.

Currently, inclusion of 15% of corn DDGS in poultry feed is recommended, but higher levels of corn DDGS can be used in poultry diet.

13.3 Vaccination of Chickens at Appropriate Time and under Ideal Circumstances

The chicks can be vaccinated in hatchery or subsequently in the poultry farms. The former is more effective as the hatchery environment is 100% sterile and the persons handling the chicks are skilled professionals. They have gone through a shower and wear sterilized cloths and a head gear.

The hatchery vaccination area should be fitted with a separated air conditioner system where the incoming air is filtered to remove dust particles which may harbour pathogenic organisms. The area should be separate from the hatchery and self contained with all facilities for ablutions, shower and restaurant for attandants. For attendants, the room should be 100% clean and sterilized every day before the start of the operation and should be no smoking zone.

Vaccination programmes vary tremendously, depending upon (i) the country and location of the farm within the country, (ii) disease situation, (iii) geographical and climatic factors, (iv) whether preference of a large commercial farm or an individual producer's farm and (v) type of production and housing system employed.

Whatever is the programme for the disease against which vaccination is to be done must follow the requisite guide-lines. The vaccination of the parent flock and immunity status should be determined every two months to ensure that the immunity level is satisfactory. In many countries, *in-ovo* vaccination is done which involves the vaccination in yet to be hatched chicks. In the setters it can be done only at the 18.5 days and a half day after the eggs are set or at the time of transfer to the hatchers. This is normally done between 17.5 day and 19.2 days with best results at 18.5 days. The egg setting time is calculated as zero hour to correspond with the hatch day. Any hatchery takes off the chicks starting in late afternoon or early morning. *In-ovo* technology has been used in USA for last 20 years and more particularly in parent stock due to high cost of the equipment used in *in-ovo* vaccination. The other advantages are that the egg containing dead embryos are left out thus saving the vaccine and the effort. It has been shown that use of a dual needle is better from sanitation point of view and reduces the risk of contamination. Currently, there is combined vaccine for Infectious Bursal Disease (IBD) or Gumboro and New Castle Disease (ND). This reduces effort of twice vaccinating. The *in-ovo* vaccination allows the chick to start building immunity 2.5- 3.0 days earlier than normal hatch chicks with less stress as in subcutaneous vaccination.

13.4 Lower Level of Feeding Protein to Broiler Females Results in Higher Lay

The body composition of broiler breeders has dramatically changed due to market demand. Genetic selection of broiler has resulted in higher efficiency of feed conversion, higher live weight gain, less fat and more breast muscle. The deposition of fat is less efficiently use of energy and due to demand of more meat and less fat. The feeding regimen needs to be better balanced in terms of energy and protein in the diet. The change in the feed composition towards higher protein levels lead to a higher development of more breast muscle and less fat results. It also improves reproduction rate. Over the last decade, the fertility and hatchability in broilers has declined. This could be due to management, ratio of males to females, health and behavior. This could also be connected with diet composition and in particular daily protein intake during laying period. The fertility and hatchability decline towards the laying period proceeds towards the terminal part. This may be due to insufficient fat reserves with the advancement in the laying period. This however, can be improved by changing the diet composition towards the lowering the protein intake during the rearing period. Little is however known about the effect of the body composition on reproduction in broiler breeders. Different feeding regimens during rearing and laying period can influence body composition. After 48 weeks breeders fed low protein diet during the rearing period produced more eggs (3.5 hatching eggs). This may be because of increased fat reserves at the end of rearing period produces more eggs. The birds were able to mobilize energy reserves during negative energy balance. To maintain the growth pattern during rearing broiler, breeders should be provided high amount of feed with higher energy : protein ratio.

It increases eating time and less unnecessary pecking during rearing which may be indicated by reduction in hunger and frustration. The low daily protein intake during rearing can lead to a poor feather cover. A 12% increase in daily feed intake due to low protein content can increase two fold increase in eating time. The eating time is inversely related to time spent on wasteful activities. Time budgeting in behavior showed that the eating time was inversely related to time spent for wasteful activities such as pecking and fighting with other birds, especially in birds raised on floor. A high energy diet during the first phase of lay increased mortality due to rupture of the tendons. This was probably caused by the lower feed intake during the initial laying period resulting in more activity and lack of uniformity. Feeding birds the standard diet as advised by breeder company produce more eggs than the birds fed the high or low energy diets.

Feeding a high energy diet during the second phase of lay lowers the protein intake with an average of 8.5% and energy intake with 2%. Even if the crude protein and aminoacid composition is the same, the total feed intake is influenced by energy content. The differential energy level have little effect on egg production except birds fed on high energy diet produced eggs with a slightly lower egg weight caused by the lower daily intake of aminoacid and Linoleic acid. A lower egg weight in the second phase of laying period is positive as these eggs cost lesser nutrients. The birds fed with high energy diet and thus relatively low protein intake showed 1.5% higher hatchability. The chicken fed the high energy feed had a lower feed available (9%), less feed intake time (16%) and a higher speed of feed intake (9%).

It is generally advised that energy : protein should be increased in broiler breeders during the rearing and second phase of lay to improve reproduction and welfare. Increased feed allowance by 10% during rearing provides a similar daily growth pattern. The energy protein ratio should not be changed in the first phase of laying period for the breeders.

13.5 Antibiotic Reduction while Containing Coccidiosis

Antimicrobial resistance has become a global public health concern in human and domestic animals. As a result many countries have decided on a sustainable policy for the use of antibiotics in the domestic animal sector.

Coccidiosis still is a major problem in broiler production and economically most important. Losses due to mortality and morbidity are high and the chemical control in addition to cost is becoming less effective due to increased resistance. Coccidiosis is one of the most important predisposing factors for bacterial enteritis. This direct effect on endemic health results in the prevalence of other enteric or systemic diseases. Vaccination against coccidiosis can also have indirect effect on gastro-intestinal related diseases such as dysbacteriosis, necrotic enteritis, and septicaemia after the gastrointestinal tract leakage. The consumption of antibiotics could therefore be altered as has been seen that the implementation of a coccidiosis vaccination programme in rotation with anticoccidiosis drug yields a significantly higher improvement. The use of vaccine against coccidiosis along with the use of antibiotics has shown an intestinal integrity. The antibiotics used for non-enteric indications have shown prevention of coccidiosis although an indirect positive effect of coccidiosis vaccine on other diseases can be expected due to improvement in intestinal integrity. It is commonly believed that more necrotic enteritis and dysbacteriosis appear in vaccinated flock due to lack of anti-clostridial effect of ionophores. No cases of necrotic enteritis are however seen after the treatment. The quantity of antibiotics used for enteric diseases declined on vaccination. The implementation of a coccidiosis vaccination in a rotation programme for control of coccidiosis could be one of the solutions to respond to the expectations concerning anti-microbial resistance.

13.6 Replacing Formaldehyde in Disinfection of Eggs

Hatcheries are on the top of poultry production pyramid with a lot of high skilled people pushing it forward. Furthermore, the poultry industry has become international where certain decisions at hatchery level can be implemented easily and quickly throughout the world.

An alternative application of formaldehyde is picking up fast as use of formaldehyde out of the hatchery is becoming a part of standard protocol in hatchery management. The adverse effect of the use of formaldehyde on people working in hatcheries is becoming a serious issue leading to banning of use of formaldehyde in hatcheries. There are two ways of defining the exposure limits to formaldehyde. Time-weighted- average (TWA) concentration over 8 hours and a short term exposure limit (STEL) during 15 minutes. The TWA varies both in concentration and maximum exposure time among countries. The STEL has more or less the same variation. The second way is the MEL, the maximum exposure limit. Alternative to formaldehyde have been used. It involves a combination of formalin and potassium per manganate ($KMnO_4$). 10 gram of paraformaldehyde per m^3 has shown a significant relationship between embryonic mortality, duration of fumigation and the concentration of formaldehyde. A significant decline (8%) was reported when formaldehyde fumigation was used for longer duration (40 min) and higher concentration (12.5 g/ m^3). Now with MEL of 0.3ppm is definitely not recommended. The problem also lies with infrastructural difficulties. The use of formaldehyde would require a bigger air evacuation system. In practice it is difficult to follow. Two hours after fumigation and air evacuation only 5g/m3 of parformaldehyde, the MEL of 0.3ppm still exceeds by 14 times. The use of lesser formaldehyde does not make it any easier and raises questions about its microbicidal efficacy.

In the last 2-3 years, alternate product and method for disinfection of hatcheries by fumigation or cold fogging with a disinfectant solution is being widely used. It ensures that the eggs do not get wet and the protocol is fully automatic. Virocid, a combination of glutaraldehyde and multichained quarternary ammonium produced by CID lines has proven to be a good alternative to formaldehyde for disinfection of hatching eggs before setting.

There is a relationship between the droplet size of the vapour, the contact angel (wettability), type and concentration of the the chemical have as a large impact on the success of the disinfection of the hatching eggs. There is a significant difference between the long reductuion of formaldehyde and virocid. In ultrasonic fogging, virocid has the same effect as the formaldehyde however, in cold foggers, virocid is significantly better than the formaldehyde.

The eggs can be swabbed with the shell rinced method using a bag containg 10 ml warm buffered salt solution. The bag is sealed and kept as such till it arrives at the lab. After fogging and air evacuation times, the air is sampled in the fumigation room to measure the remaining glutaraldehyde in the air. For glutaraldehyde (as in Virocid) the maximum exposure limit is 0.05ppm.

The eggs can be disinfected before setting starting with foggining to taking out the trolleys for setting. It is possible to replace formaldehyde with virocid for hatchery disinfection. Field trials have shown a significant lower mortality percentage during first week of the chicks' life when hatcher fumigation is being applied with 2% Virocid solution.

13.7 Nutritional Strategies to Manipulate Microbial Population of Gastro-intestinal Tract

Sustaining healthy micro-biota of gastro-intestinal (GI) tract through suppression of pathogenic bacteria with promotion of beneficial bacteria can be an alternative to use of chemical inputs. Good intestinal health is related to normal ecological equilibrium of the GI tract micro-biota. A wide range of micro-organisms are found in a normal ecological equilibrium in a healthy bird. One of the nutritional strategies used to achive this goal is direct manipulation of the microbial population. The addition of a direct fed microbial or pro-biotic provides support to the animal's defence in suppressing pathogenic micro-organisms while promoting beneficial bacteria for maintenance for GI health. Clostat is an active microbial additive containing a strain of *Bacillus subtilus* that has been developed as nutritional solution to maintain intestinal microbiota and thus GI tract integrity and animal production. *In-vitro* and *In-vivo* confirm that Clostat can reduce the population of pathogenic bacteria such as *Clostridium perfringens* while maintaining growth of beneficial bacteria such as *Lactobacili and Bifido* bacterium. Despite the benefits of improving animal performance through the use of AGPs and imbalance in the intestinal microbiota can be created. This is caused by elimination of gram positive bacteria both pathogenic and beneficial, resulting in excessive growth of gram negative bacteria. An ideal replacement per AGPs would be products that can eliminate pathogenic gram positive bacteria while maintaining beneficial bacteria properly functioning. This will have least disturbance of the intestinal microbial environment. In the absence of AGPs, *Clostridium perfingens* can be controlled with the use of a probiotics like Clostat.

The new defence is energetically expensive, therefore the rate at which animals transform energy and nutrients can be expected to be regulated as a result of immune defence activation. This means that the allocation of energy is determined by the health status of the animal. In a healthy animal only 10% of energy goes to the immune system, 30% each to maintenance, growth and reproduction. However in an unhealthy animal 80% energy goes to immune response and 20% for maintenance or there may be no energy for maintenance and growth. Threfore inflamatory responses in animals are responsible for inhibition for growth and reproduction. The Clostat improves performance through destruction of *C. perfingens*.

Efficient use of nutrients in productive animals is accomplished in a number of ways including maximizing nutrient digestibility and absorption. The digestibility is optimized through actions of efficient digestive enzyme secretion, a balanced intestinal microbial population and maintenance mucosal integrity throughout the GI tract. The GI tract is anatomically fully developed at birth but takes time for attaining full functional capability. This partially depends on genetic constitution only after 10 days of age when feed conversion efficiency reaches its best point between day of hatching and day 5. During this phase the mucosal development is based on the increase in size of villi and micro-villi, its density (number of anteriocytes and the amount of functional anteriocytes on the vilir, all of which will improve the absorption capacity as the animal grows. All the morphological and physiological changes in the intestine that take place during the post hatch period are directly meant to enlargement to the absorptive surface and the differentiation and maturatuion of the epithelial cell, enzymes and nutrient carriers. Butyrate, a short chain fatty acid produced by the microbial fermentation primarily in the large intestine has direct effect on mucosal cell proliferation, maturation and differentiation and thus improving gut health.

13.8 New Approaches for Animal Rendering

Possibility of rendering animal bi-products are enormous both for lessening environmental impact of animal protein production for pigs and poultry. When it comes to rendering, it must be a green industry and avoid any environmental impact. Rendering animal bi-products rather than composting prevents 70% of CO_2 emission. Further considering energy requirement for transport and rendering meat and bone meal, it can compete with vegetable protein. The efficient bringing an essentially waste product to value added product can reduce the cost of production as well as the negative impact of its disposal by any other means. Inclusion of 5% rendered material in feed can replace same amount of energy and protein from other sources like Soya and CO_2 from 794 to 752 kilo per tonne of feed. Since protein is scarce and costly, the use of meat and bone meal can substantially reduce the cost. However, the crisis of Mad Cow disease (BSE) must be avoided through proper rendering.

13.9 Value Added Turkey and Quail meat products

Turkey production as a component of poultry production in India contributes less than 0.5% on R&D, but gaining is important because of its use on festive occasion like Thanks Giving and Chrismas by Christian community. Further, it can be raised under back yard farming system by small and marginal farmers. There is no cultural or religious taboo in consumption of turkey meat which is a red meat but has low flavor, is tender and has higher meat : bone ratio. The cholesterol and phosphlipid content of turkey meat are slightly higher than chicken meat. Under intensive management, the meat production cost of turkey are comparatively higher than chicken and selling dressed carcasses directly to the consumers is difficult due to the large carcass size and unorganized marketing system of turkey meat. Raising turkey can be profitable if its meat is used for value added products such as turkey rolls, turkey ham, turkey breast fillets, turkey meat block, nuggets, patties, balls, kebabs, tikka, pickels and enrobed products.

Quail is another avian species which can be economically raised, has a high dressed carcass yield (70%) and breast and thighs contribute 68% to the total carcass weight. The meat is sweet, white like game meat of high quality and is considered delicious. It contains balanced protein with essential amino acids and less carbohydrates. It is rich in micro-nutrients specially vitamins (B complex, E & K). The meat has extremely low skin fat and cholesterol and is recommended for people suffering from cardio-vascular problems. Further, the bird lays a larger number of eggs which are smaller in size and can be conseumed more easily even by economically weaker section. A variety of value added products can be made from quail eggs and meat. Since the two species are not as popular as chicken, the specialized product and intrinsic food value need to be widely informed to the consumers. Quail eggs can be incorporated as whole egg liquid or cooked alone or in combination with other food sources for reducing cost and providing nutritional advantage.

13.10 Securing Carcass Quality in Chicken with Minerals

Although in India birds are sold alive for consumption of meat and the carcass quality is given little importance, here is need to ensure proper quality of chicken carcasses and this will require (i) that they are intact, including the presentation which should be clean and free from any foreign matter and any undesirable odor, (ii) free from visible blood stain except which are small and robtrusive and (iii) Protruding free from broken bones and severe contusions and (iv) the quality of blood vessels, the strength of bones and tendons indicate of better broiler carcass quality. The two major defects in the carcass are bone strength and tendons which are related to Tibial Dys-chondroplasia and perosis pathologies which impact negatively animal performance due to lameness. The two diseases are partly due to nutritional deficiency especially trace minerals. Tibial Dys-chondroplasia is a disease where growth plate cartilage accumulates in the metaphyseal region of the tibiotarsus. The disease is associated with fast growth and the lesions can increase with age. The most important cause is copper deficiency. Some deficiencies in other trace elements such as zinc have also been shown to inhibit chondrocytes (cartilage cells) resulting in proliferation and an increase in their apoptosis in broilers. It has been found that most of the trace elements intervene in bone formation as they act as co-factors of different specific enzymes involved in the process. The zinc acts through its effect on protein and nucleic acid metabolism, as a cofactor of alkaline phosphatase or collagenases or through the modification of the crystalline structure of apatite (bone mineral matrix). It also acts as a cofactor in lysyl oxidase, an enzyme which controls the regulation of collagen and elastin fibre reticulation. The manganese acts a cofactor of glycosyltransferase which is implicated in the formation of glycosamino-glycane containing chondroitine sulphate and in the synthesis of proteoglycanes present in the conjugating cartilage of avian epiphysis. Therefore, these trace elements can potentially reduce tibial dyschodroplasia through strengthening bone formation.

Perosis

Perosis is the enlargement of the tibio-metatarsel's joint resulting in the bending of the distal end of the tibia and the proximal end of the metatarsal and its displacement Achilles tenton. This seriously impairs locomotion and the bird is unable to stand. The condition is associated with a large number of trace mineral deficiencies. The omission of manganese in diets depresses growth rate and increases the incidence and severity of bone abnormality. Doses of 55 mg/kg of manganese as MnCl deceases the incidence. There is a decrease in phosphatase activity in both blood and bone and impacts carcass quality.

Paw quality

Footpad dermatitis affets the plantar region of the feet in birds. Initially there is discoloration of the skin followed by hyperkeratosis and necrosis of the epidermis. There may be inflamation and ulceration of the subcutaneous tissue. Although a large number of factors are responsible but a little moisture is a major cause. Supplementation of organic form of trace minerals reduces the incidence.

Carcass quality

Trace minerals not only cause conditions referred to earlier but also results in other pathologies due to affecting enzyme co-factors resulting in an increase in alkaline phophatase which impacts incidence of perosis in zinc deficient birds and leads to down grading of carcasses. The Zinc and Copper deficiencies induce tibial dyschondroplasia and manganese deficiencies induce perosis thus impacting locomotion and carcass quality in broiler chickens. The provision of B-TRAXIM 2C reduces negative impact of these trace element deficiency.

13.11 Role of Lysophospholipids in Nutrient Absorption Enhancement in Chicken

Both commercial layers and broilers have shown a consistant improvement in the last few decades. This has primarily occurred due to improvement in genetic potential through following intensive selection and appropriate mating systems, a more balanced nutrition, health care and management. There has been a large growth in the poultry industry, increase in size of individual farms and greater mechanisation in management. This has resulted in broilers reaching 3.0 kg at 40 days of age and layers producing 340 eggs in 52 weeks of lay. Of the management factor, nutrition has played a vital role both in quality and expenses. The provision of a good quality feed with all essential nutrients especially essential amino acids, minerals and vitamins has been ensured. This is helping in better feed intake, digestibility, absorption and assimilation. If the nutrients are not absorbed within a short time (4 h), they are attacked by the bacteria in the large intestine or excreted as fecal matter, resulting in waste of nutrients and inefficient growth and productivity. With rising feed cost, the birds' ability to absorb nutrients optimally is an important aspect of overall efficiency of production. Therefore increased emphasis has been laid on optimizing the feed efficiency and lowering the nutrient loss through droppings.

Phospholopids and fluidity of bilayer embryo are important practices affecting cell boundries and its organells and act as permeability barriers. The biological membranes have flexibility, i.e. ability to change shape witout losing their integrity and becoming leaky. The "Fluid Mosaic" model of cell memberanes indicates that membranes are made of lipid bilayer and memberane protein (peripherals and integral). The lipid component of the membrane is a two dimentional fluid in which the constituent molecules are free to move laterally. The lipid bilayer functions both as a solvent for integral proteins and as a permeability barrier. Peripheral membrane proteins are anchored at the surface of the membrane while the integral membrane proteins are contained in transmembrane regions allowing the proteins to pass completely. The two classes of membrane proteins contribute to the "mosaic" aspects of the fluid mosaic model.

Phospholipids (PLs) are most abundant lipids in membranes, and are amphipathic in nature, having hydrophilic and lypophilic properties. Phospholipids are characterized by a glycerol backbone to which a polar hydrophilic phosphodiester group and two lypophilic hydrocarbons are linked.

Alongwith phospholipid, the animal cell membrane also contains significant amount of steroid, mainly cholesterol which is necessary for maintaining and stabilizing the membrane by acting a fluidity buffer. Though the lipid bilayer structure is quite stable, its individual phospholipid and sterol molecules have some freedom of movement.

Lysophosphatidylcholine (LPC) like molecules affect the fluidity of cell membrane by changing cholesterol level in the membranes thus affecting the dynamics of the membrane. Lysophospholipid (LPL) are glycerophospholipids in which one acyl chain is lacking as compared to PLs and therefore one hydrogen group of the glycerol backbone is acylated. LPLs which induce Lysophosphatidylcholine (LPC), Lysophosphatidylethanolamine (LPE), Lysophosphatidyl inositol (LPI) and Lysophosphatidylserine (LPS) are prepared by enzymatic hydrolysis of natural Soy Lecithin by phospholipase A2.

Each memberane at equilibrium has pores and holes where phospholipids are missing from the lattice structure. Sometimes there are clusters of these vacancies of various sizes. When additional LPLs are introduced, it is their distribution that is affected and results in an increase in both in numbers and size of the pores. The exogenous LPL get quickly inter digitated into the bilayer membranes. The close packing between the layers is disrupted and the lipids go in a disorderly state and the membrane become more fluid due to increased number and size of pores. This beneficially affects the nutrient absorption in the gut due to passive flux hurdle being temporarily lowered. LPLs have the ability to change the attraction between lipids and displace calcium ions. This increases freedom of movement and lipids can aggregate closer together making the existing hole larger so that the larger molecules are easily absorbed. A pre-determined ratio between PLs and LPLs has to be maintained and also between different LPLs to have a consistent and desired end effects.

The LPLs act as a membrane fluidity moderator. They increase the number and size of pores by affecting the mechanical properties of the membranes thereby enhancing the flux rate at which the nutrients of various molecular sizes pass across the intestinal membrane and thus act as absorption enhancer.

13.12 Reducing Feed Cost, an Important Task in Commercial Poultry Production

The genetic improvement in broilers with higher growth rate, thus reducing period for which a bird is to be maintained and consequently increases the efficiency of feed conversion. The achievements of these goals require an ever increasing density of dietary nutrients, especially proteins with all aminoacids with higher digestibility. The increasing feed cost especially of protein sources with balanced aminoacids is becoming an impediment in poultry production. The meat production in poultry would have to balance the birds' growth and feed cost which amounts to essentially 60% of the total cost of broiler production. In order to balance the feed cost with achievable livewight gains, different concepts including reduction in metabolizable energy (MJ/KJ) and increasing digestible aminoacids through blending of diets with wheat or coarser grains can be implemented. An alternative is to use feed additives which promote secretion of endogenous enzymes helping in increased protein and aminoacids digestibility. The advantage of using feed additives is that their efficiency is equally high in diets with both higher or lower nutrient density. Under practical conditions, it has been observed that phytogenic digestibility enhancer has a positive impact on growth rate and efficiency of feed conversion, lowered medication cost and mortality. Managing illial digestibility efficiently results in a significant improvement in aminoacid digestibility. Higher productivity can be obtained through improved efficient feed utilization. By using soybean meal (48%), maize, wheat and soyoil in starter, grower and finisher ration so as to provide balanced nutrients results in desirable feed conversion ratio (kg feed per kg gain, FCR).

In addition to provision of balanced diet, maintenance of proper digestive and general health needs to be considered in commercial poultry production. To obtain proper efficiency of feed conversion and liveweight gains with acceptable mortality rates is essential to have more genetically superior birds supported by balanced nutrition, health and management. There is a scope for further improvement through use of digestive enhancer.

13.13 Melatonin, A Powerful Antioxidant to Ameliorate Stress in Broiler Chicken

Light is one of the essential factors in broiler production. Various physiological pathways and behavioral activity can change due to provision of light. Melatonin hormone is secreted during night and it is suppresed by light. It has various functions in the body such as affecting reproduction, metabolism and immunity. It is an effective antioxidant and is secreted by pineal gland and its secretion is affected by the light.

The high ambient temperature has a negative effect on poultry production. The feed intake and nutrient digestibility shows a declines and nutrient excretion increases, ultimately resulting in economic loss due to retardation of growth. Therefore, the birds are maintained under conditions that lower heat stress through air cooling of poultry houses. However, it is economically costly. Dietary interventions that ameliorate heat stress during production and transportation are essential. Supplementation of melatonin has a positive effect on alleviating heat stress. This increases liveweight gain, carcass yield and quality under such stressed conditions. Desreased concentration of Vitamin C, Vitamin D, Vitamin A, Fe, Zn, Cu, Cr, Cholesterol and Triglycerides can results from heat stress. The melatonin supplementation can reduce these negative effects. Hypothalamo-pitutary-adrenal-axis is activated by higher environmental temperature in response to increased level of corticosterone production which results in suppression of many immune functions and also feed intake.

Under various sress factors such as heat, transportation and psychological disturbances, there is production of reactive oxygen species (ROS) to help in normal functions of the body. Free radicals of ROS are unstable molecules and are affected by increase in temperature. Higher ROS leads to apoptosis (process of programmed cell death). Body has the mechanism to neutralize the effects of ROS i.e. antioxidant defence system both enzymatic and non-enzymatic. Antioxidants neutralize ROS efficiently but in case of excess production, it may be necessary to supplemet antioxidant from external source. Many natural feeds such as fruits contain antioxidants. Supplementation of diet with green vegetables and fruits can help in reducing the effects of ROS.

The requirement of melatonin varies with different physiological functions. The synthesis of melatonin is not limited to pineal gland and other body tissues also supplement melatonin. Under tropical environment with high temperature and humidity, the homeostatic mechanism is disturbed. There may be difficulty in dissipation of heat through evaporation leading to overloading of heat on the body. With an increase in humidity during summer, there is decrease in evaporating cooling which adds leads to oxidative stress. One of the preventative measures to ameliorate heat stress can be supplementation of melatonin or provision of cooling system.

13.14 Supplementing Diets with Acidifiers for Improving Broiler Performance

It is known that natural immune system is not properly developed in newly hatched chicken and pathogenic bacteria such as Enterobacteria and Enterococcia can multiply in GI tract and damage cell wall in intestines, adversely affecting the performance due to impaired absorption of nutrients. The feed additives which affect microbial population in GI tract are used to ameliorate the negative effect. Earlier antibiotics were used both as antimicrobial as well as growth promoters. The continuous use of antibiotics though at extremely low levels in feed to improve feed efficiency and production, has gradually led to drug resistance. Alternative to antibiotics are now been investigated and one of them are acidifiers and organic acids which can stimulate natural immune functions. The positive effect of these feed additives may be through (i) reducing colonization of pathogenic microbes, (ii) reduction in production and release of toxic components from microbial growth, (iii) protection against anti-bacterial effect, (iv) decrease in intraluminal concentration of coliform bacteria and other acid tolerant organisms which result in digestive disorders, (v) reduction in pH which limits the microbial growth, (vi) Undissociated organic acid can easily penetrate the lipin membrane of bacteria and fungi, releasing the protons in the alkaline cytoplasm through decreased intracellular pH. This alters enzymatic reactions and the nutrient transport system, forcing the bacteria to use energy to relase protons and cause an intracellular acid anion accommodation. Other benefits are improvent in digestive enzyme and increased microbial phytase activity, increased pancreatic secretion and stimulation of GI cell proliferation.

Acidifiers can be organic or inorganic or associated salts. Organic acids are widely distributed in plants and animals. They are also produced by microbial fermentation of carbohydrate and other fermentable products in GI tract. They are a variety of organic acids which include acetic acid, benzoic acid, butyric acid, citric acid, formic acid, fumaric acid, lactic acid, propionic acid and sorbic acid. Although inorganic acid such as HCl and phosphoric acid reduc the pH but are ineffective whereas organic acid even when week acids are only partly disassociated in the GI tract.

13.15 Poultry Waste Management

Most poultry units are located in peri-urban areas. This is more true for broiler production since broilers are still sold alive and dressed in the presence of customer. The concentration of large units leads to a large accumulation of poultry waste. A layer annually produces approximately 18 kg of dry matter and considering the current layer production, the waste would be around 4.5 m MT. There are two main types of wastes depending upon the rearing system. The layers are raised more on deep litre and in cages. The waste arising from deep liter does not have much nutritive value as it is mixed with litter. Cage layer waste consists of mostly excretions, spilled feed and feathers and can be used as feed and fertilizer.

Deep stocking of poultry waste produces considerable heat and destroys most of infective agents including coliforms. The maximu temperature can be reached in 4-8 days in a heaped litter and is sufficient to destroy most pathogenic organisms. Fresh poultry waste can be disposed off in an open pond when it provides nutrients for phyto- and zoo- plantons which can be used for raising fish.

Airation leads to oxidation. The droppings are collected in a continuous moving flowing trough placed under the cages. The manure is oxygenated by the paddles moving the waste, increasing the activity of aerobic bacteria which destroys the pathogens and removes bad odour. The litter is allowed to build up for 4-6 months or even longer and is used as feed especially for ruminants after proper sun drying or as organic fertilizer.

Dead birds are generally thrown on waste dump and result in spread of infection. Deep hole on the ground for disposal of carcass with some lime added to avoid bad smell and destroy infection effectively. The disposal should be atleast 150 ft away from the poultry farms. The pit should be regularly covered by fresh earth / vegetable waste.

The manure may be composted and this can allow accumulation for a long time. Aerobic bacterial action leads to destruction of pathogens. Such pits can be kept operative for several years without removal of manure. The top layer is composed of fresh manure and bottom is under anaerobic conditions and the central portion is undergoing composting. Management of deep manure disposal pit would require wet material to be adequately aerated to remove the moisture and prevent odour. Care must be taken that the drinkers donot leak and thus donot wet the accumulated manure. Poultry manure especially from the layers raised in cages can be used as 10-15% of ruminant feed and save on cost of protein feed component. The amount of nitrogen and phosphorus generated in the litter and subsequently in the manure exceeds the fertilizer requirement for crop production on adjacent crop farm. When poultry litter is applied to the soil surface about half of the N and other nutrients are available for plant production. Proper management of poultry house waste through proper storage, transportation and application to the land can help in proper nutrient management.

The use of synthetic amino acids can not only reduce dietary protein concentration but also an excretion in case of P in the form of phytic acid or phytene is largely not available to poultry so adding supplements like phytase can help in the availability of P and its excretion. The use of other enzymes can also modify feed ingredients by increasing nutritive value of diet and thereby reducing their excretion.

Poultry droppings have generally been considered organic manure in crop production but now they are being used as alternative nutrient especially in ruminant after processing resource. Dried poultry waste contains approximately 30% protein of which about 60% is NPN. The dried poultry waste has high mineral value and low metabolizable energy. Poultry droppings may contain various types of microbes, therefore before its recycling as a part of ruinant feed, it should be properly processed. Longer duration of storage can help in reducing microbial load.

13.16 Driving Forces in Poultry Economics

Egg and poultry meat are richest sources of most nutrients specially proteins, minerals and vitamins. The egg and poultry meat are still the cheapest source of high quality protein. Traditionally the birds were raised in the backyard with little feed and health inputs. This is seriously changed since 1950s and poultry industry has become highly commercialised linking different components starting from breeding farm, hatcheries and commercial chick farms, compounded feed units and processing and marketing units. Contract farming is gradually increasing with companies providing both forward and backward linkages. Since long the industry has been focusing on productivity improvement but now it is increasingly concerned with enhancing the distribution of production infrastructure, value addition and control over the supply chain. Due to low margin and almost no value addition or little processing more particularly in broilers where shelf life of meat is much lower than in case of eggs, there is need to make a large investment in processing of broilers and cold chain and educating people in accepting frozen chicken. India is now the second largest producer of broilers in Asia and fourth largest in the world. The Investment and Credit Rating Agency of India (INCRA) has projected the demand of broiler meet to grow @ 8-10% per annum.

The analysis of egg and broiler prices shows that the industry as a whole has poor margin of profits. There are a number of factors that have affected the prices of egg and broiler. The inflation in recent years has driven prices of most food commodities. The clear idea of how the prices fluctuate every year due to changes in macro-economic structure can lead to decision in production of eggs and broilers. There are seasonal variations in egg prices besides yearly variation in feed ingredients among different states. The average egg prices are generally higher during winter especially in November and December and lowest in April. Before 2005, the egg prices had stayed relatively stable inspite of large inflation; the demand has not grown significantly since that time. There has been a high inflation in egg prices in the year 2008 which was attributed to a decline in egg production and growth of layer units as well as increase in cost of production because of rise in prices of poultry feed. Further the incidence of bird flu in 2010 led to a lowered egg production. Subsequently there has been an increase in prices because of higher demand, higher transportation cost and higher input cost.

For the broiler industry, year 2012 had been experienced serious difficulties. Growth slipped to 9%, much lower than in the preceeding years. Some larger farms had to continue their production inspite of the fluctuating market prices. The prices of eggs and poultry meat have recently seen an increase due to high feed prices and poor crop harvest world wide.

Currently it is common to achieve a hen house production of 310 eggs in 52 weeks in layers and 3.0 kg live weight in less than 6 weeks with a feed conversion ratio between 1.8 and 1.9 in broilers. There is an increasing consumption of poultry meat and eggs and if the trend continues, it will triple to 9.0 kg broiler meat per year by 2030. The feed which represents almost 70% of the total production cost has resulted in higher than the returns from the sale of eggs and broilers is rising faster than the prices of eggs and broiler meat but the poultry production is still growing phenomenally inspite of poor market sustainability and zoonotic infectious disease problems in addition to feed cost. In addition to feed, the cost of other inputs like labour and electricity has also increased. In addition to general inflation, these are major factors which have been driving the prices for eggs and broiler meat.

The profit margin for broiler industry is declining due to increased number of enterprises. It has also declined with the lowering of share following share of local production of broilers. This has been as a result of higher impact of imports indicating greater choice for quality. This calls for increasing investment in infrastructure for the poultry industry to make it more productive domestically. It is prudent that an investor would make higher investment in smoothening the supply chain in poultry business which will take care of compounded feed cost, other input costs and transportation cost. There is need for developing strategies to address the demand and supply imbalance arising from time to time. It will also ensure that inflation fluctuations are under control. Adequate investment is also needed in diversifying products and improved economics of poultry production and finally improving the broiler and egg quality. This is required creating big brands providing quality products. This will further a way to attract better government efforts in FDI, better technology and low cost capital.

13.17 Rural Poultry Production

Rural poultry production is generally synonymous with free range grazing of indigenous (unselected/selected) / their crosses with exotic layer / broiler breeds. Since independence the Government of India (GOI) and State Governments have been encouraging rural poultry production through distributing male of exotic layer/ dual purpose and providing health cover and compounded feed. The backyard poultry production essentially involves free range maintenance of birds during the day so that they can pick up any organic matter and meet their nutrient requirement. At night they may be provided with simple protection from predators. The GOI and State Governments are promoting the rural poultry production to provide economic sustainability, nutritional security especially alleviating protein deficiency. In addition to chicken, other avian species especially duck (mostly in coastal areas), turkeys, quail, gunea fowl and emu are involved.

Back yard poultry production thus required little investment on infrastructure and is primarily meant for providing supplementary income and nutrition. There is a large demand for indigenous chicken eggs and live birds as most people consider these to be more nutritious. For example the eggs have deep yellow yolk. A number of egg, broiler and dual purpose chicken strains have been evolved which are suitable for extensive rearing in rural areas. There are some commercial producers of such chicken and are promoting their large scale production.

The back yard poultry needs care during brooding and during initial six weeks of age. Although backyard poultry germplasm is more resistant to most infectious diseases, they should be vaccinated against Ranikhet and Fowlpox. To improve their production and survival, supplementary feed especially upto six weeks of age will be desirable. Green leaves such as from Subabool and Malberry and some broken grains or household waste food can be provided. Azola and white ant can be used as supplementing protein requirement.

Organizing rural poultry production into farmers group such as cooperatives for providing production inputs and marketing facilities for eggs and live birds can help in improving returns from the enterprise. There is a possibility of creating a large number of small intensive poultry production units on the pattern of dairy cooperatives/ producer companies where the cooperative/ producer company maintains collectively the input and marketing facilities, giving a large marketing output and a large supply input which can be more economical and in addition to providing high quality eggs and chicken meat. It can provide remunerative employment.

13.18 Egg shell- An Economic By-product

The outer hard covering / shell protect the inner contents of the egg. It takes around 20 hours to form. The egg consists of egg shell, air pocket/ cell, shell membrane, thin albumin, thick albumin, chalazae which is another yolk, viteline membrane, next cornea, the germinal disc and egg yolk. Egg shell serves to protect the egg against damage and microbial contamination, desiccation, regulation of gas and water exchange for the growing embryo and provides calcium for embryogenesis. It makes 9-12% of the egg weight and contains 27 essential microelements, primarily calcium with some magnesium carbonate, calcium phosphate and organic matter, small amounts of sodium, potassium, zinc, manganese, iron, copper and sulphur. It also contains some water, protein, crude fat, ash, alanine, arginine, asparticacid, cystine, histidine, leucine, isoleucine, lysine, tyrosine, valine, phenylalanine, proline, serine and threonine.

Inspite there is limited processing of eggs and thus availability of large quantity of eggshell at a few places but it is advisable not to consider eggshell as waste and sending it as a land fill. It can increase the soil fertility and quickly decomposes and provides calcium and some other minerals. Crushed eggshell can be used in potted plants and house hold raised flower, vegetables and fruits trees. It can also be used as eco-friendly pesticides. It can also be further used as a coating pigment for inkjet printing paper, various decorative purposes, as a food additive to filter coffee and to reduce its bitterness. It is biodegradable and can be used for raising seedlings. It is also used as eco-friendly household abrasive in the crushed form and with a little soapy water can be used to clean thermoses and vessels. It is non-toxic and can be used as a natural drain cleaner especially sinks in the kitchen. It traps additional solids and gradually brakes up and naturally cleans pipes as it passes down the drain. It has important medicinal values such as healing cuts, treating grown toe nails, skin irritation and skin tightening specially on the face. It can be used as a source of calcium in animal feed.

❑❑❑

CHAPTER-14

Summary and Conclusions - Current Status, Strengths, Weaknesses, Opportunities and Threats (SWOT) Analysis in Poultry Production in India and Way Forward

14.1 Current Status

Currently poultry production has emerged as the most dynamic and rapid growing component of Domestic Animal (DA) sub-sector of the agriculture in India with an average annual growth of about 5% in layer production and 10% in broiler production. This has happened in the last 10 years. The Indian poultry industry contributes Rs. 400 billion to the national GDP which is 0.058% and is 10% of the GDP from DA. The success of poultry production is due to its transformation from backyard rural and peri-urban production utilizing indigenous avian genetic resources, essentially non-descript production types, with little emphasis on their sustainable management and conservation and developing approaches for improvement through breeding, improved nutrition, appropriate health cover and adequate housing and management. Most information is available on indigenous avian genetic resources under free range scavenging conditions with little production and protection inputs. At present 5 million people are directly or indirectly engaged in the poultry sector and in addition there are a large number of people engaged in processing and marketing. The major development of commercial poultry production is in urban and peri-urban areas and is in the hand of few multi-national and national poultry breeding farms which produce commercial layers and broilers from grandparent lines or pure-lines/strains imported from large international poultry breeding concerns. These have very large poultry breeding research and development facilities with best poultry geneticists, nutritionists, management specialists and health specialist employed. The availability of high producing commercial chicks without any difficulty and at reasonable price has led to a large expansion of commercial egg and broiler farms in the country. However they are essentially located in urban and peri-urban areas as they do not depend on regular production of feed inputs like in ruminant DA and meet essentially the requirement of urban neo-rich who have better education, employment opportunities, nuclear families, and realization of the importance of animal protein and the taste and satiety factors it provides. The rural areas produce less than 30% of eggs and hardly any broiler and primarily depend on indigenous birds of different avian species mostly chicken and in limited areas ducks. Other avian species like quails, guinea fowl, turkey and emu are of more recent introduction and have only small regional importance. As far as the commercial sector is concerned, it is fully integrated in provision of day old chicks, housing and management equipments, compounded feed and health cover and also take up processing and marketing of eggs and broilers. The National Egg Coordination Committee (NECC) and Broiler Marketing Cooperative Society (BROMARK) are engaged in declaring the whole sale prices of eggs and broilers respectively, but their areas of operation are highly restricted and following their advice is not mandatory. Compared to egg marketing because of longer shelf life and relative ease of packaging and transport, the trade in broiler because of its high perishability and further the general feeling of the people who consume broiler meat that dressed broiler whether hot or frozen is a dead chicken. They, therefore and want the live chicken to be slaughtered in their presence, which results in serious problems in sale of birds due to mortality and loss of weight during their keeping in captivity at the point of sale and during long distance transport. Further, both the egg and broiler trade is in the hands of private traders and a number of links in the chain are involved from production to consumption which adds to the losses in quantity and decline in quality as well as increases the prices for the consumer. Poultry Farmers' Cooperatives, State Poultry Development Corporations, NECC and BROMARK are playing a relatively minor role in ensuring remunerative prices through sale of eggs and broilers and the interest of the consumer is also being adversely affected in price and quality of product.

Among the avian species, layer and broiler chicken dominate the poultry industry and have acquired commercial proportion and have placed India at a reasonably high position in the world in poultry production. This is due to the availability of genetically superior layer and broiler stocks with higher production and superior efficiency of feed conversion and survival than other domesticated avian species. The contribution of layer to employment and incomes, and food and nutrition is still small and is confined essentially to peri-urban and rural areas. The indigenous chicken accounts for 30% of the total poultry population. Of the other avian species, ducks accounts for 7% and other avian species excluding chicken and ducks 3%. The major production and consumption of eggs and broilers is in urban and peri-urban areas. The live bird sale and manual slaughter in the market / village meat shop is wet marketing and leads to lot of wastage of poultry slaughter byproducts being of poor quality because the male live birds are maintained for sale resulting in loss of weight and condition and further the meat is consumed without its proper setting resulting from rigor mortis. The vast rural market because the 68.5% of the Indian population still lives in villages, remains unprovided with eggs and poultry meat of improved birds and only locally available desi chicken and birds of other avian species, spent hens and ducks and to a limited extant broilers are marketed. The eggs available are also of the indigenous chicken and ducks.

International trade in eggs and poultry meat accounts for 10% and 2.5% of their global annual output, respectively. India also exports table eggs, hatching eggs and frozen broilers mainly to Gulf, SAARC countries and South East Asian countries as well as dehydrated and frozen egg products mainly to Japan and some European countries. It however, in terms of volume constitute about 0.6% of the global trade. The value of India's export of poultry products has steadily increased to about Rs. 441 crores in 2007-08 from a meager figure of Rs. 88 crore only 10 years back. This has further increased in the recent years. Export of egg powder alone accounts for 45% of the total export value of poultry products from India.

14.2 Major Constraints and Future Prospects in India

India's poultry subsector of the agriculture sector is characterized by a mixture of small and marginal production with zero input (ZIP), low output, low input (LIP) and High input (HIP)- high output. While layer farms are more widely distributed especially in rural and peri-urban areas, the commercial broiler farms are mainly concentrated around metropolitan and large cities and other urban and peri-urban areas. There are differences in the constraints faced by large and small farmers. The large farmers have large throughput and high efficiency of production, processing and marketing and suffer less than the small producers who mostly depend on middle man for the disposal of their produce which results in uncertain and fluctuating prices.

Inspite of the success of the Indian poultry industry, low volume of processing and rapid escalating prices of poultry feed and its un-assured quality. The feed accounts for 60-65% of the egg and broiler production cost and is seriously impacting growth of the poultry subsector of the DA sector. The prices of maize and soybean meal have almost doubled in recent years, partly due to stagnation in maize production and its diversion to starch industry and export of soybean meal and even wheat bran and rice polish to earn foreign exchange. There has always been a demand by the DA productivity that export of maize and oilcakes/meals should be avoided but to earn foreign exchange and to have a balance of trade, the Government is always increasing the export of oilcakes/meals and bran / polish. There is a diversion of molasses for alcohol industry and of the grains for ethanol production to meet the energy needs in light of the growing fossilized fuel prices especially petroleum products and the negative environmental effects due to use of fossil fuels.

The standards of quality of feed supplements inspite of their having been laid down by Bureau of Indian Standards (BIS), are hardly followed except by large feed manufacturers which are members of CLFMA. In addition to ensuring the quality of compounded feed, detoxification of feed from aflatoxins, improving digestibility and bio-availability of nutrients from non-conventional feed resources, establishing nutrient requirements for diversified and non-commercial poultry production, utilizing alternative avian species are some of the areas needing considerations of the planners of poultry production in the country. Furthermore dietary interventions to produce designer eggs rich in omega-3 fatty acids, low in cholesterol and improved egg shell quality deserve R&D considerations to meet the growing demand of the quality poultry products.

Appropriate breeding approaches involving selection and appropriate mating systems, so as to provide faster genetic gains for improving productivity and profitability of layers and boilers are required. The earlier R&D efforts, both in the public and private sector, has paid rich dividends in India as in rest of the world through improving productivity and profitability. There is however a need to evolve breeding strategies for increasing adaptability to tropical environment especially under relatively low input extensive production conditions generally prevailing in rural areas. Concern must be shown towards the possible impact of various systems of poultry production on environment and to prevent the adverse effects of climate change associate with DA production. The problem of ascites and leg weakness in broilers under intensive management need to be researched so as to prevent them but not at the cost of rapid growth. There are serious concerns shown on ethical grounds as well as the effects of intensive housing and management and the way broiler chicken are handled during transportation from farm to the slaughter house and during slaughter are becoming important as they are likely to affect the quality of produce and may result in serious health hazard to the consumers.

Sustainable use and conservation of indigenous poultry genetic resources involving different species, especially farmed under more extensive management conditions and especially because of their higher adaptability to environmental stresses and prevalent diseases and identifying genes responsible for the superiorities and their introgression into commercial stocks deserves immediate R&D efforts. Some efforts have been made in the past in this direction using some of the tropically adapted avian genetic resources in improving the adaptability to stressful environment and avian diseases in more productive layer and broiler stocks. The modern techniques for identifying such genetic variants at molecular level and using biotechnological (molecular biology and genetic engineering) approaches, identifying quantitative trait loci (QTL) for economic traits especially those which are not easily recordable or require slaughter of birds such as carcass fatness, muscling, egg shell strength and resistance to disease. The use of QTLs in Marker Assisted Selection (MAS) to achieve the desired goal needs to be strengthened. Candidate gene polymorphism and approach for detection of gene and genotyping and sex chromosome expressed diversty, component analysis of complex traits and identification of QTLs and use of mitochondrial DNA (mDNA) as a marker for studies on genetic diversity and evolution in avian genetic resources are some of the newer approaches which are now being extensively persued in understanding genetic variation related to quantitative traits and their utilization in developing breeding plans. Some of these markers can be available even before the birth of the chick and at an early life or can provide more accurate estimate of genetic variation.

Extensive research has been undertaken on genetics and breeding of chicken both under intensive and extensive and a number of strains such as NIRBHEEK, UPCARI, HITCARI, SHYAMA, VANRAJA, GRAMPRIYA, NANDAM, GIRIRAJA, KRISHNA-J, CHB have been developed by various research and development organizations and are being popularized for rural poultry development especially to assist small and marginal farmers, landless laborers and unemployed youth in maintaining smaller units of chicken for egg and meat production using a dual purpose bird. The Government of India has taken rural poultry production to increase rural employment and incomes and provide supplementary nutritious food to rural people. It seems not correct to consider that it is not possible to establish commercial layer and broiler units in rural areas and they should be restricted to utilizing low producing birds with low inputs for meat and egg production. In 60s the Government of India had taken program for increasing egg and poultry meat production in peri-urban areas to provide employment to unemployed educated youth and improve nutrition through eggs and poultry meat. Smaller units were established for which sheds were provided in addition to day old chicks, compounded feed and health cover. There were also some efforts in encouraging collective marketing. These units however were not economically viable as they did not function for production and marketing as a single large cooperative unit, as in case of dairy cooperatives and now dairy producer company.

The experience of these under the National Dairy Plan of the GOI instituted in 2013 need to be considered along with the earlier experience of enhancing rural poultry production through government programs and a new model similar to the rural dairy production wherein a large number of smaller layer/broiler units are established but constituting a large production group and undertake collectively provision of day old chick through establishing their own poultry breeding units to produce layer and broiler chicks, have their own manufacturing units for poultry equipments for housing, feeding and watering, provision of compounded feed from its own compounded feed plant which may purchase feed ingredients during harvesting season when prices are low and the government may provide other feed inputs such as coarse grains and wasted grains from FCI and National Seed Corporation and molasses on priority basis and they may also collectively process and market eggs and poultry meat.

Heat stress in tropical poultry production especially in case of boilers is one of the major impediments in more efficient production due to relatively higher mortality and morbidity. Identification of physiological mechanism for regulation of atrisia of ovarian follicles and cost effective ways of replenishment of bicarbonate ions and carbon di oxide may help in the alleviation of ovarian follicle atrisia. Similar emphasis needs to be laid on shelter management to ensure comfort and reduce environmental stress and evolving suitable semen diluents in turkey where because of heavier breast to produce large quantity of breast meat has led to reduced mating capacity and fertility. Other avian species such as emu quail, ducks, geese, would require special R&D attention. Some of it has been studied under the ICAR under avian research facility viz. CARI, PDP and AICRPs centres located in major agro-ecological regions. These were earlier directed toward high yielding layer/ broiler commercial chicks through utilizing different components of genetic variance available in different exotic breeds/ stains/ lines. However, now the greater emphasis on R&D is on rural production under extensive and intensive production systems.

Increased profitability in poultry enterprises through reducing nutritional, environmental and disease stresses and ensuring proper storage, transport, processing and marketing of eggs, their processed products and broilers, can help the small and medium poultry producers both in improving their economic returns and provision of poultry products at a reasonable price to the consumers. Bio-security to ensure poultry and human health and increased export of live chicks and poultry products would require priority attention. Rapid response to events like outbreaks of infectious diseases, especially of zoonotic importance is required. More effective utilization of poultry byproducts in ruminant feed, fuel and fertilizer are areas which require attention so as to improve economics of poultry production and reduce negative environmental impacts. Strengthening technology transfer through various programs like KVKs needs to be given priority attention. KVKs in addition to providing solutions to the problems of poultry producers through suitable call centers, trainings and visits can help in improve economics of rural poultry production.

There is a serious regional imbalance in production and consumption of eggs and chicken meat. The long distance transports of live broilers and even shell eggs, has serious limitations. Expanding poultry production in areas where, it has a relatively lower presence as well as ensuring proper movement of eggs and broilers from areas with excess production to the areas with shortages and also diversification of poultry production especially in rural areas and under extensive management through utilization of species like ducks, guinea fowl and quail need to be propagated.

A large demand-supply mismatch exists because of the egg and broiler production is concentrated in a few areas and there is a large increase in demand throughout the country. This will require a better market intelligence related to demand forecast and ensuring faster movement of eggs and broilers. It is estimated that a 5% increase in supply of egg and chickens leads to 25% reduction in the market prices and conversely a similar decline in supply results in a similar increase in prices. The projections of demand of eggs and broilers in different seasons and in different regions of the country and linking the production centers with demand centers through providing cold storage and rapid transportation facility can help in mitigating these problems. Tremendous efforts have been made in case of dairy, where milk is being transported by road and rail transport over a long distance to provide milk in areas with chronic or seasonal shortages. It is easier for the eggs to be sold and transported long distances but not in case of live broilers. However, if the broilers are slaughtered and the carcass is frozen, their storage and long distance transport can be facilitated. This will also have a positive economic impact on broiler production.

The Bureau of Indian Standards (BIS) and Agriculture Produce Marketing Federation lay standards for poultry products but they are not strictly enforced and thus the consumer does not get the requisite product for the price he pays. Agricultural and Processed Food Export Development Authority (APEDA) and NABARD are involved in marketing of eggs and broilers and can ensure more equitable marketing in quantity, quality and prices throughout the country and throughout the year.

Except for some efforts of the NECC to promote egg consumption and BROMACH working through mass media, no serious public or private efforts in promoting egg and broiler consumption through removing some of the myths such as about non-vegetarianism of eggs and adverse effects on health of consumption of poultry meet have not been made and are urgently required.

Following the removal of quantitative restrictions (QR) by India on import of poultry products from April 2001 under obligations of

WTO, there is likelihood of large scale dumping of cheaper poultry products of uncertain quality in Indian market and depressing the prices of Indian poultry produce. Indian standards on poultry products should conform to standards of Codex Alimentarius and application of appropriate level of protection so as to safeguard poultry trade within the country under WTO agreement.

There is a rising concern of pollution caused by poultry farm waste and from hatchery and poultry dressing plants which require proper disposal, preferably through recycling as ruminant feed after proper processing. Lot of research and development has already been made in rendering poultry house waste and slaughter byproducts. But a collective efforts both in their utilization and promoting their use as a component of poultry feed has not been made at an appropriate level in India. The arising concerns with respect to zoonotic diseases spread from chicken are causing a depression in the consumption of eggs and poultry meat.

The global egg production was projected to increase to approx. 63 m mt. in the year 2009 to 73 m mt in 2015 with the bulk of increase occurring in developing countries particularly in India and China which has almost 1/3rd of the world population and have a faster rate of growth both in production and GDP. Further both the countries are developing industrially and the population in the urban areas is fast growing. This will fuel the demand both for eggs and chicken meat. The projected output is expected to be 106 bn eggs and 4.2 m mt. of poultry meat thereby increasing the per capita availability to 81 egg and 3.2 kg poultry meet by the year 2020, in India.

Poultry processing in general and egg processing in particular are gradually evolving in India as in some other developing countries like China, Brazil, Mexico and Thailand. Both these processing sectors particularly the latter, have enormous growth potential owing to either stagnant or slow growth rate in egg production in economically developed countries but high demand for processed products. Based on projections of rapid increase in egg production upto 2015 which may be difficult to achieve because of the number of limitations due to feed prices and outbreaks of avian influenza variety H5N1, special efforts would be required to achieve the production goals. Further, the feed prices are expected to rise due to major diversion of feed resources for fuel production alternative to petroleum products. Ethical concentrations among certain ethnic and religious segments of the society are likely to break and consumption of poultry eggs and meat may further increase. In India, there is a growing feeling among vegetarian population that since the eggs are infertile and there is no loss of life in their consumption and the eggs are an important source of high quality protein with all essential amino acids, vitamins and minerals and being available throughout the country and throughout the year at affordable prices, the consumption of egg is likely to increase which may give impetus to raising chicken for egg production. Rising pollution concern from disposal of poultry waste both from poultry housing, hatcheries and poultry dressing plants will need serious attention for to be effective and not creating environmental pollution through disposal preferably as ruminant feed, bio-fuel and fertilizer. It may be mentioned that as stated earlier, poultry has a relatively lesser contribution to environmental degradation when compared relative to ruminant and food crop production. Further raising poultry under more extensive or semi-intensive systems especially in rural areas can reduce its impact on environment and provide valuable organic manure for growing food and cash crops.

It is hoped that adequate attention will be paid by authorities in public and private sector to various problems associated with increased demand in eggs and broilers and attention to intensify R&D and training in poultry production, protection, processing and marketing and larger investment will have to be made in research and development of various components of poultry production specially in rural areas which have so far been bypassed. Larger attention would be required to rural poultry production both through encouraging utilization of genetic resources of Indian avian species but with better production inputs and also ensuring availability of high producing tropically adapted and nutritionally efficient layer and broiler stocks of chicken and other avian species especially ducks and quails. The Central Institutes viz. CARI and PDP and SAUs/SVUs will have to strengthen their research and training facilities to re-orient towards intensified rural poultry production pertinent to agro-ecological and socio-economic conditions prevelant in different regions of the country. Diversification in terms of species, production system, product processing and marketing are areas which would require priority R&D attentions.

❑❑❑

Annexures

Annexure-I Central Avian Research Institute and Project Directorate on Poultry- Their Major Mandates, Achievements and Future Programmes

A. Central Avian Research Institute, its achievements, present and future programmes

The remarkable growth achieved in the Indian poultry sector is due to several factors like initiation of pure line breeding within the country in both public and private sectors leading to availability of elite commercial layer and broiler germ plasm; and introduction and improvement of other avian species such as duck, guinea fowl, quail, turkey and emu. The parallel development of other input sub-sectors like non-conventional and cheaper feed resources, hatchery, poultry housing and farm appliances, poultry biological (diagnostics and prophylactic measures and medicines), feed analytical laboratories, modern mechanized poultry and egg processing plants, vertical and horizontal integration in poultry production, availability of institutional credit facilities on relatively low interest rates and above all ever-increasing demand of poultry products, have significantly contributed to the growth and sustainable development of poultry in India. There has been a large development research, education and training infrastructure and manpower developed especially since 1970s. This saw the initiation of two All India Coordinated Research Projects on Poultry for eggs and poultry for meat with coordinating units at the Indian Veterinary Research Institute, Izatnagar and research centers located in major agro-ecological regions and operated by the State Agricultural Universities. In 1978 considering greater need for independence of the imports of commercial layers and broiler and intensification of research and educational facilities, the Division of Poultry Science of the IVRI was upgraded into an independent research initiative in the form of Central Avian Research Institute at Izatnagar utilizing the existing facilities of offices, laboratories and breeding farm. These facilities were strengthened during the subsequent plans and the institute is now one of the important R&D facility in the tropics. Considering the additional research, educational and development facilities and especially maintenance of layer and broiler pure lines which were used at the institute and supplied for R&D to the other AICRP centers along with the random controlled population and since the institute was to undertake research on all economically important avian species and expand its research in other areas on production, health and product technologies, an independent initiative in the form of Project Directorate on Poultry (PDP), Hyderabad was taken.

After the establishment of the PDP, the responsibilities of coordination, maintenance of pure lines except those which were included in its breeding programme, and random bred control population meant for comparisons with the selected lines was maintained by the CARI.

Poultry science education and research initiatives in conjunction with the development efforts of the Union and State Ministries of Agriculture and now the Central Poultry Development Organization are playing a key role in providing highly qualified man-power, for training to poultry entrepreneurs both large and small and technology support to the poultry sector. The Institute with its main campus and a subsequently established regional centre at Bhubaneswar, Odisha is dedicated to Poultry Science research, education and extension in the Country with the following objectives.

1) To undertake basic, applied and adaptive research in all disciplines relating to production of different avian species.
2) To develop processing technologies for value addition, improving quality through processing and proper disposal / utilization of poultry by-products.
3) To impart education in Poultry Science at different level and in different specialized disciplines.
4) To transfer technologies developed at the institute after they have been field tested for studying their economic and social acceptability.
5) To provide referral and consultancy services in all aspects of production, processing and marketing (value chain) of different avian species.

To fulfill the above objectives the major research programmes related to following were undertaken :

i) *Genetic improvement*: Since 1970 the country has made large efforts for developing genetically superior stock of layer and broiler chicken and also of other avian species. This was done to make the country self sufficient in the availability of superior germ plasm and develop production, protection and processing technologies relevant to the country's need. The institute has made a significant progress in developing germ plasm of different avian species in the country and developed associated improved production technologies and transferred them to the public and private poultry agencies. SAUs/ SVUs, KVKs, State Animal Husbandry Departments and NGOs etc. are also providing superior germ plasm to the poultry farmers in their respective command areas. The institute has over the time introduced a number of other avian species such as quail, ducks, guinea fowl and more recently has introduced emus. The high performing improved indigenous fowls have very high demand in rural/tribal areas as they are highly suitable for production under extensive/ semi-intensive management. The pure lines of various exotic / indigenous breeds / strains of different avian species have been provided to various development agencies and directly to the poultry farmers.

ii) *Poultry Biotechnology*: The challenges that poultry industry is facing have been addressed to through biotechnological approaches which are being used for enhancement of productivity, disease resistance, tropical adaptability, as well as sustainable management and conservation of avian genetic resources.

iii) The germ plasm of layer and broiler chicken, ducks, quails, guinea fowl, turkey have been characterized using RAPD, AFLP and microsatellite markers. QTL and candidate gene analysis for identifying molecular markers related with economic traits, disease resistance and tropical adaptability has been carried out. PCR based techniques have been standardized for sex differentiation in different poultry species.

iv) The expression, genomic analysis and epigenetic modifications of various candidate genes involved in heat shock response have been studied in broiler strains. Various physiological and haemo-biochemical parameters have also been evaluated under different stress conditions. The naked neck broiler developed at institute has better production and heat tolerance capabilities.

v) The work on gene driven technologies like transgenesis (transgenic sperms and silencing of myostatin gene), RNA interference (RNAi), in-vivo embryo-culture system using single and double window approach etc. has been carried out for augmenting productivity and disease resistance. The *in-vivo* silencing of myostatin (~70%) has been achieved in chicken by administrating shRNA targeting myostatin cloned in lentivector with GFP at day old stage. rDNA technology for production of poultry cytokines for their use as vaccine adjuvant, immune modulator and growth promoter has been utilized.

vi) Nucleotide variations and SNPs among different avian species/ strains have been analysed. Critical genes involved in forced moulting have also been identified.

vii) Immuno-divergent lines for humoral and cell mediated immune responses have been developed. Identification of an SNP associated with ND vaccine response and development of new MHC genotyping procedure and selection criteria for enhanced immunocompetence have been achieved. Analysis of TvB locus to find ALV resistant/susceptible alleles among WLH, Kadakanath and Aseel highlight the scope of molecular breeding for ALV resistance.

viii) Techniques of in-ovo nutrient supplementation based on gene expression analysis has been standardized to improve early chick growth and development of vital organs. Technique of in-ovo procedures for multiple vaccine delivery has also been standardized for better post hatch immunity.

ix) Key factor influencing parthenogenetic development in unfertilized turkey and chicken eggs has been identified through micro array, real time PCR and chromosomal analysis.

Poultry Nutrition and Feed Resource Development: Faced with the challenges of ever increasing feed cost and reducing availability of quality feeds, the institute has devised methods to determine precise nutrient requirement and their availability and in relation to the requirements of different nutrients (amino acids, energy, minerals, protein and vitamins) for different avian species, production types and age groups under different production conditions to optimize feed cost. Several alternate feed resources have been identified, evaluated for their nutritional value and efficiency of utilization by different production types. Since maize and soybean meal are becoming costly and are in short supply because of export and diversion to other industrial uses, alternative feed ingredients which are more readily available and relatively cheaper but can replace maize and soyabean have been identified. Some of these feed resources are pearl millet, sorghum-red, brown and white, undersized wheat, finger millet and small millets, cereal by-products such as maize germ meal, maize gluten meal, rice polish, broken rice, deoiled rice bran, wheat bran, oilcakes such as sunflower, mustard/rapeseed-expeller and solvent extracted, cottonseed, sesame, karanja, neem seed, sunflower and castor seed and gum-industry residues such as guar meal, high protein roasted guar korma, fruit processing waste such as apple pomace and animal protein supplements from slaughter house poultry byproducts such as meat meal, meat-cum-bone meal, earthworm meal and other feed ingredients viz. dried yeast, azolla meal. The effective combinations of cereal and protein meals have also been established. The database of nutrient contents, digestibility, particularly availability of amino acids and minerals and safe/effective level of inclusion of different feed ingredients have been developed. Different processing techniques like acid/alkali treatment, autoclaving, fermentation, fungal treatment, roasting, water washing and soaking (reconstitution), supplementation/addition of enzymes, prebiotics, probiotics, acidifiers, water and feed sanitizers and supplementation of critical nutrients (amino acids, minerals, energy) have been used to augment the nutritive value of different feeds. Low cholesterol and ù-3 fatty acid enriched eggs have been developed through dietary intervention. The efficacy of different herbs, additives and nutritional agents, and dietary manipulations have been established for climate resilience poultry production. The Institute has made significant achievements in developing technologies to deal with the anti-nutritional factors, adulterants and toxicants in various feeds.

MakeFeed Poultry, the Windows (R) based software developed to design cost-efficient feed formulae for different classes and age groups of various avian species, has been immensely popular in the poultry industry.

Shelter Management: The institute has pioneered the rearing and management practices of different avian species under diverse systems of rearing. Entire range of rearing appliances such as battery brooders, feeders, incubation trays, laying and rearing cages, waterers, etc. for different avian species have been designed and got fabricated. The institute has also designed low cost poultry houses utilizing locally available materials for semi-intensive or small scale poultry rearing.

Effective floor space requirement for cage and floor rearing of turkey and quail have been standardized. Package of practices for high altitude poultry farming has been standardized.

Stress Management and Reproduction Technology: Several technological interventions have been developed for mitigation of various stresses in poultry production. The techniques of artificial insemination in various avian species have been standardized. Semen storage techniques and semen dilutor for AI in various avian species have been developed. Moreover, several physiological mechanisms have been studied to evolve suitable interventions aimed at enhancing productivity of different avian species.

Processing, Value-Addition and Assuring Product Quality: A number of value-added products have been developed utilizing poultry eggs and meat. Slaughter waste has been utilized for production of pet food and other foods for human consumption. The effective and economical techniques of preservation and extending shelf-life including suitable packaging of poultry products have also been standardized. The efficacy of natural preservatives for shelf-life extension of poultry products has been evaluated. The techniques of meat tenderization have been standardized for effectively utilization of tougher meat of old and culled birds. Database on product safety parameters such as occurrence of potent pesticides' residues, presence of aflatoxin and heavy metals in poultry products as well as surveillance of the microbial quality including food pathogens in poultry products have been standardized.

Market Surveillance: The institute regularly studies market trends and developments taking place in the poultry sector in India as well as globally. Institute also provides consultancy services for establishing poultry units and for raising institutional finance. The cost and returns from quails, turkeys, guinea fowls, ducks, broilers and layers under different systems of production are continuously monitored. Economics of raising parent lines, production of commercial broilers and layers has also been studied.

Technology Transfer and HRD: The institute has made a significant progress in disseminating the proven technologies developed by it. The germ plasm of species like quail, turkey and ducks has been widely disseminated in the Country. Quails and turkeys have already gained substantial popularity in the Country. But for the restrictions of the Wild Life Act 1972, the Japanese quails would have grown exponentially in the country and would have become a viable alternative to layer and broiler chicken, as both pickled quail eggs and meat are considered as elite food and a delicacy. Similarly, the Institute has also made a significant contribution to redevelop rural poultry production. The indigenous dual purpose improved chicken has been improved through selection and crossing with exotic layer and broiler breed and a number of high yielding and adapted to less intensive management in rural areas have been developed. Similar activities have been under taken by PDP centers of AICRP on poultry and by poultry breeding farms of Central and State Governments and a few commercial poultry breeding farms. These varieties are being further propagated by the NGOs, social organizations to provide self employment and incomes to small and marginal farmers and land less labourers and other economically and socially deprived people in rural and peri-urban areas.

The availability of technical manpower both in the public and private sector is less than adequate at present. The human resource development and capacity building have been taken up by this Institute, PDP and a number of state teaching and development organizations through specialized trainings programmes on various aspects of poultry production and management. Besides, the Institute, in collaboration with the deemed university, IVRI, Izatnagar also imparts postgraduate education in various sub-disciplines of Poultry Science. Other modes of capacity building such as summer/winter schools, farmers' fair, conferences, seminars and symposia are also organized by the Institute from time to time.

B. The Project Directorate on Poultry (PDP)

The Project Directorate on Poultry (PDP) was established by the ICAR on March 1, 1988 on the pattern of other PDs in crops and livestock to coordinate the AICRPs on Poultry for meat and eggs. The earlier mechanism of coordinating and servicing the project units was with the Division of Poultry Science of IVRI and subsequently with the CARI. With the expansion of research activities both involving other disciplines and Avian species, the coordination and servicing activity, which involved major staff and facilities would not have allowed the expansion of the facilities at CARI because of space and manpower limitation and it was decided to establish a separate PD. The activities of PD involved maintenance of pure lines of layers and broilers used in breeding research programmes at different units of the AICRP but also maintain random bred controlled population and supply them to the various units of the AICRP. It had to carry out ancillary studies on nutrition, health and management of the pure lines maintained by it. Over the time, the activities of the project directorate have expended to undertake more detailed studies in other disciplines. More recently with the emphasis of GOI on poultry production, the ICAR has been mandated to develop technologies for rural poultry production and some emphasis has given both by CARI and PDP on developing technologies for rural poultry production.

The earlier research programmes both of CARI and AICRPs have made tremendous contribution to basic knowledge on different aspects of poultry production and its use in the development of technologies for improving layer and broiler production. The layer and broiler pure lines currently available hold the promise for further improvement. These also have been used in developing improved varieties for rural poultry products. The limitations in R&D institutional farms has been the limitations of financial manpower and space facilities relative to commercial breeding farms which could make a larger impact on commercial poultry production. The pure lines have been tested not only for their production efficiency but also immune competence.

A number of high yielding strains, mostly dual purpose (egg and meat) have been developed by the two ICAR poultry institutes as well as by the SAUs /SVUs and through some private initiatives. There is need to continue the activities with emphasis on plumage colour and type like in case of indigenous chicken, increase shank length, moderate body weight, low feed intake, health and management inputs and high immune competence. These birds should lay efficiently in terms of egg number and egg size.

Study of molecular mechanism of higher efficiency of adaptation to nutritional, environmental and health problems need to be studied. Some efforts have already been made and through the use of modern genetic approaches especially at molecular level improvement can be made in the indigenous genetic variance through selection or introgression of superior genes from exotic breeds.

Nutritional optimization is most essential because of the cost involved and variation in the production traits accompanied for by nutrition. Particular reference is required to limiting amino acids and minerals. There is also a need to reduce the fat and cholesterol content of eggs and chicken meat and enhance the concentration of specific nutrients in poultry products. The increased content of pesticides, mycotoxins and antibiotics in feed which not only adversely affect the production but also pose health hazards to their consumers.

Studies on the consumer preference of the indigenous chicken meat and eggs needs to be studied with respet to their chemical and organo-lactic properties so that these characters can be introduced into commercial layers and broilers both for urban and rural poultry production.

Rural areas have least facilities for processing and storage of poultry products leading to large loses. Studies on rural processing, storage and transport to the central consumption needs to be researched.

Animal welfare issues especially lead to their housing and provision of health care need serious concentration. The rural poultry production should not only be confined to indigenous low producing birds maintained under free rage, low input production but improved birds specialized in egg or meat production and maintained in relatively smaller units but live together for supply of all inputs and services. These may collectively be able to produce large enough numbers of eggs / chicken for meat that necessarily require breeding facilities, feed compounding facilities, manufacturing of materials for sheds, health services and processing and marketing facilities can be created through linking different production units in a number of contiguous villages so that the eggs/broilers or their processed products are large to be competitive to the commercial poultry producers.

Management poultry waste is not a problem in extensive management especially in rural areas but is becoming a matter of concern in large intensive poultry production units in urban and peri-urban areas. Proper disposal of the poultry waste which not only involve excretions / droppings but also bedding in floor raised birds, carcasses of dead birds and slaughter house waste. Proper bio-balancing of nutrients can reduce excretion of uric acid and other ammonical mineral waste. The proper treatment of liter and hatchery waste can be treated using physical, chemical and biological methods and transform into high quality organic fertilizer.

Human Resource Development and Technology Management and its transfer to its end user is important in all research organizations and efforts should be made to strengthen the facilities so that the knowledge and material generated by the PDP reaches the end user.

Annexure-II Indian Standard

Poultry Feeds – Specifications (Fifth Revision)

1. Scope

This standard prescribes requirement, sampling and methods of test for chicken (*Gallus domesticus*) feeds.

2. References

At the time of publication, the editions indicated were valid. All standards are subject to revision, and parties to agreements based on this standard are encouraged to investigate the possibility of applying the most recent additions of the standards.

3. Types

Chicken feeds shall be of the following fifteen types:

a) *Broiler Pre-starter Feed (BPSF)* - a ration to be fed to chicks, intended for meat production and to be used from 1 to 7 days.

b) *Broiler Starter Feed (BST)* - a ration to be led to growing chickens, intended for meat production, from 8 to 21 days.

c) *Broiler Finisher Feed (BFF)* - a ration to be fed to growing chickens, intended for meat production, from 22 days to finish.

d) *Chick Feed for Layer (CFL)* - a ration to be fed to chicks, intended for egg production, from 0 to 8 weeks.

e) *Grover Chicken Feed for Layer (GFL)* - a ration to be fed to growing chickens, intended for egg production, from 9 to 20 weeks or until laying commences.

f) *Layer Feed for Phase I (LFP-I)* - a ration to be fed to laying birds from 21 weeks to 45 weeks.

g) *Layer Feed for Phase II (LFP-II)* - a ration to be fed to laying birds from 46 weeks to 72 weeks. Phase II and I feed in layer cycle is necessary because there are changes in production, egg size, requirement of calcium, efficiency of digestion, age, etc.

h) *Breeder Chick Feeding for Broiler (BCFB)* - a ration to be fed to chicks, intended for broiler breeding, from 0 to 4 weeks.

j) *Breeder Grower Feed for Broiler (BGFB)* - a ration to be fed to chickens, intended for broiler breeding, from 5 to 22 weeks.

k) *Breeder Layer Feed For Broiler (BLFB)* - a ration to be fed to laying birds, intended for broiler breeding, from week 23 onwards.

m) *Breeder Broiler Feed for Male (BBFM)*- a ration to be fed to male birds, intended for broiler breeding, from week 23 onwards.

n) *Chick Feed for Layer Breeder (CFLB)* - a ration to be fed to chicks, intended for layer breeding, from 0 to 4 weeks.

p) *Grower Feed for Layer Breeder (GFLB)* - a ration to be fed to chickens, intended for layer breeding, from 5 to 22 weeks.

q) *Breeder Layer Feed (BLF)* - a ration to be fed to laying birds, intended for layer breeding, from week 23 onwards.

r) *Breeder Layer Feed For Male (BLFM)* - a ration to be fed to male birds. Intended for layer breeding, from week 23 onwards.

4. Requirements

4.1. Description: Chicken feed shall be in the form of pellets, crumbs or mash. The feed shall be free from rancidity, musty odour, toxic ingredients, adulterants, moulds and insect infestation.

4.1.1. Ingredients: The ingredients listed shall only be used for manufacturing chicken feeds.

4.1.2. The chicken feeds shall also conform to the requirements given in Tables 1 and 2.

4.1.3. Chicken feeds shall also contain the following vitamins, fatty acids, amino acids and minerals obtained either from the natural source or from any added source, in quantity not less than shown against each in Table 3.

4.1.4. The compound poultry feeds shall also conform to the maximum limits of harmful substances as given in Table 4.

4.2. Optional Requirements

4.2.1. It is recommended that chicken feeds may contain feed additives.

4.2.2. The composition of commonly used poultry feed ingredients is given in Table 5.

4.2.4. The specification of poultry feed raw material is given in Tables 6 and 7.

4.2.5. The expected performance of chickens are given in Tables 8 and 9.

5. Packing and marking

5.1 Packing: The material shall be packed in clean, dry and sound, plain or polyethylene lined jute or laminated paper bags. The mouth of each bag shall be machine stitched.

*5.2 Marking:*Each bag shall be suitably marked so as to give the following information legibly:

a) Name and the material and brand name, if any;

b) Name and type of the poultry feed;

c) Name and address of the manufacturer; Net mass when packed, in kg; and

d) Year and month of manufacture.

5.2.1 In addition to the information listed in 5.2, each bag shall have a label or tag attached to it or contain a leaflet giving the following information:

a) Type of poultry feed;

b) Name and quantity of the antibiotic or coccidiostates added, if any;

c) Crude protein content;

d) Crude fibre content;

e) Aflatoxin B, content;

f) Metabolisable energy (calculated), in kcal/kg; and

g) The declaration that minerals, vitamins, fatty acids and amino acids are present in the material as per the specification.

Note: The manufacturer may declare the values of minerals, vitamins, fatty acids and amino acids from the record showing the quantities of these added to each batch.

5.3. BIS certification marking: The product may also be marked with the Standard Mark.

5.3.1. The use of the Standard Mark is governed by the provisions of the Bureau of Indian Standard Act, 1986 and the Rules and Regulations made there under. The details of conditions under which the licence for the use of the Standard Mark may be granted to manufacturers or producers may be obtained from the Bureau of Indian Standards.

6. Sampling

Representative samples of the material shall be drawn according to the prescribed method.

7. Tests

7.1 Tests shall be carried out as prescribed in col 1 8 of Tables 1, 2 and 3.

7.2 Quality of reagents: Unless specified otherwise, pure chemicals and distilled water (see IS 1070) shall be employed in tests.

Note-'Pure chemicals' shall mean chemicals that do not contain impurities, which affect the results of analysis.

Table 1. Requirements for chicken feeds (Classes 4.1.2,7.1 E-4.2 and E-5)

Sl No.	Characteristics	Requirements for															
		Broiler feed			Layer feed				Broiler breeder feed				Layer breeder feed				Method of test ref to clause
		Pre-starter	Starter	Finisher	Chick	Grower	Layer Phase I	Layer Phase II	Chick	Grower	Layer	Male	Chick	Grower	Rom	Male	
(1)	(2)	(3)	(4)	(5)	(6)	(7)	(8)	(9)	(10)	(11)	(12)	(13)	(14)	(15)	(16)	(17)	(18)
(i)	Moisture, percent by mass, Max	11.0	11.0	11.0	11.0	11.0	11.0	11.0	11.0	11.0	11.0	11.0	11.0	11.0	11.0	11.0	4 of IS 7874(Part 1) or IS 14830
(ii)	Crude protein (N x 6.25), percent by mass, Min	23.0	22.0	20.0	20.0	16.0	18.0	16.0	20.0	16.0	16.0	15.0	20.0	16.0	17.0	16.0	5 of IS 7874 (Part 1) or IS 14825
(iii)	Ether extract, percent by mass, Min	3.0	3.5	4.0	2.0	2.0	2.0	2.0	2.5	2.5	2.5	2.5	2.0	2.0	2.0	2.0	7 of IS 7874 (Part 1)
(iv)	Crude fibre, percent by mass. Max	5.0	5.0	5.0	7.0	9.0	9.0	10.0	7.0	9.0	9.0	9.0	7.0	9.0	9.0	9.0	8 of IS 7874 (Part 1) or IS 10226 (Part 1)
(v)	Acid insoluble ash, percent by mass, Max	2.5	2.5	2.5	4.0	4.0	4.0	4.5	4.0	4.0	4.0	4.0	2.5	2.5	2.5	2.5	10 of IS 7874 (Part 1) or IS 14826
(vi)	Salt (as Na Cl), percent by mass, Max	0.5	0.5	0.5	0.5	0.5	0.5	0.5	0.5	0.5	0.5	0.5	0.5	0.5	0.5	0.5	4 of IS 7874 (Part 2)

Notes

1. The values specified for characteristic at Sl. No. (ii) to (vi) are on dry matter basis.
2. Earlier the broiler cycle was for eight weeks. It has now reduced to 6 week. The split is therefore 0 to 3 weeks starter and 4 to 6 weeks finisher. The starter period is further split into pre-starter 0 to 7 days and starter 8 to 21 days. This optimizes the performance. Therefore it is advised that prestarter feed to be used from 1 to 7 days, starter feed from 8 to 21 days and finisher feed from 22 days to finish.
3. An expected broiler performance as on current status if given in Table 8 and 9. It must be noted that the performance parameter may change with the input of high genetic material in future. These values are applicable as on current basis and may only be viewed guidelines.
4. It has been observed that with the increasing usage of essential amino acids such as lysine and methionine the need for high protein has come down significantly. This has resulted into lower of protein content in the broiler feed lines.
5. Studies are being conducted on the role of threonine and tryptophan. If they are available commercially to improve performance. The protein value can be further changed in future.
6. The energy values have been increased as compared to exiting Indian Standards because of current feed efficiency of 1.8 as compared to previous 2.2. The feed being manufactured now-a-days is denser with high energy.
7. Ether Extract means all ether soluble materials which include oil alcohol cholesterol pigments etc. Since the method for estimation exclusively for oil is not available either extract annotation is being used.
8. In earlier feeds use methionine and choline was limited. This incorporation has gone up and since both help as lypolytic factors. It is felt that the role of biotin is limited, hence the biotin value been reduced compared to existing Indian Standards.
9. Chick stage is 0 to 8 weeks. Grower stage is 9 to 20 weeks. Phase I is from 21 weeks to 45 weeks and Phase II is from 46 weeks to 72 necks of age of the bird. It is therefore advised to use the respective feeds accordingly.

10. Phase I and Phase II in layer cycle is necessary because there are changes in production, egg size, requirement of calcium, efficiency of digestion, age. etc.

11. Extra calcium source in the form of shell grit/limestone at about 4-3 g per bird pee da) is advised in case of laying stage both in Phase I and Phase II feeds.

12. Expected performance of layers has been furnished in Table 9, which may be used as guideline, depending upon the present genetic potential of the bird.

13. It is advised to use chick feed from 0-4 weeks, grower feed from 5-22 weeks and layer breeder feed and male breeder feed from week 23 onwards.

Table 2. Requirements for chicken feeds
(Clauses 4.1.2 and 7.1)

Sl No.	Characteristics	Requirements for															
		Broiler feed			Layer feed				Broiler breeder feed				Layer breeder feed				Method of test ref to
		Pre-starter	Starter	Finisher	Chick	Grower	Layer Phase I	Layer Phase II	Chick	Grower	Layer	Male	Chick	Grower	Rom	Male	
(1)	(2)	(3)	(4)	(5)	(6)	(7)	(8)	(9)	(10)	(11)	(12)	(13)	(14)	(15)	(16)	(17)	(18)
(i)	Calcium (as Ca), percent by mass, Min	1.0	1.0	1.0	1.0	1.0	3.0	3.5	1.0	1.0	3.5	1.0	1.0	1.0	3.5	1.0	IS 13433 (Parts 1 and 2)
(ii)	Total phosphorus, percent by mass, Min	0.7	0 7	0.7	0 7	0 65	0.65	0.65	0.7	0.7	0.7	0.7	0.65	0.60	0.60	0.60	Clause 6 of IS 7874 (Part 2) or IS 14828
(iii)	Available phosphorus, percent by mass, Min	0.45	0.45	0.45	0.45	0.40	0.40	0.40	0.45	0.45	0.40	0.40	0.45	0.40	0.40	0.40	Annex F
(iv)	Lysine, percent by mass, Min	1 3	1.2	1 0	1.0	0.7	0.7	0.65	1.0	0.8	0.85	0.80	0.95	0.70	0.70	0.80	Annex G
(v)	Methionine, percent by mass, Min 0.5	0.5	0 5	0.45	0 40	0 35	0.35	0.30	0.45	0.40	0.45	0.40	0.40	0.40	0.40	0.40	Annex H
(vi)	Methionine + Cystine percent by mass, Min	0.9	0.9	0.85	0.70	0.60	0.60	0.55	0.70	0.70	0.70	0.70	0.70	0.60	0.60	0.60	IS 1374
(vii)	Metabolizable energy (Kcal/kg), Min	3000	3100	3200	2800	2500	2600	2400	2800	2750	2800	2750	2800	2600	2600	2600	Annex J
(viii)	Aflatoxin B_1 (ppb), Max	20	20	20	20	20	20	20	20	20	20	20	20	20	20	20	Annex K or IS 13427

Notes

1. The values specified for characteristics at Sl No. (ii) to (vi) arc on dry matter basis.

2. IS 14828 shall be the referee's method. In case of dispute.

3. In case of dispute, HPLC method shall be the referee's method.

4. Earlier the broiler cycle was for eight weeks. It has now reduced to 6 weeks. The split is therefore 0 to 3 weeks starter and 4 to 6 weeks finisher. The starter period is further split into pre-starter 0 to 7 days and starter 8 to 21 days. This optimizes the performance. Therefore it is advised that pre-starter feed to be used from 1 to 7 days, starter feed from 8 to 21 days and finisher feed from 22 days to finish.

5. An expected broiler performance as on current status is given in Tables 8 and 9. It must he noted that the performance parameters may change with the input of high genetic material in future. These values are applicable as on current basis and may only be viewed as guidelines.

6. It has been observed that with the increasing usage of essential amino acids such as lysine and methionine, the need for high protein has conic down significantly. This has resulted into lowering of protein content in the broiler feed lines.

7. Studies are being conducted on the role of threonine and tryptophan. If they are available commercially to improve performance, the protein values can be further changed in future.

8. The energy values have been increased as compared to existing Indian Standards, because of current feed efficiency of 1.8 as compared to previous 2.1. The feed being manufactured now-a-days is denser with high energy.

9. Ether Extract means all ether soluble materials, which include oil, alcohol, cholesterol, pigments etc. Since the method for estimation exclusively for oil is not available, ether extract connotation is being used.

10. In earlier feeds, use of methionine and choline was limited. This incorporation has gone up and since both help as lypolytic factors, it is felt that the role of biotin is limited. Hence the biotin values have been reduced compared to existing Indian Standards.

11. Chick stage is 0 to 8 weeks. Grower stage is 9 to 20 weeks. Phase I is from 21 weeks to 45 weeks and Phase II is from 46 weeks to 72 weeks of age of the bird. It is therefore advised to use the respective feeds accordingly.

12. Phase I and Phase II in Layer cycle is necessary because there are changes in production, egg size, requirement of calcium, efficiency of digestion, age etc.

13. Top dressing of extra calcium source in the form of shell grit/ limestone at about 4-5 g per bird per day is advised in case of laying stage both in Phase I and Phase II feeds.

14. The expected performance of layers has been furnished in Table 9, which may be used as guideline, depending upon the present genetic potential of the bird.

15. It is advised to use chick feed from 0-4 weeks, grower feed from 5-22 weeks and layer breeder feed and male breeder feed from week 23 onwards.

Table 3. Requirements for minerals, vitamins, amino acids and fatty acids per kg of chicken feeds (Clauses 4.1.3 and 7.1)

Sl No.	Characteristics	Requirements for															
		Broiler Feed			Layer Feed				Broiler Breeder Feed				Layer Breeder Feed				Method of Test Ref to
		Pre-starter	Starter	Finisher	Chick	Grower	Layer Phase I	Layer Phase II	Chick	Grower	Layer	Male	Chick	Grower	Rom	Male	
(1)	(2)	(3)	(4)	(5)	(6)	(7)	(8)	(9)	(10)	(11)	(12)	(13)	(14)	(15)	(16)	(17)	(18)
(i)	Manganese, mg/kg, Min	100.0	100.0	100.0	70.0	60.0	60.0	60.0	100.0	100.0	100.0	100.0	100.0	100.0	100.0	100.0	IS 15121
(ii)	Iodine, mg/kg, Min	1.2	1.2	1.2	1.0	1.0	1.0	1.5	1.5	1.5	1.5	1.5	1.5	1.5	1.5	1.5	IS 15121
(iii)	Iron, mg/kg, Min	80.0	80.0	80.0	70.0	60.0	60.0	60.0	80.0	80.0	80.0	80.0	80.0	80.0	80.0	80.0	IS 15121
(iv)	Zinc, mg/kg, Min	80.0	80.0	80.0	60.0	60.0	60.0	60.0	80.0	80.0	80.0	80.0	80.0	80.0	80.0	80.0	IS 15121
(v)	Copper, mg/kg, Min	12.0	12.0	12.0	12.0	9.0	9.0	9.0	12.0	12.0	12.0	12.0	12.0	12.0	12.0	12.0	IS 15121
(vi)	Selenium, mg/kg, Min	0.15	0.15	0.15	0.15	0.15	0.15	0.15	0.15	0.15	0.20	0.15	0.15	0.15	0.20	0.15	IS 15121
(vii)	Vitamin A, IU/kg, Min	11000	11000	10000	9000	8000	8000	8000	12000	12000	15000	12000	12000	12000	15000	12000	IS 15121
(viii)	Vitamin D_3, IU/kg, Min	3000	3000	3000	1800	1600	1600	1600	2500	2500	3000	2500	2500	2500	3000	2500	Annex L
(ix)	Vitamin B_1, mg/kg, Min	2.5	2.5	2.5	2.0	1.5	1.0	1.0	2.0	2.0	3.0	2.0	2.0	2.0	3.0	2.0	IS 5398
(x)	Vitamin B_2, mg/kg, Min	6.0	6.0	6.0	6.0	5.0	5.0	5.0	5.0	5.0	6.0	5.0	5.0	5.0	6.0	5.0	IS 5399
(xi)	Pantothenic acid, mg/kg, Min	15.0	15.0	15.0	10.0	9.0	7.0	7.0	15.0	15.0	25.0	15.0	15.0	15.0	25.0	15.0	IS 9840
(xii)	Niacin, mg/kg, Min	40.0	40.0	40.0	40.0	20.0	20.0	20.0	40.0	40.0	50.0	40.0	40.0	40.0	50.0	40.0	IS 5400
(xiii)	Biotin, mg/kg, Min	0.15	0.15	0.15	0.10	0.10	0.10	0.10	0.20	0.20	0.20	0.20	0.20	0.20	0.20	0.20	IS 9820
(xiv)	Vitamin B_{12} mg/kg, Min	0.015	0.015	0.015	0.010	0.008	0.008	0.008	0.025	0.025	0.030	0.025	0.025	0.025	0.030	0.025	IS 7529
(xv)	Folic acid, mg/kg, Min	1.0	1.0	1.0	1.0	0.50	0.50	0.50	3.0	3.0	4.0	3.0	3.0	3.0	4.0	3.0	IS 7234
(xvi)	Choline, mg/kg, Min	500.0	500.0	500.0	500.0	200.0	400.0	400.0	850.0	850.0	700.0	500.0	850.0	850.0	700.0	500.0	IS 7874
(xvii)	Vitamine E, mg/kg, Min	30.0	30.0	30.0	15.0	10.0	10.0	10.0	20.0	20.0	50.0	20.0	20.0	20.0	50.0	20.0	Annex M
(xviii)	Vitamin K, mg/kg, Min	1.5	1.5	1.5	1.5	1.5	1.5	1.5	2.0	2.0	3.0	2.0	2.0	2.0	3.0	2.0	IS 7874
(xix)	Vitamin B_6, mg/kg, Min	5.0	5.0	5.0	3.0	3.0	3.0	3.0	5.0	5.0	6.0	5.0	5.0	5.0	6.0	5.0	IS 7530
(xx)	Linoleic acid, percent by mass, Min	1.1	1.1	1.1	1.0	1.0	1.0	1.0	1.0	1.0	1.0	1.0	1.0	1.0	1.0	1.0	IS 7874

Notes

1. The values specified for characteristics at Sl No. (i) to (xx) are on dry matter basis.
2. Earlier the broiler cycle as for eight weeks. It has now reduced to 6 weeks. The split is therefore 0 to 3 weeks starter and 4 to 6 weeks finisher. The starter period is further split into pre-starter 0 to 7 days and starter 8 to 21 days. This optimizes the performance. Therefore ills advised that Pre-starter Feed to be used from 1 to 7 days. Starter feed front 8 to 21 days and Finisher Feed from 22 days to finish.
3. An expected broiler performance as on current status is given in Tables 8 and 9. It must be noted that the performance parameters may change with the input of high genetic material in future. These values are applicable as on current basis and may only be viewed as guidelines.
4. It has been observed that with the increasing usage of essential amino acids such as lysine and methionine the need for high protein has come down significantly. This has resulted into lowering of protein content in the broiler feed lines.
5. Studies are being conducted on the role of threonine and tryptophan. If they are available commercially to improve performance, the protein values can be thither changed in future.
6. The energy values have been increased as compared to existing Indian Standards, because of current feed efficiency of 1.8 as compared to previous 2.2. The feed being manufactured now -a-days is denser with high energy.
7. Ether Extract means all ether soluble materials, which include oil, alcohol, cholesterol, pigments. etc. Since the method for estimation exclusively for oil is not available, ether extract connotation is being used.
8. In earlier feeds use of methionine and choline was limited. This incorporation has gone up and since both help as lypolytic factors, it is felt that the role of biotin is limited. Hence the biotin values have been reduced compared to existing Indian Standards.
9. Chick stage is 0 to 8 weeks. Grower stage is 9 to 20 weeks. Phase I is from 21 weeks to 45 weeks and Phase II is from 46 weeks to 72 weeks of age of the bird. It is therefore advised to use the respective feeds accordingly.
10. Phase I and Phase II in Layer cycle is necessary because there are changes in production, egg size, requirement of calcium, efficiency of digestion, age, etc.

11. Top dressing of extra calcium source in the form of shell grit/ limestone at about 4-5 g per bird per day is advised in case of laying stage both in Phase I and Phase II feeds.

12. The expected performance of layers has been furnished in Table 9, which may be used as guideline, depending upon the present genetic potential of the bird.

13. It is advised to use chick feed from 04 weeks, grower feed from 5-22 weeks and layer breeder feed and male breeder feed from week 23 onwards.

Table 4. Maximum prescribed limit for harmful substances and test methods in compound poultry feeds
(Clauses 4.1.4, E-2.3 and E-3.1)

S.No.	Substance	Feed	MAX content in mg/kg referred into a moisture pcontent of 11 Percent	Test methods
(1)	(2)	(3)	(4)	(5)
(i)	Arsenic	Complete feed for poultry	2	A.O.A.C.
(ii)	Fluorine	Complete feed for poultry	30	A.O.A.C.
(iii)	Lead	Complete feed for poultry	5	A.O.A.C.
(iv)	Mercury	Complete feed for poultry	Nil	A.O.A.C.
(v)	Nitrite (Na nitrite)	Complete feed for poultry	15	A.O.A.C.
(vi)	Aflatoxin B_1	Complete feed for poultry	0.02	A.O.A.C.
(vii)	Castor	Complete feed for poultry	10	A.O.A.C.
(viii)	Free gossypol	Complete feed for poultry	20	A.O.A.C.
(ix)	Hydrocyanic acid	Complete feed for poultry	10	A.O.A.C.
(x)	BHC	Complete feed for poultry	20 ppb	A.O.A.C.
(xi)	DDT	Complete feed for poultry	5 ppb	A.O.A.C.
(xii)	Endosulphan	Complete feed for poultry	10 ppb	A.O.A.C.
(xiii)	Aldrin	Complete feed for poultry	1 ppb	A.O.A.C.

Notes

1. Based on the adequate information available on all other mycotoxins such as Ochrataxins, Citrinine, T2 Toxin, Fusarium, Zearaleoone etc. Their limits in the existing Indian Standards will be considered later

Table 5. Composition of commonly used ingredients in poultry feed (Clause 4.2.3)

Sl. No.	Ingredient	ME	Proximate specification (%)					Amino acids specification (%)										
			Crude	Crude	Crude	Total	Sand	Lysine		Methionine		Methionine + Cystine		Tryptophan		Threonine		Linoleic Acid
		Kcal/kg	Protein	C. Fat	Fibre	Ash	Silica	Total	DigD	Total	Digest	Total	Digest	Total	Digest	Total	Digest	
	Energy Ingredient																	
i)	Maize	3300	9	4	2	1.5	1	0.27	0.22	0.17	0.16	0.37	0.34	0.08	0.06	0.31	0.25	1
ii)	Jowar	3000	10	3	4	3	1	0.22	0.16	0.17	0.15	0.38	0.28	0.1	0.07	0.31	0.24	1.1
iii)	Bajara	2640	12.7	4.9	2.2	2	1	0.42	NA	0.24	NA	0.38	NA	0.18	NA	0.44	NA	NA
iv)	Rice (broken)	2600	7.9	1.7	1.4	4	2	0.26	0.21	0.2	0.17	0.37	0.31	0.09	NA	0.26	0.21	0.6
v)	Wheat	3100	14	2.6	2.5	2	1	0.38	0.31	0.21	0.18	0.5	0.44	0.15	NA	0.38	0.32	2
vi)	Barley grain	2640	11.5	1.9	5	2.5	1	0.44	0.34	0.18	0.15	0.42	0.34	0.12	NA	0.53	0.45	1
vii)	Rice polish	2700	12.7	14	5	8	2.5	0.54	0.4	0.24	0.18	0.5	0.36	0.14	NA	0.45	0.31	4.4
viii)	Ragi	2950	12.6	1.85	2.8	1.45	0.5	0.36	0.24	0.15	0.2	0.36	0.26	---	---	0.32	0.3	---
ix)	Tapioca flour	3300	2	0.7	12.9	8.5	---	0.06	---	0.006	---	0.01	---	---	---	---	---	---
x)	Vegetable fat	8800	---	99.4	---	---	---	---	---	---	---	---	---	---	---	---	----	31.0
	Protein source																	
xi)	Soy extract	2500	48	1	3.5	5	2	2.98	2.68	0.69	0.63	1.41	1.24	0.61	0.57	1.89	1.68	0.4
xii)	Soy meal	2250	44	0.8	6.5	6	2.5	2.75	2.48	0.64	0.59	1.31	1.15	0.57	NA	1.76	1.57	0.4
xiii)	Groundnut extract	2690	48	1.5	6.8	7.2	2.5	1.77	NA	0.42	NA	1.15	NA	0.5	NA	1.16	---	0.19
xiv)	Groundnut meal	2400	44	1	10	8	2.5	1.39	1.07	0.42	0.37	1.1	0.9	0.41	NA	1.12	0.94	0.19
xv)	Rapessed extract	1900	36	1.7	11.5	7	2	2.02	1.61	0.73	0.65	1.64	1.33	0.47	0	1.58	1.26	0
xvi)	Sunflower extract	1540	28	1	24	7.7	2	1.06	0.86	0.67	0.62	1.15	0.99	0.34	0	1.05	0.89	0.5
xvii)	Seasame extract	2200	44	0.5	6.1	11.5	2	1.01	0.83	1.16	0.98	1.97	1.6	0.54	0	1.44	1.05	1.9
xviii)	Fullfat soy	3300	38	18	5	4.6	2	2.37	1.9	0.51	0.4	1.16	0.83	0.69	0.45	1.57	1.21	7.7
xix)	Maize gluten 42	3150	.42	2	4	3	1.5	0.8	0.63	1.0	0.85	1.6	1.33	0.2	0.17	1.1	1.06	---
xx)	Maize gluten 60	3650	60	2	2.5	1.3	0.5	1.1	0.85	1.5	1.3	2.3	2.0	0.3	0.25	1.6	1.32	---
xxi)	Fishmeal	2180	45	7	1	22	5	2.5	2.8	0.84	0.7	1.15	0.86	0.7	---	1.4	1.2	---
xxii)	Meat and Bonemeal	1848	45	8.6	2.1	38	---	2.48	2.12	0.65	0.59	1.16	0.94	0.29	0.23	1.6	1.36	0.3
Others																		
xxiii)	Ricebran doc	1800	16	0.5	14	12.5	5	0.66	0.48	0.31	0.23	0.64	0.44	0.17	---	0.54	0.37	---
xxiv)	Wheat bran	1400	14.5	3	11	7	2	0.63	2.12	0.23	0.19	0.56	0.44	0.28	0.21	0.52	0.38	1.7
xxv)	Salseed extract	2500	9	1	3	---	1.5	0.5	0.38	0.32	0.24	0.52	0.4	0.1	0.07	0.3	0.23	0.3
xxvi)	Molasses	2000	3	---	---	9.5	---	---	---	---	---	---	---	---	---	----	---	---

Table 6. Consumption of commonly used feed ingredients : Natural Vitamins (Clause 4.2.2)

Raw Material	Riboflavin	Niacin	Panto-thenic acid	Thiamin	Choline	Biotin	Folic acid	Pyri-doxine	Carotine	Xantho-phil	Alfa Toco-pherol	Vit. A IU/kg
Energy ingredient												
Maize	1.10	19.80	3.96	3.3	506	0.07	0.29	4.62	1.98	15.4	11.00	3300
Jowar	1.20	42.70	11.00	3.9	678	0.18	0.02	NA	NA	NA	NA	0
Bajara	1.60	52.60	7.40	6.6	789	NA	NA	NA	NA	NA	NA	NA
Rice (broken)	0.88	28.60	7.92	2.64	792	0.07	0.18	4.40	0	0	8.80	0
Wheat	1.10	48.40	9.02	4.4	1078	0.11	0.42	2.20	0	0	8.80	0
Barley grain	1.54	52.80	7.92	4.84	1100	0.04	0.66	2.86	0	0	7.04	0
Rice polish	1.76	407.00	46.20	19.8	1232	0.62	NA	13.20	NA	NA	90.20	NA
Ragi	1.50	15.60	9.20	4.4	0	0.05	0.60	0.00	0	0	0	0
Tapioca flour	0	0	0	0	0	0	0	0	0	0	0	0
Vegetable fat	0	0	0	0	0	0	0	0	0	0	0	0
Protein source												
Soy extract	2.86	26.40	15.40	4.62	2640	0.33	0.66	5.94	---	---	1.96	---
Groundnut extract	7.70	165.00	46.20	5.94	1892	0.37	0.40	8.8	---	---	2.86	300
Rapeseed extract	3.52	158.40	9.46	5.06	6699	0.88	2.20	7.04	---	---	---	---
Sunflower extract	2.2	198.00	28.60	2.86	2860	0.66	1.32	11.00	---	---	11	7
Sesame extract	3.30	28.60	5.50	2.64	1496	0.33	0.00	12.54	---	---	---	---
Fullfat soy	2.64	22.00	11.00	4.62	2860	0.29	4.18	10.78	---	---	9.24	0
Maize Gluten 42	1.50	54.50	9.60	0.22	330	0.15	0.22	3.6	16.2	---	---	25
Maize Gluten 60	2.20	81.00	2.90	0.28	2200	0.22	0.23	2.8	44	---	---	60
Fish meal	6.60	66.00	8.80	1.32	3060	0.09	0.20	0	---	---	---	---
Meat and Bone meal (50%)	1.98	35.20	4.62	0.44	1320	0.04	0.22	---	---	---	---	---
Others												
Ricebran Doc	0.88	28.60	7.92	2.64	792	0.07	0.18	4.4	---	---	8.8	---
Wheat Bran	3.08	184.80	28.60	6.60	1870	0.22	1.19	6.82	0	0	13.2	0
Salseed extract	NA	NA	NA	NA	NA	NA	NA	NA	NA	NA	NA	NA
Molasses	2.86	33	37.4	0.88	748	0.66	0.09	4.18	NA	NA	7.04	NA

Table 7. Poultry feed raw material specification: macro and micro minerals (Clauses 4.2.4)

Raw Material	Macro Minerals (%)							Micro Minerals (mg/kg)					
	Calcium	Total Phosph.	Avail. Phosph.	Sodium	Chloride	Potassium	Magnesium	Copper	Iron	Manganese	Zinc	Sulphur	Selenium
Energy Ingredient	Mg/kg	Mg/kg	Mg/kg	Mg/kg	Mg/kg	Mg/kg	Mg/kg	Mg/kg	Mg/kg	Mg/kg	Mg/kg	Mg/kg	Mg/kg
Maize	0.01	0.25	0.08	0.01	0.04	0.42	0.11	2	40	7	10	1100	0.04
Jowar	0.04	0.40	0 13	0 01	0 1	0.4	0 13	10	40	10	10	900	0
Bajara	0.13	0.72	0.36	0.04	0	0.43	0.16	21.6	40	29	13.9	1300	0
Rice (broken)	0.11	0 48	0.24	0.04	0	0.34	0.14	3.3	40	17.6	1.8	50	0
Wheat	0.05	0.28	0.14	0.02	0.05	0.35	0.15	5	50	38	30	1400	0.065
Barley Grain	0.08	0.42	0.21	0.03	0.18	0.56	0.12	10	70	16	15	1500	0.35
Rice Polish	0.27	1.37	0 14	0 06	0 07	1.7	0 95	13	190	130	30	1800	0
Ragi	0.08	0 30	0.00	0.00	0.00	0.00	0.00	0.00	0.00	0 00	0.00	0 00	0 00
Tapioca Flour	0.58	0 12	0.00	0.00	0.00	0.00	0.00	0.00	0.00	0 00	0.00	0 00	0 00
Vegetable Fat	0.00	0.00	0.00	0.00	0.00	0.00	0.00	0.00	0.00	0.00	0.00	0.00	0.00
Protein Source													
Soy Extract	0.40	0.60	0 14	0 02	0 05	2.00	0 27	21	100	27	40	4300	0.01
Groundnut Extract	0.10	0 60	0.20	0.07	0.00	1.15	0.33	0	0	26	21.7	2800	0
Rapeseed Extract	0.60	1 10	0.25	0.03	0.10	1.20	0.64	6	160	53	71	2500	0 98
Sunflower Extract	0.35	0.90	0.300.01	0.05	1.00	0.62	35	140	34	100	3800	1.5	
Sesame Extract	2.00	1.30	0 24	0 04	0 00	1.39	0 00	0	0	48	0	0	0
Fullfat Soy	0.25	0.59	0.20	0.04	0.08	1.20	0.21	15	75	30	40	3000	0.1
Maize Gluten 42	0.16	0 40	---	0.10	---	0.03	0.06	28.2	400	73	---	600	1
Maize Gluten 60	0.02	0 70	---	0.03	---	0.45	0.15	22	167	4 4	41	600	1
Fishmeal	7.16	1.67	1.67	0.19	0.60	---	---	21.7	320	38.9	---	---	0
Meat and Bonemeal (45%)	10.00	5.10	5 10	0 60	0 00	1.30	1 00	0	500	10.1	0	2600	0.25
Others													
Ricebran Doc	0.37	1 80	---	0.06	0.07	1.70	0.95	13	190	130	30	1800	0
Wheat Bran	0.08	1 15	0.40	0.02	0.06	1.23	0.50	14	170	100	9.5	2200	1
Salseed Extract	0.24	0.16	0.00	0.00	0.00	0.00	0.00	0.00	0.00	0.00	0.00	0.00	0.00
Molasses	0.80	0.80	0.04	0.16	2.31	2.8	0.35	50	180	40	20	3500	0
Minerals													
Limestone Powder	38.00	0 00	0.00	0.05	0.03	0.10	2.10	0	3.5	0	0	0	0
Dicalcium Phosphate	23.00	18.00	18.00	0.06	0.01	0.10	0.60	70	500	120	380	11100	0
Sodium Chloride	0.30	0.00	0.00	39.00	60.00	0.00	0.01	0	50	0	0	2000	0
Soda Bi Carb.	---	0.00	0.00	27.00	0.00	0.00	0.00	0	0	0	0	0	0
Shell Grit	38.00	0.10	0.10	0.20	0.01	0.10	0.30	0	2.9	100	0	0	0
Bone Meal	29.80	12.50	12.50	0.04	0.00	0.20	0.30	0	5	0	100	24000	0

Table 8. Expected performance of broilers (typical body weights, feed requirements and energy consumption of broilers) (Clause 4.2.5, and Table 1,2 and 3)

Sl No.	Age (Weeks)	Body Weight			Weekly Feed Consumption			Cumulative Feed Consumption			Weekly Energy Consumption Cal ME/Bird			Cumulative Energy Consumption ME/Bird		
		Male	Female	Avg.	Male	Female	Avg.	Male	Female	Avg.	Male	Female	Avg.	Male	Female	Avg.
(1)	(2)	(3)	(4)	(5)	(6)	(7)	(8)	(9)	(10)	(11)	(12)	(13)	(14)	(15)	(16)	(17)
i.	1	152	144	148	134	131	132.5	135	131	133	395	386	391	395	386	391
ii.	2	376	344	360	290	273	281.5	425	404	414.5	856	805	830	1251	1191	1221
iii.	3	686	617	651.5	487	444	465.5	912	848	880	1437	1310	1373	2686	2501	2594
iv.	4	1085	965	1025	704	642	673	1616	1490	1553	2077	1894	1985	4765	4341	4579
v.	5	1576	1344	1046	960	738	849	2576	2228	2402	2925	2251	2590	7693	6592	7169
vi.	6	2088	1741	1915	1141	1001	1071	3717	3229	3473	3480	3503	3267	11173	9645	10436
vii.	7	2590	2134	2362	1281	1081	1181	4998	4310	4654	3907	3297	3602	15080	12972	14038

Table 9. Expected Performance of Commercial Layer Flocks
(Clause 4.2.5, and Tables 1, 2 and 3)

S.No.	Age in Weeks	Production (Percent)	Egg/HII (Weeks)	Egg (III)	Cumulative Daily
(1)	(2)	(3)	(4)	(5)	(6)
i.	19	5	0.35	0.35	75
ii.	20	15	1.05	1.40	62
iii.	21	38	2.66	4.06	90
iv.	22	64	4.48	8.54	93
v.	23	83	5.60	14.34	96
vi.	24	80	6.22	20.55	102
vii.	25	92	5.43	26.99	104
viii.	26	94	6.57	33.56	106
ix.	27	94	6.56	40.12	108
x.	28	95	6.63	46.75	108
xi.	29	96	6.69	53.44	109
xii.	30	97	6.76	60.20	111
xiii.	31	97	6.76	66.96	111
xiv.	32	97	6.76	73.20	115
xv.	33	96	6.68	80.40	115
xvi.	34	96	6.67	87.07	115
xvii.	35	96	6.67	93.73	114
xiii.	36	96	6.66	100.39	114
xix.	37	95	6.58	106.98	114
xx.	38	95	6.58	113.55	113
xxi.	39	95	6.58	120.13	113
xxii.	40	95	6.58	126.69	113
xxiii.	41	94	6.59	133.18	113
xxiv.	42	94	6.68	139.66	113
xxv.	43	94	6.47	146.13	113
xxvi.	44	93	6.40	152.53	113
xxvii.	45	93	6.39	158.92	113
xxviii.	46	93	6.39	165.31	113
xxix.	47	93	6.38	171.69	113
xxx.	48	93	6.37	178.06	113
xxxi.	49	92	6.30	184.36	113
xxxii.	50	92	6.29	190.65	112
xxxiii.	51	91	6.22	196.87	112
xxxiv.	52	90	6.14	203.01	112

xxxv.	53	89	6.07	209.06	112
xxxvi.	54	89	6.07	215.15	112
xxxvii.	55	89	6.06	221.21	112
xxxviii.	56	89	6.06	227.27	112
xxxix.	57	89	6.06	233.33	112
xl.	58	86	5.98	239.31	112
xli.	59	89	5.98	245.29	112
xlii.	60	60	5.97	251.26	112
xliii.	61	68	5.97	257.22	110
xliv.	62	87	5.90	263.12	110
xlv.	63	87	5.89	269.02	110
xlvi.	64	86	5.82	274.84	110
xlvii.	65	86	5.81	280.65	110
xlviii.	66	86	5.81	285.46	110
xlix.	67	85	5.74	292.20	110
1)	68	84	5.66	297.86	110
(i)	69	84	5.66	303.52	110
(ii)	70	83	5.59	309.11	110
(iii)	71	82	5.52	314.63	110
(iv)	72	81	5.44	320.07	110

□□□

Further Readings

Acharya R M, Dhillon J S and Tiwari M S. 1969. Age at first egg and egg production- their inheritance and expected response to different methods of selection. *British Poultry Science* 10: 175-181.

Acharya R M and Kumar J. 1971. Collection and evaluation of native fowl germplasm. V. Age at first egg and egg production in desi, Rhode Island red and their reciprocal crosses. *Indian Journal of Animal Science* **41**(4): 277-282.

Acharya R M, Dhillon J S and Biswas D K. 1971. Part *vs* full-year record- selection in breeding chicken for annual criterion egg production. *Indian Journal of Poultry Science* **6**(2): 7-11.

Aggarwal C K, Kumar J and Acharya R M. 1971. Collection and evaluation of native fowl germplasm. Part VII- growth, feather score and mortality in Rhode Island Reds (RIR), desi and their reciprocal crosses. *HAU Journal of Research* **1**(3): 122-126.

Aggarwal C K, Kumar J and Acharya R M. 1971. Collection and evaluation of native fowl germplasm. Part VIII- Studies on egg production characteristics of four Indian breeds of chickens. *HAU Journal of Research* **1**(3): 127-129.

Acharya R M, Dhillon J S and Biswas D K. 1972. Selection for egg production in poultry. *Indian Journal of Poultry Science* **7**(2): 19-25.

Alexander D J. 1998. Historical aspect. In: Newcastle disease (Ed. Alexander, D.J.) Kluwer Academic Publishers, Boston, pp. 1-10.

Arora C L, Dharamarajan M. 1970. Sex chromatin and nuclear sexing in birds. *Cytologica* **35**(4): 601-608.

Arora K L, Arneja D, Acharya R M. 1971. Fertility, hatchability and embryonic mortality in four indigenous breeds of poultry. *Indian Journal of Poultry Science* **6**(3): 13-16.

Australian Agricultural Consulting and Management Company (AACMC) 1984. Livestock Sub-sector Review, Volume 1, Annexure 3.

Balaraman S and Kaul P N 1985. Adoption of improved practices by traditional fisherman in Kerala. *Indian Journal of Extension Education* **21**(3 and 4): 80-88.

Bessei W 1993. Lessons from field experience on the development of poultry production. Strategies for sustainable animal agriculture in developing countries. Proceedings of the FAO expert consultation, Rome, Italy, 10-14 December 1990. http://www.fao.org/DOCREP/004/T0582E/T0582E25.htm

Darwin, C. (1896). The origin of species by means of natural selection, or the presentation of favoured races in the struggle of life. Published by D. Appleton and Company, New York, USA.

Dhaliwal J S and Acharya R M. 1972. Efficiency of selection based on part-year egg production. *Journal of Research (PAU)* **IX** (1 Suppl.) : 229-232.

Dhaliwal J S and Acharya R M. 1972. Relationship of egg weight and egg quality with hatchability. *Journal of Research (PAU)* **IX** (1 Suppl.): 224-228.

Dana S S. 1998. Animal husbandry practices among Santal and Lodha tribes of Medinipur district of West Bengal. Ph.D. Thesis, Division of Extension Education, IVRI, Izatnagar.

Fakhruddin 1996. The livestock and poultry wealth. NBS Publishers and Distributors, Bikaner.

Ho, P.T. (1979). The indigenous origin of Chinese agriculture. In: Reed, CA (Ed). Origin of Agriculture. Mouton, The Hague, pp. 413-484.

Iqbaluddin 1998. Poultry production through rural development. Scientific proceedings of second Pan Commonwealth Veterinary Conference, Volume 1, Bangalore, India.

Jain G L, Acharya R M and Sundaresan D. 1968. Heritability of egg production in chickens. *Journal of Research (PAU)* **5**: 272-275.

Jain G L, Acharya R M and Sundaresan D. 1968. Evaluation of individual, family and combined selection for egg production in chickens. *Journal of Research (PAU)* **5**: 424-428.

Kaushal M L, Biswas D K, Acharya R M and Sandhu J S. 1973. Impotance of heterosis for broiler traits in chicken. *Indian Journal of Poultry Science* **8**(4): 213-217.

Kumar J and Acharya R M. 1975. Effect of feathering on the performance of desi, White Leghorn and Rhode Island Red chickens. *Indian Journal of Animal Science* **45**(9): 660-663.

Kumar J and Acharya RM. 1975. Fertility and hatchability of indigenous and exotic breeds of chickens. *H.A.U. Journal of Research* **2**(2): 188-193.

Kumar J, Aggarwal, C.K. and Acharya, R M. 1971. Collection and evaluation of native fowl germ plasm. Part II. Efficiency of feed conversion, egg production and egg size in desi, Rhode Island red and their reciprocal crosses. *H.A.U. Journal of Research* **1**(2): 146-149.

Kumar J, Acharya R M and Aggarwal C K. 1971. Collection and evaluation of native fowl germ plasm. Part VI. Studies on egg quality in desi, Rhode Island Red and their reciprocal crosses. *Indian Journal of Animal Science* **41**(5): 381-385.

Kumar J, Acharya, R.M. and Tamhan SS. 1971. Collection and evaluation of native germplasm. 10. Carcass yield and carcass quality of indigenous breeds, exotice breeds and their reciprocal crosses. *Indian Journal of Animal Science* **41**(12): 1138-1143.

Mohanty G. 1987. Poultry health programme for rural poultry development. Paper presented at the FAO expert consultation on rural poultry development in Asia, Dhaka, 23-28 March 1987.

National Commission on Agriculture 1976. Report, Government of India. Ministry of Agriculture and Irrigation, New Delhi, Part VII (Animal Husbandry).

Panda B K and Nanda S K. 2000. Some observation on tribal poultry keeping in Orissa state. Paper presented in XX annual conference and symposium of Indian Poultry Science Association, 'Challenges to Poultry Industry in the New Millennium', 12-14 October, Chennai, pp. 188.

Peters, J.P. (1913). The Cock. *J.Am.Oriental Soc.* **33**: 363-401.

Randhawa M S. 1946. Role of domesticated animals in Indian history. *Science and Culture,* Volume XII, No. 1.

Rangnekar D and Rangnekar S. 1996. Traditional poultry production system - A need for fresh look from rural development perspective. XX World's Poultry Congress, New Delhi, 2-5 Sept., pp. 405-408.

Rao G V and Thomas P C. 1984. The breed characteristics of Kadaknath breed of indigenous chicken. *Avian Research* **68**(1 and 2): 55-57.

Rashid N, Barua A and Bulbul S M. 1995. A study on the performance of Khaki Campbell, Desi and Khaki, Campbell X Desi ducks with and without extra feeding under rural conditon of Bangladesh. *Asian-Australiasian Journal of Animal Sciences* **8**: 375-378.

Rehman S. 1995. A study of social and economic aspects of livestock owning Gujjar and Bakarwal tribe of Jammu and Kashmir. Ph.D. Thesis, Division of Extension Education, IVRI, Izatnagar.

Saha D. 2003. Status of rural poultry production in North 24 Parganas district of West Bengal. M.V.Sc. Thesis, Division of Extension Education, IVRI, Izatnagar.

Sapra K L, Acharya R M, Biswas D K. 1970. Diurnal variation and some environmental aspects of egg production in chicken. *H.A.U. Journal of Research* **1**(2): 130-135.

Sasaki M. 1996. Policies and strategies of rural poultry development with particular references to Asian developing countries. In: Proceedings of XX World's Poultry Congress, Vol. III, New Delhi, 2-5 September 1996.

Sharma D P, Acharya R M and Kumar J. 1971. Collection and evaluation of native fowl germplasm. IV. Comparative studies on body weights and carcass yield of Rhode Island red, indigenous (desi) and their reciprocal crosses. *Indian Journal of Animal Science* **41**(3): 185-191.

Singh H. 1994. Prospects for broiler integration. In: Indian poultry industry year book 1994 (editor) Gupta, S.K. Bata Barka Nath Printers, New Delhi, pp. 221-225.

Singh D P. 2000. Thrills and challenges for backyard poultry production. In: Proceedings of recent advances in rural poultry farming, October 7-16, CARI, Izatnagar.

Singh D P and Johari D C. 1990. Kadaknath the native fowl needs to be conserved. Indian Farming, March 1990, pp. 29-32.

Singh D P and Pani P K. 1986. Aseel's background and foreground. Poultry Guide, Feb. 1986, pp. 53-60.

Smith A J. 1990. Poultry- Tropical Agriculturist Series. CTA, Macmillan Publishers, London, pp. 179-184.

Somasekharan A P. 1980. Factors influencing adoption of selected animal husbandry practices by milk producers. M.V.Sc. Thesis, Department of Extension, Trichur, Kerala.

Swain P and Mohanty T. 1996. Poultry farming: A means for self-employment. *Poultry Guide*, **33**(12): 71-73.

West, B and Zhou, B.X. (1988). Did chicken go north? New evidence for domestication. Journal of Archeological Science **15**: 515-33.

□□□

About the Authors

Dr. R.M.Acharya
B.V.Sc. & A.H. (Pb), M.S. (Ohio), Ph.D. (Iowa)
Former Deputy Director General (A.S.), ICAR
784, Sector-9, Faridabad, 121 006, Haryana, India

Dr. R. M. Acharya was associated with National Commission on Agriculture as Member Secretary on the groups on Small Ruminant Production, and Veterinary, Animal Science and Dairy Education and prepared the reports and the recommendation for consideration and acceptance of the commission. The long experience in teaching at undergraduate and postgraduate level in the Punjab/ Haryana Agriculture Universities, research and research management experience at the Universities and under the Indian Council of Agricultural Research as Director, Central Sheep and Wool Research Institute from 1970-1980, which saw tremendous growth of infrastructure and initiation of new initiatives such as AICRPs on Goat for Meat. In position as Deputy Director General (Animal Sciences) was responsible for planning, evaluation and co-ordination of projects in Animal Production, Animal Health and Animal Products Technology, Fisheries Sciences, Social Sciences and Economics and Forage Research. He was member of the FAO expert panels on Animal Genetic Resource Conservation, Biotechnology, Small Ruminant Production and prepared technical bulletins on Sheep and Goat Breeds in India and State of Indian Livestock Genetic Resources. He Was also associated with UNDP, SDC, IDRC, World Bank, Ford Foundation and Rockefeller Foundation on preparation/ evaluation of research and development projects in Animal Husbandry.

Dr. Puneet Kumar
Ph.D.; PGD in Technology Management in Agriculture
Principal Scientist, Animal Physiology and Incharge, Zonal Technology Management Centre, Indian Veterinary Research Institute (IVRI), Izatnagar-243 122, Bareilly (UP), India

Dr. Puneet Kumar served as scientist at Central Institute for Research on Goats, Makhdoom, P.O. Farah, Mathura (UP) for 25 years. There he worked on economical and comfortable animal housing for different agro-climatic conditions, micro-climate and its effect on animal production. He also worked extensively on thermoregulatory mechanisms of goats in different thermal, solar radiation environment coupled with water scarcity. Presently he is working in the area of climate change and its impact on livestock production and diseases at the Indian Veterinary Research Institute, Izatnagar. In addition to research work in Animal Physiology, he is actively engaged in a new initiative of Indian Council of Agricultural Research in the area of Technology Commercialization, Entrepreneurship Development, Intellectual Property Management, Contract and Consultancy Projects through Zonal Technology Management Centre.

About the Authors